C0-ATP-193

THE COMPLETE BOOK OF

DIET DRUGS

Everything You Need to Know
About Today's Prescription
and Over-the-Counter
Weight Loss Products

Steven R. Peikin, M.D.

Recipes by
Liz Zorzanello Emery

KENSINGTON BOOKS
KENSINGTON PUBLISHING CORP.
http://www.kensingtonbooks.com

KENSINGTON BOOKS are published by

Kensington Publishing Corp.
850 Third Avenue
New York, NY 10022

Copyright © 2000 by Steven R. Peikin, M.D.
Recipes Copyright © 2000 by Liz Zorzanello Emery

"Body Mass Index Chart" and illustrations titled "Goal Weight in the Treatment of Obesity" and "Exercise for Weight Maintenance" reprinted by permission of the publisher from *Current Approaches to the Management of Obesity* by F. Xavier Pi-Sunyer, M.D., pp. 31, 43, 179 Copyright © 1996 by Dannemiller Memorial Foundation, 12500 Network Boulevard, San Antonio, TX 78249-3302.

All Kensington titles, imprints and disrtributed lines are available at special quantity discounts for bulk purchases for sales promotion, premiums, fund raising, educational or institutional use.

Special book excerpts or customized printings can also be created to fit specific needs. For details, write or phone the office of the Kensington Special Sales Manager: Kensington Publishing Corp., 850 Third Avenue, New York, NY, 10022. Attn. Special Sales Department. Phone: 1-800-221-2647.

Kensington and the K logo U.S. Pat. & TM Off.

First Kensington Trade Paperback Printing: May, 2000
First Kensington Paperback Printing: January, 2002
10 9 8 7 6 5 4 3 2 1

Printed in the United States of America

For Scott

ACKNOWLEDGMENTS

First and foremost, I want to thank Lori Snodgrass for her enormous contribution to the creation of this work. I applaud her ability to make complicated, technical information an easy read.

I would also like to thank Diane Barton, M.D. (Department of Medicine, Cooper Hospital/University Medical Center, Camden, New Jersey) for her assistance in reviewing the manuscript. Also thanks to Marni Bevan for her assistance in editing the manuscript. Many thanks to my agent, Barbara Lowenstein, and the excellent group at Kensington.

As always, it was a pleasure working with Liz Emery, M.S., R.D., who edited the entire nutrition section and created the wonderful recipes in Part II. I respect her professionalism and global knowledge of nutrition. Vicki Schwartz, M.S., R.D., an outstanding clinical dietician and college professor, deserves credit for her contribution to Chapter 9, "The Complete Book of Diet Drugs Diet Plan," and Chapter 11, "Weight Maintenance (After Weight Loss)." It was also a pleasure working with Myra Santiago, Ph.D., who was a major contributor to Chapter 10, "Exercise for Faster, Easier Weight Loss."

A special thanks to Marjorie Varneke, who helped put it all together. A final thanks to Monica Vesci and Cynthia Hunter for their technical assistance.

A NOTE TO THE READER

In the new millennium we will witness a renewed enthusiasm for drugs to help people lose weight. Outstanding research has shown us that whether we use the same old tried-and-true diet drugs or the drugs just recently approved by the FDA, significant, sustained weight loss can be achieved even in previously unsuccessful dieters.

With so many options now available, the field of weight management has become quite complex, leaving the dieter confused as to how to proceed.

In *The Complete Book of Diet Drugs,* the reader is given information on current approaches to drug-assisted weight loss. Although the material is based upon standard obesity management practices, all views expressed in *The Complete Book of Diet Drugs* should be considered solely those of the author and may differ from those of your personal physician. *The Complete Book of Diet Drugs* is intended to make you an informed consumer, but the book is not intended to replace your doctor, who should remain an integral part of and fully responsible for your weight management program. If you intend to self-medicate using over-the-counter (OTC) diet drugs, it is still necessary to notify your doctor since you may have medical problems that could make OTC drugs dangerous for you.

Most individuals who use diet drugs do not experience serious side effects. In fact, for most people the health risks of remaining obese far exceed those of the drugs used to treat obesity. In rare cases, certain diet drugs can cause serious medical problems. Even diet alone without drugs can cause side effects and medical problems, including gallstones. The *Complete Book of Diet Drugs* and careful physician monitoring can help you reduce those risks, but not entirely eliminate them.

As information such as that contained in *The Complete Book of Diet Drugs* gets more widely disseminated, more and more significantly overweight people will use diet drugs to achieve their weight goals and a giant step will have been taken to control the biggest killer of the Western world, after smoking.

CONTENTS

* Only the most popular brand names of each category of drug are used.

Part II. *The Complete Book of Diet Drugs* Meal Plan and Recipes

INTRODUCTION

S o . . . how many times have you tried to lose weight? How many *more* times are you going to try to lose weight? Don't get me wrong. I'm not asking you to admit defeat at the weight-loss game. Almost everyone, at one time or another, has tried to lose weight. Maybe it worked. You chose a path and followed it . . . for a while. And then what happened? You gained weight. Sometimes even more weight than you lost in the first place. Sound familiar? It's a struggle that many, *many* people battle all of their lives. Are you tired of losing the battle? Well, now you can win it for good.

The latest research indicates that drug therapy is the most effective method to help most people lose weight and keep it off. People who have never had a significant weight problem may be able to keep their weight in check with just diet and exercise. But for tens of millions of obese individuals who can't lose weight, or can lose weight but can't keep it off, or have weight-associated risk factors such as heart disease or diabetes, drugs can be a highly effective solution. These drugs usually enable an individual to restrict eating without feeling deprived. They allow weight loss at a relatively fast but safe pace.

How fast and how much? The average person using diet drugs will lose 1 percent of his or her initial body weight per week. That means that someone who weighs 170 pounds will weigh approximately 156 pounds within 8 weeks, and 144 pounds within 12 weeks. While the average rate of weight loss is 1 percent per week, you should also know that many individuals lose only 5–10 percent of their starting weight before reaching a plateau, where continued weight loss becomes problematic.

Be that as it may, always remember this: *Losing even small amounts of weight dramatically and immediately reduces many health risks.*

About a year ago, for example, a young woman named Sarah came to see me about her weight problem. Although she was only moderately obese (5 feet 2 inches and 162 pounds), she was extremely self-conscious about her appearance. Sarah always wore black, loose-fitting clothes. She loved the beach but she refused to wear a bathing suit. She had never been a successful dieter. She had tried everything from Weight Watchers to Dr. Atkins' Diet Revolution with nothing to show for her efforts. Her doctor discouraged her from trying diet drugs because she was only moderately obese. When Sarah came to see me, she was convinced that she was a hopeless case.

It was obvious to me that diet and exercise tips alone were not going to make a substantial impact on Sarah's weight problem. From what she had heard about diet drugs, she assumed that only weak people with drug-seeking behavior or the most severely obese used them. She was also worried that the drugs might be the same as phen/fen or Redux and would cause heart and lung disease. After I talked with her about the drugs—the benefits as well as the potential risks—she agreed to try medication. Sarah now takes 15 mg of Ionomin™ (phentermine) every other day. After 10 weeks of medication and following recommendations for diet and exercise, she has maintained her weight at 140 pounds. She experiences very little in the way of side effects, and needless to say, she is absolutely thrilled. Sarah has bought two bathing suits, neither one is black, and she's happy to wear them whenever she goes to the beach.

For every Sarah who uses a diet drug, however, there are many people who are reluctant to use drugs despite the known risks of remaining obese. Pulmonary hypertension and serious valvular heart disease in phen/fen users, although rare, did frighten many potential diet drug users. In September 1997, 9 million phen/fen users had the rug pulled out from under them when fenfluramine was withdrawn from the market due to safety concerns. The combination of fenfluramine, which increases brain serotonin, with phentermine, which increases brain norepinephrine, was highly effective in controlling weight. As a result, some phen/fen users switched to "herbal phen/fen," a combination of ephedrine and St. John's wort (discussed in Chapter 8), but the majority just stopped taking their medication and gained all their weight back.

The valvular heart disease and pulmonary hypertension seen in some phen/fen and Redux users was caused by high levels of a chemical called serotonin. While serotonin suppresses appetite and slows down stomach emptying, resulting in weight loss, in high concentrations the chemical can produce a white plaque on heart valves, impeding their function. The same thing probably occurs in the blood vessels supplying the lungs, making it difficult for blood to pass through branches of the pulmonary artery. The resulting pressure backup (pulmonary hypertension) damages the right side of the heart and eventually the patient succumbs to lung and heart failure.

Redux and Pondomin (fenfluramine) have been taken off the market. The diet drugs on today's market do not cause valvular heart disease and primary pulmonary hypertension. But because of these recent recalls, many people assume that all diet drugs must be dangerous. Most experts, including me, believe that kind of reasoning is wrong.

It is now thought that only drugs that cause the *release* of serotonin from nerves cause valvular heart disease and pulmonary hypertension. A newly available drug, Meridia™ (sibutramine), does not cause serotonin release. It works by preventing the *reuptake* of serotonin into the nerve terminal. Its action is very similar to the antidepressant drugs Prozac™ and Effexor™, which do not cause the chemical to be released on a continuing basis, thus preventing damage to the heart and blood vessels. *Specific serotonin reuptake inhibitors* (SSRIs), the more technical name of the drugs in question, only augment serotonin levels when the nerve naturally releases the chemical. Again, under these conditions, no vascular damage appears to occur.

Although phentermine was the "phen" of the phen/fen regimen, this drug does not release serotonin and there is no convincing evidence that phentermine causes valvular heart disease and pulmonary hypertension. In fact, phentermine has been used to treat obesity for more than 20 years and is still considered safe and effective.

Xenical™ (orlistat), another drug recently approved by the FDA for long-term treatment of obesity, also has no potential to cause valvular heart disease or primary pulmonary hypertension. Xenical™ interferes with lipase, a pancreatic enzyme that digests dietary fat. While taking Xenical™, your body absorbs only two-thirds of the fat you eat while the other one-third passes through you.

Although the complications associated with fenfluramine were unfortunate, we cannot let that experience send us back to the Dark Ages in obesity treatment. Shortly after the recall of fenfluramine, a leading Johns Hopkins researcher put it this way: "To abandon the pharmacotherapy of obesity at this point would be throwing the baby out with the bathwater."

There is no going back. The treatment of obesity must remain enlightened and state-of-the-art. It is fortunate that patients and physicians say they are still eager for new diet drugs and the pharmaceutical companies are clearly forging ahead with obesity research. Several new drugs are currently in development, including a drug that actually burns up fat by increasing body metabolism.

In *The Complete Book of Diet Drugs* you will find detailed explanations of the current treatment alternatives for obesity. The information is intended to be balanced, responsible, up-to-date, and representative of the conventional medical wisdom of bariatric experts (weight loss specialists). The book is not intended to replace or diminish the role of your family doctor. On the contrary, you are encouraged to consult your physician prior to initiating any diet drug regimen whether or not a prescription is required in order to maximize safety.

Should we practice caution? Yes. Inertia? No! In a recent issue of *Fortune,* a journalist wrote, "We're spending $33 billion a year to get thin and still gaining weight. Maybe it's time to roll out new weapons in the war on fat." Thank goodness new treatments that will revolutionize the management of obesity have arrived and *this time* drug companies and the FDA are listening.

In 1997 Knoll Pharmaceutical Company brought Meridia™ to the United States market, and in 1999 Roche Laboratories launched Xenical™. The launching of Meridia™ and Xenical™ was extremely important for the field of obesity management. These produces have put drug treatment of obesity back on track, replacing the loss of fenfluramine with safer yet very effective drugs. Meridia™ and Xenical™ are only the first of many new patent-protected diet drugs that will soon be available. In light of the recall of Redux and fenfluramine, the FDA exhaustively scrutinized these drugs before their approval.

With so many diet drugs, you now face a bewildering number of exciting options. You will want to know:

- What drugs are best for you.
- What dosage is best for you.
- How long you will need to take the drugs.

The Complete Book of Diet Drugs provides this information and more to answer all of your questions about drug treatment for weight loss and weight control.

After reading *The Complete Book of Diet Drugs* you will likely:

- Overcome any anxiety you may have about the use of diet drugs.
- Decide whether drugs are right for you (in many cases, the answer is *yes*).
- Learn how the drugs work and which are the most appropriate.
- Be aware of possible side effects.
- Review a timetable for staying on the drugs.

More and more overweight people are becoming aware of the drug option as an answer to their weight problem. Although many people are interested in trying diet drugs, they also worry about side effects (especially after the negative press generated by the recall of fenfluramine) and are skeptical that drugs will be helpful. They may also have little or no knowledge about how to proceed with diet drug therapy.

The Complete Book of Diet Drugs will help you determine if you are a candidate for diet medication and, if so, help you get started on a state-of-the-art, medication-assisted diet program. As this is the *first* book to include an in-home, complete weight control program fully compatible with the use of prescription or over-the-counter diet drugs, you hold in your hand a key to future health.

One woman, for instance, who has been using Meridia™ to manage her weight problems says, "This is the first time I've been able to keep weight off without going crazy. I don't understand the thinking that it's okay to treat the problems caused by being overweight with drugs but not to treat the obesity itself." Even if you are not a candidate for diet drugs or decide against the diet medication option, the book contains excellent calorie-reducing meal plans, behavioral modification techniques, and an exercise program that will help you realize *your* weight goals.

The Complete Book of Diet Drugs will assist you in achieving the goal you never thought possible: *rapid, easy,* and *lasting weight loss* with all its attendant values of living a longer, healthier life. Thus, in the first few chapters I address any concerns you may have. You will learn why obesity is a real disease—one that should be treated, in many cases, with currently available drugs and drug combinations. I will indicate the recommended dosages and specify when to take the medication. I will also discuss side effects that may possibly arise and how to remedy them. In addition, I will instruct you on how to ask your physician the right questions regarding a drug-assisted weight loss program. For those of you who would like to take a peek at future treatments for weight loss and obesity as we enter the new millennium, in Chapter 6, I will describe the newest drugs yet to be released for public consumption.

While drugs will make it much easier to reduce the number of calories in the diet by suppressing appetite and reducing food cravings, or by preventing dietary fat absorption, they will not do all the work necessary to lose weight successfully and permanently. As a result, in *The Complete Book of Diet Drugs* I incorporate the three other components necessary for weight loss and control:

- A sensible eating plan
- An exercise program
- Behavior modification

All of you must pay attention to diet and exercise to reap the full benefits of any weight loss medication you take. In fact, the FDA is quite clear on this issue, insisting that companies who market diet drugs inform consumers that the drugs should be used only in conjunction with a nutritionally balanced, low-calorie diet; exercise; and behavior modification. *The Complete Book of Diet Drugs* offers you a 1,200–1,500 calorie diet based on the American Dietetic Association Exchange Lists for Meal Planning. The majority of registered dieticians use the Exchange List when they counsel their overweight patients. Delicious, original recipes and prearranged meal plans written by Liz Emery, R.D., are also included in Part II of the book.

Exercise is important in everyone's life. The more you exercise, the more you can eat and still lose weight. Most importantly, exercise will prevent you from regaining the weight you have lost. Dr. Myra Santiago, a well-published professor of exercise physiology from Temple University in Philadelphia, created the original exercise program in *The Complete Book of Diet Drugs*. It is an excellent program, as many of my patients have agreed.

For instance, there is George, a 38-year-old with a sedentary job as an account executive. Over the years, he acquired quite a "gut." George wanted to do something about it once and for all. After failing with diet and exercise, he decided to try Xenical™ along with diet and exercise. Over a three-month period, George's weight dropped 25 pounds, from 190 to 165. Now, his walk/slow job routine has helped him maintain his weight at

165 by incorporating exercise into his lifestyle. George is able to stay svelte without remaining on the medication.

Unfortunately, because weight problems usually last forever, treatment must follow suit. Although studies show that the new diet drugs are safe and effective for long-term weight control, the FDA has not yet approved any diet drug for use beyond two years of treatment. Chapter 11, which details weight maintenance after weight loss, explains how behavior modification, in addition to exercise, may also allow you to stop diet medication, at least for a while, without regaining the weight you have lost. Eating behavior is key here, and I will tell you about the latest tried-and-true ways to change how and why you eat the way you do. In fact, some recent studies have demonstrated that when behavior modification is combined with diet drugs, the outcome is even better! Did your mother tell you to chew your food slowly and to eat only while sitting at the table? In Chapter 9, which includes information on behavior modification, you will find out why "Mom's always right." For those of you who prefer not to cook, I have included a list of the best choices in prepared, frozen entrées. Included as well are suggestions for supplementing these entrées with fresh fruits and vegetables to ensure a nutritionally balanced meal.

I have written Appendix I as an informational aid specifically for your personal physician. Many primary care doctors are not up-to-date on the most current information concerning diet drugs. I include a summary of the program, as well as a review of the "nuts and bolts" of prescribing various drug regimens. Your doctor will learn to recognize when to start diet drugs, situations where diet drugs are advisable, dosing schedules, and recommended ways to monitor your progress. You can photocopy this part or cut it out and give it to your doctor. I also provide a short list of references if your doctor would like to learn more about diet drug therapy—an excellent idea for any concerned physician.

Appendix II includes various meal plans ranging from 1,300 to 3,000 calories per day along with the American Dietetic Association's Exchange List for Meal Planning. These lists, based on a special grouping of foods, allow you to create your own individualized meal plans after you have reached your goal weight.

Appendix III includes a list of common foods and their nutrient values. So when you feel like eating something, say a cinnamon-raisin bagel, you can determine how many calories and grams of fat it contains and omit food of equal caloric value from that day's meal plan.

Let's take a glance at a typical person who is following the program outlined in *The Complete Book of Diet Drugs*.

Jill is taking a diet drug along with the nutritionally balanced meals, exercise, and behavior modification. She begins her day with a 10 mg dose of Meridia™. Twenty minutes later, she eats a breakfast of Baked Apple French Toast (see Chapter 18). She drives to work and parks in the farthest corner of the lot (no dings in her car)! She walks a quarter-mile to her office building and takes the stairs to her floor. At noon, she lunches on soup, salad, a tuna sandwich (no mayo), and a diet drink. After work, Jill goes home and prepares dinner. She eats a Stouffer's Lean Cuisine Hearty Portions Oriental Glazed Chicken microwave entrée accompanied by fresh fruit and vegetables. By the end of the day she has consumed 1,350 calories. Is she starving? *No!* She feels completely full and satisfied, and is well on her way toward achieving her goal weight.

PART I

Putting
The Complete Book
of Diet Drugs
Program
to Work for You

1

Diet Drugs Are Here to Stay

Giving up smoking is easy. I've done it hundreds of times.
—MARK TWAIN

Substitute the words "losing weight" for "giving up smoking" and Twain's adage applies just as well. Most people are able to lose some weight—they do it every time they go on a diet. But the results are short-lived. Only 5 percent of all dieters succeed at keeping their weight off for at least two years because weight maintenance requires constant exercise and dicting. The majority of people regain every ounce and then some. Despite calorie counting, fat gram counting, exercise, and behavior modification, 34 million Americans are obese. (Obesity is often defined as 20 percent above ideal body weight. I'll discuss obesity in detail in the next chapter.) Seventy million people think that they need to lose weight. Furthermore, 80 percent of all women diet and 50 percent are on a diet at any one time.

The problem isn't just lack of willpower. Most overweight people didn't get that way because they lack the strength to walk past a bakery without stepping inside, or because they've eaten more double cheeseburgers than the rest of the world. In most cases, overweight people with chronic weight problems have an inherited disease, much like diabetes and hypertension. And many obese people appear to have a body metabolism disorder as well. Like diabetes and hypertension, obesity cannot be cured. Although this fact is well documented, most obese people—and their doctors—don't accept this fact.

Those of us who are experts in treating obesity have long recognized that cutting calories is not our only treatment option any more than cutting back on sugar alone is the treatment for diabetes or restricting salt the "cure" for hypertension. The solution for many people is drugs—drugs that are highly effective in causing and maintaining weight loss; drugs that I use for the majority of my obese patients.

In my own private practice, I have seen sensational results with diet drugs in patients of all weights and circumstances. For example, Betty came to me after her second pregnancy. Although thin as a child, Betty struggled with her weight most of her adult life. She was also unprepared for the effects that her two pregnancies would have on her weight. At 5 feet 4 inches and 120 pounds before her first child was born, Betty gained 50 pounds with each pregnancy. Her postpartum weight after her first child was 130 pounds and reached 158 pounds after her second baby. Betty's mother was obese and Betty was devastated to think that now she would be, too. Those extra pounds were enough to put her at a weight that justified prescribing phentermine. The result: For the first time in years, Betty had control over her eating and was able to steadily lose weight. Within 2 months she had lost 20 pounds.

Another patient, Nora, a 25-year-old schoolteacher, had tried "every diet in the book." And although she lost weight with each new diet, within a few months she would quickly regain it, and more. With her latest attempt, she had succeeded in losing 20 pounds on the Weight Watchers program. After a few months though, Nora found it difficult to adhere to the maintenance plan. She hoped medication could help, but her family doctor told her that she didn't weigh enough yet to justify drug-assisted weight control. Nora could see the writing on the wall; she had already gained back 5 pounds and knew that she was in danger of gaining more. Not wanting all of her hard work to go for naught, Nora came to me for help.

My philosophy is this: What is the sense in forcing someone to become overweight again before using diet drugs? It was clear to me from her history that maintenance diet and exercise alone were not going to work for Nora. She had tried and failed time and time again. I put Nora on 15 mg of phentermine a day and, for the first time in her dieting history, she has maintained her goal weight for six months and counting.

It is important to note that each patient must be evaluated individually. Certainly, not all of the people I treat use phentermine. For example, Laura was 5 feet 2 inches and weighed 146 pounds. She was generally dispirited and feeling hopeless about losing weight. After careful evaluation, I realized a large part of Laura's problem was depression. I prescribed for Laura a drug called Effexor™. Effexor™ is an antidepressant that tends to suppress appetite by increasing brain serotonin. (Serotonin is a chemical produced by the brain that suppresses appetite, in addition to having an effect on mood.) Although I prescribed the drug for her depression, I anticipated the drug would have an effect on Laura's weight as well as her spirits. Within 6 weeks, Laura lost 15 pounds and had taken a new interest in both her appearance and her life. I am keeping her on drug therapy, and so far she is maintaining her lower weight. What's more important is that Laura is no longer depressed.

It is amazing to me that so many severely overweight people have never tried drug therapy even after diet alone has failed them many, many times.

Martha offers us another example of success. Martha was a 35-year-old single mother of four. At 5 feet 5 inches, she weighed 300 pounds. Her weight was not just an issue of vanity or her health; it affected every aspect of her life. Martha had been turned down for several jobs and she felt her rejections were a direct result of her obesity. Her social life was nonexistent and she thought that her children were embarrassed by her weight.

Exercising was difficult because walking any distance was arduous and climbing stairs required taking "rest stops." When she came to see me, her ankles were so large she couldn't fit into shoes. At one point, she had no choice but to wear flip-flops in the snow. Martha had tried dieting, but she was never able to lose more than 50 pounds. When she came to our office, she was initially prescribed the phen/fen regime. She lost 150 pounds. Her life was improved beyond measure. Along with the undeniable health benefits of losing the weight, she was offered a wonderful new job that involves meeting the public and she became engaged to be married. When fenfluramine was withdrawn from the market because of potential heart and lung problems, Martha stopped her medication and regained 50 pounds within several months. She was desperate for an alternative to fenfluramine. I prescribed Meridia™ (sibutramine). Meridia™ acts like phen/fen but does not cause the serious side effects seen in phen/fen. Her weight is dropping once again and she now feels in control of her life.

Like Martha, Jean was also obese. She was 5 feet 7 inches, and as a young bride, she weighed 145 pounds. When she came to us, Jean weighed in at 350 pounds. Again like Martha, Jean's weight hindered her ability to function normally. Exercising was out of the question. Jean's husband was distressed by her appearance and worried about her health. By taking 30 mg of phentermine per day, Jean lost 100 pounds. At this weight she is able to exercise, and is motivated to lose even more weight. Her faded sex life has become active again, and Jean feels good about herself.

Betty, a 48-year-old woman, could not wait for Xenical™ (orlistat) to be available in the United States. She had read very positive articles about how the drug had helped so many people in Europe. She liked the fact that Xenical™ does not get absorbed into the body, making it a very safe drug. Betty was 5 feet 3 inches and weighed 152 pounds. She had been recently diagnosed with diabetes and was told to lose weight. She'd had a lifelong weight problem. While some of her friends had a "sweet tooth," she always joked that she had a "fat tooth." Betty had trouble staying away from fatty foods like pasta sauce, salad dressing, hamburgers, and pizza. All the diets she had previously followed restricted these foods, which had made them difficult to follow. Even her diabetes doctor wanted her to eat more fat and less sugar.

With Xenical™, dietary fat is not severely restricted. In fact, it works better if you do not cut too far back on your fat intake. By taking Xenical™ before each meal, Betty was able to eat 14 grams of fat at breakfast, 20 grams of fat with lunch, and another 20 grams of fat at dinner. When she had followed the Nutri/System program, she was able to eat only 23 grams of fat in an entire day. Her 1,500-calorie diet along with exercise and Xenical™ enabled her to lose 15 pounds in 10 weeks. She did notice a slight change in the consistency of her bowel movements, but she felt it was a small price to pay for her dieting success.

Bill is an anesthesiologist with a hectic work schedule. Many times he is called in to work in the middle of the night, and his meals used to consist of fast food. Bill frequently snacked when he was stressed, and he found himself eating his way to an extra 50 pounds. With that extra weight, he was huffing and puffing at the end of the day. He was so tired after work that he often fell asleep watching the evening news. After getting approval from his family doctor, he started taking Dexatrim (phenylpropanolamine), an over-the-counter (nonprescription) diet drug along with an 1,800-calorie diet. Bill lost 50 pounds and is now at his ideal body weight. He has so much more energy that he regularly awakens at 4:00 A.M. to work out on his treadmill.

You will read many case histories throughout *The Complete Book of Diet Drugs* that illustrate how drug therapy has helped people lose weight. Not everyone benefits from diet medication. It is not unusual to find individuals who have tried using a diet drug without significant results. Furthermore, the right plan for one person may not be right for you. You need to know which drug or drugs will work best for you, what dosage you should take, and how long you should take them. These are topics we will explore in the upcoming chapters. But now, let's find out what caused your weight problem in the first place. By knowing what causes obesity, we are in a better position to treat this vexing problem the best way possible.

2

Obesity: A Very Treatable Disease

What Is Obesity?

Thirty-four million Americans, and nearly an equal number of Europeans, are obese. Now, you may be thinking: "I might have a weight problem, but I'm not obese." When we think of the "O" word, we conjure up images of people who can't make it through doorways or fit into airline seats. But these unfortunate individuals are not just obese, they are what we term "morbidly obese." Morbid obesity is defined as being 100 pounds or 100 percent above ideal body weight.

The term "morbid obesity" has recently been renamed "serious" or "extreme" obesity. The change in wording, however, does nothing to affect the health risks associated with the disease. Clearly, people who are seriously obese have reason to be grim. Consider this: Once you become seriously obese, your risk of death from heart attack, stroke, and cancer *more than doubles* compared to normal-weight individuals.

Are you seriously obese? Find your height in Table 2.1. If you weigh more than the corresponding weight, you are seriously obese.

Table 2.1   How to Determine If You Are *Seriously* Obese

Height (inches)	Weight (pounds)
58	190
60	200
62	210
64	220
66	230
68	240
70	250
72	260
74	270
76	280

Table 2.2   How to Determine If You Are Obese

	Females			Males	
Height (feet/inches)	Range (*medium frame*)	20% *Overweight*	Height (feet/inches)	Range (*medium frame*)	20% *Overweight*
4'8"	96–107	122	5'1"	118–129	149
4'9"	98–110	125	5'2"	121–133	152
4'10"	101–113	128	5'3"	124–136	156
4'11"	104–116	132	5'4"	127–139	160
5'0"	107–119	136	5'5"	130–143	164
5'1"	110–122	139	5'6"	134–147	169
5'2"	113–126	144	5'7"	138–152	174
5'3"	116–130	148	5'8"	142–156	179
5'4"	120–135	154	5'9"	146–160	184
5'5"	124–139	158	5'10"	150–165	190
5'6"	128–143	163	5'11"	154–170	194
5'7"	132–147	168	6'0"	158–175	200
5'8"	136–151	173	6'1"	162–180	205
5'9"	140–155	178	6'2"	167–185	211
5'10"	144–159	182	6'3"	172–190	217

Based on the 1959 Metropolitan Height/Weight Tables using the medium frame.

Okay, what if you're not seriously obese? Are you obese? There are many medical definitions and formulas for obesity. Each formula is an attempt to determine a number above which there is an increased risk of developing medical problems such as diabetes, coronary artery disease, or even death. Below are a few formulas that can help you determine if you are obese:

You are obese if:

1. You are more than 20 percent above your ideal body weight. Table 2.2 can help you determine if you are 20 percent above ideal body weight.
2. If you're a man and your BMI is >27.8, or if you're a woman and your BMI is >27.3.

Using more recent guidelines, a BMI greater than 25 and less than 30 is considered overweight, while a BMI equal or greater than 30 is considered obese (see NHLBI report findings below). Body mass index (BMI) evaluates your weight relative to your height. Most experts now use BMI instead of percentage ideal body weight to assess obesity because it correlates well with body fat and risk for obesity complications.

How to Calculate Your BMI

$$\text{BMI} = \frac{\text{weight (kilograms)}}{\text{height (meters)}^2}$$

a. Determine your weight in kilograms by multiplying your weight in pounds by .45.
b. Determine you height in meters by multiplying your height in inches by .0254.
c. Multiply your height in meters by itself.
d. Divide your answer in "a" by your answer in "c" to get your BMI. For your convenience, Table 2.3 will give you your approximate BMI.

Table 2.3
How to Determine BMI

Height (Feet/Inches)

Weight (pounds)	5'0"	5'1"	5'2"	5'3"	5'4"	5'5"	5'6"	5'7"	5'8"	5'9"	5'10"	5'11"	6'0"	6'1"	6'2"	6'3"	6'4"
100	20	19	18	18	17	17	16	16	15	15	14	14	14	13	13	12	12
105	21	20	19	19	18	17	17	16	16	16	15	15	14	14	13	13	13
110	21	21	20	19	19	18	18	17	17	16	16	15	15	15	14	14	13
115	22	22	21	20	20	19	19	18	17	17	17	16	16	15	15	14	14
120	23	23	22	21	21	20	19	19	18	18	17	17	16	16	15	15	15
125	24	24	23	22	21	21	20	20	19	18	18	17	17	16	16	16	15
130	25	25	24	23	22	22	21	20	20	19	19	18	18	17	17	16	16
135	26	26	25	24	23	22	22	21	21	20	19	19	18	18	17	17	16
140	27	26	26	25	24	23	23	22	21	21	20	20	19	18	18	17	17
145	28	27	27	26	25	24	23	23	22	21	21	20	20	19	19	18	18
150	29	28	27	27	26	25	24	23	23	22	22	21	20	20	19	19	18
155	30	29	28	27	27	26	25	24	24	23	22	22	21	20	20	19	19
160	31	30	29	28	27	27	26	25	24	24	23	22	22	21	21	20	19
165	32	31	30	29	28	27	27	26	25	24	24	23	22	22	21	21	20
170	33	32	31	30	29	28	27	27	26	25	24	24	23	22	22	21	21
175	34	33	32	31	30	29	28	27	27	26	25	24	24	23	22	22	21
180	35	34	33	32	31	30	29	28	27	27	26	25	24	24	23	22	22
185	36	35	34	33	32	31	30	29	28	27	27	26	25	24	24	23	23
190	37	36	35	34	33	32	31	30	29	28	27	26	26	25	24	24	23
195	38	37	36	35	33	32	31	31	30	29	28	27	26	26	25	24	24
200	39	38	37	35	34	33	32	31	30	30	29	28	27	26	26	25	24
205	40	39	37	36	35	34	33	32	31	30	29	29	28	27	26	26	25
210	41	40	38	37	36	35	34	33	32	31	30	29	28	28	27	26	26
215	42	41	39	38	37	36	35	34	33	32	31	30	29	28	28	27	26
220	43	42	40	39	38	37	36	34	33	32	32	31	30	29	28	27	27
225	44	43	41	40	39	37	36	35	34	33	32	31	31	30	29	28	27
230	45	43	42	41	39	38	37	36	35	34	33	32	31	30	30	29	28
235	46	44	43	42	40	39	38	37	36	35	34	33	32	31	30	29	29
240	47	45	44	43	41	40	39	38	36	35	34	33	33	32	31	30	29
245	48	46	45	43	42	41	40	38	37	36	35	34	33	32	31	31	30
250	49	47	46	44	43	42	40	39	38	37	36	35	34	33	32	31	30

For individuals not covered by this table, calculate BMI by converting pounds to kilograms (1 pound = 0.45 kilogram) and inches to meters (1 inch = .0254 meter).

The equation for BMI is weight (in kilograms) divided by height (in meters) squared [kg/m^2].

Source: *Shape Up America!*, 6707 Democracy Blvd., Suite 107, Bethesda, MD 20817.

Table 2.3
How to Determine BMI
(cont.)
Height (Feet/Inches)

Weight (pounds)	5'0"	5'1"	5'2"	5'3"	5'4"	5'5"	5'6"	5'7"	5'8"	5'9"	5'10"	5'11"	6'0"	6'1"	6'2"	6'3"	6'4"
255	50	48	47	45	44	42	41	40	39	38	37	36	35	34	33	32	31
260	51	49	48	46	45	43	42	41	40	38	37	36	35	34	33	32	32
265	52	50	48	47	45	44	43	42	40	39	38	37	36	35	34	33	32
270	53	51	49	48	46	45	44	42	41	40	39	38	37	36	35	34	33
275	54	52	50	49	47	46	44	43	42	41	39	38	37	36	35	34	33
280	55	53	51	50	48	47	45	44	43	41	40	39	38	37	36	35	34
285	56	54	52	50	49	47	46	45	43	42	41	40	39	38	37	36	35
290	57	55	53	51	50	48	47	45	44	43	42	40	39	38	37	36	35
295	58	56	54	52	51	49	48	46	45	44	42	41	40	39	38	37	36
300	59	57	55	53	51	50	48	47	46	44	43	42	41	40	39	37	37
305	60	58	56	54	52	51	49	48	46	45	44	43	41	40	39	38	37
310	61	59	57	55	53	52	50	49	47	46	44	43	42	41	40	39	38
315	62	60	58	56	54	52	51	49	48	47	45	44	43	42	40	39	38
320	62	60	59	57	55	53	52	50	49	47	46	45	43	42	41	40	39
325	63	61	59	58	56	54	52	51	49	48	47	45	44	43	42	41	40
330	64	62	60	58	57	55	53	52	50	49	47	46	45	44	42	41	40
335	65	63	61	59	58	56	54	52	51	49	48	47	45	44	43	42	41
340	66	64	62	60	58	57	55	53	52	50	49	47	46	45	44	42	41
345	67	65	63	61	59	57	56	54	52	51	50	48	47	46	44	43	42
350	68	66	64	62	60	58	56	55	53	52	50	49	47	46	45	44	43
355	69	67	65	63	61	59	57	56	54	52	51	50	48	47	46	44	43
360	70	68	66	64	62	60	58	56	55	53	52	50	49	47	46	45	44
365	71	69	67	65	63	61	59	57	55	54	52	51	50	48	47	46	44
370	72	70	68	66	64	62	60	58	56	55	53	52	50	49	48	46	45
375	73	71	69	66	64	62	61	59	57	55	54	52	51	49	48	47	46
380	74	72	70	67	65	63	61	60	58	56	55	53	52	50	49	47	46
385	75	73	70	68	66	64	62	60	59	57	55	54	52	51	49	48	47
390	76	74	71	69	67	65	63	61	59	58	56	54	53	51	50	49	47
395	77	75	72	70	68	66	64	62	60	58	57	55	54	52	51	49	48
400	78	76	73	71	69	67	65	63	61	59	57	56	54	53	51	50	49

For individuals not covered by this table, calculate BMI by converting pounds to kilograms (1 pound = 0.45 kilogram) and inches to meters (1 inch = .0254 meter).

The equation for BMI is weight (in kilograms) divided by height (in meters) squared [kg/m²].

Source: *Shape Up America!*, 6707 Democracy Blvd., Suite 107, Bethesda, MD 20817.

3. Your waist/hip ratio is greater than 0.8 if you are a woman, or greater than 1.0 if you are a man.

Why is this important? Studies show that it not only matters how much you weigh, but where your fat is located. Being fat in your waist (male or android pattern obesity) is associated with heart disease and diabetes more often than carrying extra pounds in your hips (female or gynoid pattern obesity).

To determine your waist/hip ratio, use a flexible tape measure and measure your waist. Hold the tape snugly but don't pull it tight. Write down the number. Using the same technique, measure your hips at the fullest point and record the number. Divide your waist measurement by your hip measurement to get your waist/hip ratio.

Because a man's waist/hip ratio is considered abnormal if it's >1.0, men can perform a shorter version of this test that is sometimes called "the 30-second heart attack test."

Take a tape measure, belt, string, or ribbon and wrap it around your hips. With your fingers, pinch the point on each end where the tape meets. With your fingers still marking the place where the tape meets, move the tape to your waist. Wrap the tape around your waist to see if the two pinched ends meet (or overlap) on your hips. If the ends don't meet or overlap, your waist is bigger than your hips and your waist/hip ratio is greater than 1.0.

Women can consult Table 2.4 to find their maximum allowable waist size for any given hip measurement, in inches.

Table 2.4

Waist	Hip	Waist	Hip
28	35	34.5	43
29	36	35	44
29.5	37	36	45
30.5	38	37	46
31	39	37.5	47
32	40	39	48
33	41	40	49
33.5	42	40	50

Some experts feel that waist circumference is a more accurate indicator of abdominal or visceral fat than waist/hip ratio. Men with a waist circumference >40 inches (102 cm), and women with a waist circumference >35 inches (88 cm) have an increased risk of heart disease and diabetes.

Now, if any of the above obesity formulas describe you, you are considered to be medically obese. If you are obese, you are not alone. In fact, 45 percent of all men and women have a BMI over 27. Serious obesity is also on the rise with 2 percent of all men and 4 percent of all women having a BMI over 40. This is twice the rate it was 10 years ago.

Why Is Obesity Considered a Disease?

Webster's Dictionary defines disease as "an impairment of the normal state of the living animal that affects the performance of the vital functions." Obesity *can* and often *does* affect vital body functions. Conditions related to obesity cause over 300,000 deaths a year in the United States. Only smoking causes more preventable deaths. It is estimated that obesity results in $68 billion per year in excess medical costs. An additional $33 billion is spent on diet-related programs and products. Table 2.5 is a partial list of medical problems associated with obesity:

Table 2.5
Diseases Associated with Obesity

Coronary artery disease
Cancer
Stroke
Diabetes
Arthritis
Gallstones
Gastroesophageal reflux (heartburn)
Fatty liver with or without hepatitis
Sleep apnea and other respiratory problems
Gout
Menstrual irregularity and infertility
Hyperlipidemia (high blood fat level)
Hypertension (high blood pressure)

Heart attack, cancer, and *stroke* are the three most common causes of death in the United States. Obesity increases your risk of being afflicted by these problems. In fact, obesity is associated with *half* of the ten leading causes of death in the United States. While not all cancers are more likely in the obese, cancers of the breast, colon, prostate, and uterus are more commonly seen in overweight people. Thus, two of the three most common causes of death from cancer (breast and colon in women, prostate and colon in men) are associated with obesity.

Many overweight people also have more than one complication. In fact, Dr. Theodore Van Italie, when he was professor of medicine at Columbia University Medical School, coined the term "the deadly quartet" for people with obesity, hypertension, hyperlipidemia, and diabetes. Individuals afflicted concurrently with these conditions have a very high mortality rate. If you fit this description, your doctor has probably prescribed a slew of prescription medications. These may include a calcium channel blocker (Calan SR™, Procardia™) and/or ACE-inhibitor (Accupril™) for high blood pressure, Mevacor™ or Pravachol™ for high cholesterol, and Glyburide™ and/or Glucotrol™ for diabetes. But for your obesity, your doctor may have given you only an admonishment to lose a few pounds. This approach to patient care makes no sense to me. What you also need is treatment for the single problem that is aggravating the other three —namely, obesity.

Sam was a 48-year-old restaurant owner. At 6 feet tall and weighing 220 pounds, Sam had a family history of obesity, diabetes, and high blood pressure, all three of which he inherited. After three months on 120 mg of Xenical™ three times a day, he weighed 198 pounds and no longer needed insulin to control his diabetes, or medication for hypertension. But Sam's story is not unique. Most complications of obesity will improve or completely reverse after a person loses just 10 percent of his or her starting weight, or about 25 percent of his or her excess weight. Losing 10 percent of your starting weight may not seem like a lot, but a 10 percent weight loss translates into a 30 percent loss of fat stores.

Obesity also causes or worsens diseases that, while not life-threatening, commonly bring pain and disability with them. Even people who have a BMI over 25 (overweight but not necessarily obese) are at a higher risk for the diseases listed in Table 2.5 and outlined below.

Arthritis

Obesity aggravates arthritis by putting extra pressure on the joints, especially the weight-bearing joints such as the hips and knees. Constant wear and tear on the joints, however, can also cause osteoarthritis to develop prematurely. The result is a self-defeating cycle that can further aggravate obesity in some people. The cycle goes something like this: The more weight you gain, the more stress you place on the joints, intensifying the pain of your arthritis as you do so. As your mobility becomes restricted, your life turns more sedentary. Add to this a reduction in exercise and fewer calories burned, and your weight gain will increase. Without appropriate weight reduction, many people in this situation will finally require total hip or knee replacements.

Gallstones

Overweight people have an increased risk for gallstones. In fact, if you are 20 percent above your ideal body weight, you have a twofold increased risk of developing gallstones compared to normal weight individuals. A seriously obese person (BMI>40) has a sixfold increased risk. On the other hand, you may have heard that dieting actually causes gallstones. This is true with certain very low-fat diets, such as the all-liquid diets

Optifast™ and Medifast™. These diets can increase your risk for developing gallstones while you are actively losing weight. However, once you achieve and maintain your goal weight with any diet, your risk of gallstones dramatically reduces. In addition, while losing weight on a diet of 1,200 or more calories supplying over 20 grams of fat per day, there appears to be only a small risk or no risk at all of developing symptomatic gallstones. Thus, I recommend to my dieting patients that they consume at least 10 grams of fat in a single meal at least once a day. Why? Research has shown that a meal with 10 grams of fat will contract the gallbladder as well as a Big Mac. And one single forceful gallbladder contraction once a day has been shown to prevent gallstone formation in some scientific studies. You can also greatly decrease your chance of forming gallstones during weight loss by taking the drug ursodeoxycholic acid (Actigall, Urso) as part of your diet regimen.

Heartburn

Many of my patients complain to me about heartburn. If you have experienced heartburn, you know how painful it can be. That burning feeling in your chest is caused by acid from your stomach flowing backward (refluxing) into your esophagus. Under normal circumstances, your stomach contents are usually prevented from entering your esophagus by a one-way valve at the bottom of your esophagus called a sphincter. If the pressure below the valve becomes too high, the valve fails, and acid enters the esophagus. Extra fat in the abdomen can exert the pressure that causes the sphincter to fail. For this reason, overweight people frequently experience heartburn and even regurgitation.

A recent study demonstrated that the extra acid reflux in obese individuals leads to a higher incidence of esophageal cancer. Do you find yourself taking Pepcid AC before dinner most evenings? By losing weight and restricting dietary fat (dietary fat actually relaxes the sphincter), you may reduce the occurrence of gastroesophageal reflux and eliminate your heartburn.

Fatty Liver

When you are obese, your body fat isn't only under your skin. Body fat can infiltrate many important organs, including the liver. A fatty liver, often seen in obesity, diabetes, and alcoholism, is usually not a serious condition. Nonetheless, fat in the liver sometimes causes an inflammatory reaction—a condition called "nonalcoholic steatohepatitis" (NASH). If left untreated, the inflammation can cause scarring of the liver (cirrhosis). Have you ever been turned down when donating blood because a liver enzyme was elevated, yet tested negative for viral hepatitis B and C? You may have NASH, which you can treat with weight loss. Some doctors also recommend vitamin E supplementation and ursodeoxycholic (Urso or Actigall) as part of your weight-loss program.

Sleep Apnea

Do you snore? Does your partner keep rolling you over in the middle of the night, or grab a pillow and head for the opposite side of the house? Are you chronically tired? Have you ever fallen asleep at work or felt yourself drifting off while driving? If you answer "yes" to these questions, you may have a potentially serious condition known as "sleep apnea." Many overweight people experience a partial blockage of their airway during sleep, caused in part by fat-infiltrated soft tissue in the back of the throat. This blockage causes a snoring sound. The sound may be unhealthy not only for your relationship, but may also signal the onset of potential health problems. More specifically, the blockage can reduce oxygen levels in your blood, which can result in cyanosis (bluish skin discoloration), high blood pressure, and even irregular heart rhythms. Sleep apnea can be treated with a special breathing device, but losing weight may be all you need to correct the problem.

Hypertriglyceridemia

Overweight patients are frequently found to have high blood levels of fat (triglycerides) and bad (LDL) cholesterol and low levels of good (HDL) cholesterol. This is even more common in people whose extra weight is emphasized in their waist (male pattern or android pattern of obesity). Hypertriglyceridemia (high levels of fat in the blood) is a condition that can cause a host of cardiovascular problems.

Hypertension (High Blood Pressure)

Obesity is also an important risk factor in the development of hypertension. Obesity alone can put extra stress on your heart, and adding high blood pressure to the equation causes even more stress. Thus, it's important to maintain a normal weight as well as treat the hypertension. Many people assume that having high blood pressure means you cannot take diet medication. It is true that some of the drugs used today (e.g., Meridia™, Ionomin™, Fastin™) can raise blood pressure slightly. But as long as your blood pressure is controlled with medication, the diet drugs can be used with your doctor's supervision. Xenical™ is ideally suited for hypertensive obese individuals since the drug has no direct effect on blood pressure.

Noninsulin-Dependent (Type II) Diabetes

Adult-onset diabetes is often associated with obesity. Excess weight makes the body resistant to the hormone insulin, which regulates blood sugar. By reducing body weight (especially around the waistline), sensitivity to insulin is restored and blood sugar often becomes normal, eliminating the need for oral hypoglycemic drugs (e.g., Glucotrol, Glyburide) or supplemental insulin shots.

Preventing or Reversing Disease by Weight Loss

Let me emphasize again the importance of controlling your weight in the management of health disorders. With most diseases associated with obesity, losing even a small portion of excess weight may be the best remedy. If you have one or more of the previously mentioned weight-related diseases, you need to make every effort to achieve and maintain a healthier weight. If you have tried and failed to do this, consider diet drugs to assist you in that goal.

In September 1998, the National Heart Lung and Blood Institute (NHLBI) of the National Institutes of Health (NIH) published the report of the Obesity Education Initiative Expert Panel on the Identification, Evaluation, and Treatment of Overweight and Obesity in Adults. The panel concluded there was strong evidence to recommend weight loss to lower elevated blood pressure, blood glucose (sugar), triglycerides, total cholesterol, and LDL-cholesterol (and raise good HDL-cholesterol).

Many people wonder if thinner people live longer. Scientific evidence indicates that thinner animals (including humans) *do* live longer. Rats that are thin live an average of *one-third longer* than obese rats. The evidence in humans is striking as well. In a study of women ages 25 to 55 published in the *New England Journal of Medicine*, the lowest mortality rate was observed in those women who weighed 15 percent less than the average weight of women of a similar age. Even a weight gain of just 22 pounds after age 18 is associated with increased mortality by the time the person reaches middle age. As expected, the study showed that women with a BMI greater than 32 had greater than a fourfold increased risk of death from heart disease than women with a BMI below 19. What researchers were *not* expecting to find was:

- 20 percent increased risk of death from all causes in women with a BMI between 19 and 25
- 30 percent increased risk of death from all causes in women with a BMI between 25 and 27
- 60 percent increased risk of death from all causes in women with a BMI between 27 and 29

There was no difference found in mortality between normal weight and heavyweight smokers. The above findings were true only for nonsmoking women. Smoking is so unhealthy that even smokers who are at their ideal weight have a high mortality.

If you view this information as a scare tactic or a ploy to launch you into taking control of your weight problem, then I apologize beforehand; it is certainly not my intent. The truth is that negative reinforcement rarely *encourages* people to take action. With overweight people, and especially with those people subjected to nagging and other efforts to push them into losing weight, the accompanying anxiety and depression will only work against them.

Positive reinforcement is certainly a better motivator here than constant criticism. So why do you need to know these dismal statistics? Knowledge of the significant health risks associated with obesity will allow you to justify taking the small risk of experiencing diet drug side effects. As you will see, in most cases the potential risks of diet drugs are more than outweighed by the much greater risks in remaining obese.

The Cause of Obesity (It's Not What You Think)

In our "thin is in" world, the societal pressure from being overweight is enormous. Magazines, television, and fashion dictate that a thin body is ideal. Now, take a moment to consider the psychological stresses of being obese. Low self-esteem, depression, and feelings of isolation (real and imagined) can result. If you are overweight, you are no stranger to the comments: "If only she would exercise some willpower," or "He is such a nervous eater," or the famous "Her face is so pretty . . . if only she would lose some weight." These remarks hurt, and it is easy for people to believe them.

Gina, a 35-year-old receptionist and a mother of two, knows all too well how difficult it was for her. Overweight as a child, the neighborhood children used to call her "fat thing." During adolescence, the pressure on her to be thin became overwhelming. In high school, her best friend, who was naturally thin, used to badger Gina just to practice some willpower to lose weight. She experimented with fasting and single food diets, but they were too restrictive and impossible to sustain. Even while depriving her body of essential nutrients, Gina never lost much weight. She spent much of her time obsessing about her weight, and her self-confidence was shaky. For years she suffered misplaced guilt and shame. Gina's family history should have clued her into her problem: Her mother and older sister were both overweight. She called her obesity "the family curse."

Ultimately, Gina heard about the benefits of taking diet drugs. Her doctor prescribed Meridia™ (sibutramine), and Gina started to lose weight. She has maintained her weight for almost a year now, and her self-confidence has really blossomed. She feels so good about her experience that she wants to help others. Gina recently formed a support group in her town to aid others with similar weight problems. Gina said to me, "It's hard enough to be overweight and feel we repulse other people, but to feel guilt and shame for something that isn't our fault is intolerable." Bravo, Gina!

The truth is, most people believe that overweight people should be able to control their problem. Yet, if it were so simple, obesity would have been eliminated years ago. In my experience, overweight people are highly motivated to lose weight. They spend billions of dollars every year in an attempt to reduce. Often they are able to lose a few pounds, but as I mentioned earlier, the weight usually is gained back along with a few *additional* pounds.

Most obese people will explain that they love to eat. Realistically, most people love to eat. Eating is not just a physiological need, it is a social activity, and much of life revolves around it. Deals are made over "power breakfasts" and business lunches; dates are frequently centered on going out to dinner; and parties almost always include food. Remember—thin people love to eat, too. Loving to eat doesn't make people overweight.

My patients also tell me they have no willpower, and can't stop eating before they are full. I assure them that thin people do not stop eating before they are full, either. The body is designed to eat when it feels the hunger signal and to stop when it feels the full signal. But for many overweight people, the signal for fullness may become distorted. As a result of overeating, fullness may actually feel more like *pain* than pleasure. This is because it's recognized too late.

Some of my patients *are* able to resist eating until they are full, and they lose weight this way. Unfortunately, the struggle that they endure to continue to lose weight by not eating so much is rarely successful for long. These patients frequently experience feelings of hunger, weakness, lightheadedness, irritability, and fatigue. Because they can't sustain their "willpower," they regain the weight they've lost. Although willpower may be necessary to treat obesity in most diets, lack of willpower is not responsible for obesity. The fact is, in many cases, *obesity is an inherited metabolic disease.*

Genetic Factors

As readily as we acknowledge other inherited traits, it is time to accept that heredity plays a large part in determining your weight. No one questions, for instance, that your blue eyes are from your grandmother or that your curly hair is inherited from your father. I have one patient who tells me when she looks in the mirror she shouts, "Mom, how did you get in my mirror?" Yet many people still blame learned eating and exercise habits as the sole cause of obesity in children of obese parents. Science, however, has now proven that favoring your mother's body type is not a coincidence.

To illustrate this, let me tell you about some of the research that has been done on this subject. Studies of identical twins indicate a strong genetic component to obesity. If one twin is obese, *nearly 90 percent of the time* the other twin is also obese. The correlation with fraternal twins or nontwin siblings is less than 50 percent and much lower for adopted siblings. A study of adopted children, performed by Albert Stunkard at the University of Pennsylvania, found the weight of adopted children was much more likely to correlate with the weight of their biological mother than their adoptive parents. This is the case even when a child never lived with his or her biological mother.

Another scientist named Bouchard was interested in the same phenomenon. To find out whether or not genetics played a role in weight gain, he studied identical twins. By overfeeding pairs of identical twins, he found that each twin pair gained approximately the same amount of weight. He also found a wide disparity in the amount of weight gained between the twin pairs. Some twin pairs gained just a few pounds, while others gained a large amount of weight. Bouchard's study gives us two important "take home" messages:

- Heredity has a strong influence on weight.
- Body metabolism differs greatly between unrelated people.

New technology has allowed us to add additional proof to the genetic link. Genes that code for obesity have now been cloned. Certain obese mice inherit a defective gene called the "Ob gene," and are unable to produce a protein called "leptin." This protein regulates body fat. When leptin is injected into the obese mouse, the mouse loses weight. But doctors at Thomas Jefferson University in Philadelphia have reported that, unlike obese rodents, obese humans actually have *too much* leptin in their systems. Does this mean leptin is not important in humans? The answer is, no. Higher than normal levels of leptin in overweight individuals suggest that obese people can make the protein but do not respond to it as effectively as do normal weight individuals.

At least six obesity-related genes have now been identified, and thanks to the Human Genome Project, we now know of over a hundred genes that are responsible in some way for our weight. The MG (Mahogany) gene, discovered in mice, appears to regulate the burning of calories. Scientists at Millennium Pharmaceuticals in Massachusetts found that mice with a mutated MG gene do not gain weight on a high-fat diet. These and other genes that play a role in the regulation of body weight give scientists a specific target. Drugs are currently being developed to manipulate these genes.

Environmental Factors

After emphasizing the metabolic and genetic abnormalities that cause obesity, let's not completely discount the impact that society has on our weight. Certainly, the popular notion of what an attractive weight is has varied throughout the centuries. There was a time when looking full-figured, or "Rubenesque," was popular. In the 1960s, Twiggy and her super-thin, shapeless body was the rage. Later we had Jane Fonda and her fit, aerobicized body to emulate. And today, Calvin Klein, with the help of Kate Moss, has many of us feeling ashamed to be a healthy, normal weight. Fashion magazines bombard us (targeting mostly young women) with the gold standard for weight. You may be surprised to know that the average fashion model is 5 feet 9, weighs 110 pounds, and has a BMI of 16.6. The average woman is 5 feet 4, weighs 145 pounds, and has a BMI of 24.

In contrast, consider how other cultures view their bodies. In some third world countries like Nigeria, having a rotund wife is a status symbol suggesting affluence. Many American Samoans are happy to be overweight. Members of societies where food is scarce do not worship at the "Temple of Thinness." After all, having enough to eat is their objective. A few extra pounds can indicate wealth and health. Other cultural attitudes may be more familiar to us. Many households, for example, include a member who admonishes the children to clean their plates. "Remember all those starving children?" And how can we forget Grandma, who insists on second helpings for growing boys —except that "growing boy" is now 42 years old and is growing only wider. These external influences can certainly compound weight problems.

Lifestyles are also at work on our weight. Not all of us in today's society are plowing fields or physically exerting ourselves as we once were. We are not expending as many calories during the day at our jobs. Yet eating patterns and food choices that can contribute to being overweight are now more abundant than ever. Fewer of us are sitting down at the table to eat freshly prepared foods. A more typical scenario is grabbing a quick burger as we drive to our next meeting. The trend is to eat on the run and snack in between. And what do we choose to eat as we run? The choices are varied, but many quick and easy meals are loaded with fat, sugar, and salt.

While obesity is usually considered an adult problem, children are also at risk. Studies have shown that more children are overweight than ever. The latest government statistics show that the number of seriously overweight children and teens has doubled in the past 30 years, and most of this increase has occurred in the past 15 years. Experts suggest that lack of physical activity is mostly to blame. Today more children are sedentary, watching television or playing video and computer games. Add to that the fast food many children consume and you're left with a whole lot of excess pounds.

So, the good news is clear: Your weight problem isn't entirely your fault. There are social and genetic factors that contribute to your weight problem. Now that you have shed your guilt about being overweight, however, it's best to try shedding those extra pounds. In addition, you may ask yourself, "If I am genetically programmed to be overweight, am I doomed? Can I really become thin and stay thin even though my genes say I should be fat? Is there any way to reprogram my body, or am I to be fat forever?"

How Can Genetic Diseases Be Controlled?

It is nearly impossible to cure genetic diseases. High-tech futuristic gene therapy may someday be routine, but for now we rely on drugs to control genetic diseases. Table 2.6 lists common diseases that have strong genetic influences, including obesity, schizophrenia, hypertension, coronary artery disease, and breast cancer.

Table 2.6   The Importance of Inheritance

Disease	r Value*
Obesity	.88
Schizophrenia	.80
Hypertension	.57
Coronary artery disease	.49
Breast cancer	.45

*Relative relationship between heredity and the disease. If r value is 1.00, the disease is 100% genetically linked. If r value is 0.00, genetics play no role in the disease.

Whether you have high cholesterol, hypertension, diabetes, or schizophrenia, medication can control most, if not all, of your symptoms and prevent complications. This is true of obesity as well. *Hooray!* Are you shocked? Is it *really* true? We have all heard of diet drugs, but do they really work? And what about the side effects? In Chapter 3, we will separate fact from fiction and learn the truth about diet drugs.

3

A New Look at Diet Drugs

Diet drugs are one of the most maligned classes of medications available on the U.S. market. Only THC, the active ingredient in marijuana, as a treatment for nausea caused by chemotherapy, or megavitamins for the prevention of cold, heart disease, and cancer are more controversial. This attitude also prevails in Europe and the United Kingdom, where doctors treat a very small percentage of the obese with medication. You may be surprised to learn, however, that some diet drugs have been available to doctors for over 20 years! And the information demonstrating their effectiveness in treating obesity has been known for just as long. Why have these drugs been ignored by the vast majority of family physicians and internists since their advent in the 1970s? Even the new drugs Xenical™ and Meridia™ have not been given to the majority of obese individuals seeking advice from their doctors about ways to control weight. In this chapter, we'll explore the reasons the medical community has failed to embrace diet drugs as a treatment for obesity, and why their negative attitude has contributed to a "Dark Age" in obesity treatment. By dispelling the myths surrounding diet medication, we can move from the Dark Ages to a renaissance in the management of weight problems.

Myth 1: Diet drugs can cause heart valve problems and pulmonary hypertension.

Reality: Only the drug fenfluramine has been shown to cause these complications. fenfluramine hydrochloride (Pondomin), the "fen" of the popular Phen/fen combination drug regimen, and dex-fenfluramine hydrochloride (Redux), brought on the U.S. market in 1996, were voluntarily withdrawn from the market in 1997 after these fenfluramine compounds were discovered to cause serious heart and lung disease in a minority of people using them for weight control. No one has ever been shown to develop a heart valve problem or pulmonary hypertension from *any* of the drugs currently available to treat obesity. With FDA scrutiny for diet drugs at an all-time high, medication-assisted weight loss is safer now than it has ever been in the past.

Myth 2: Diet drugs only help you get started on a weight loss program. After a few weeks, their effectiveness wears off.

Reality: The only effects that wear off are some of the side effects. While it's true that the stimulant feeling associated with phentermine tends to lessen with time, the appetite suppressant effect persists. Conclusive information proves that phentermine and Meridia™ suppress appetite and control weight for as long as the medication is taken. Likewise, Xenical™ has been shown to maintain weight loss for as long as the drug is administered to the patient. In fact, the FDA has approved Xenical™ as safe and effective for two years' use. Weight loss is likely to be maintained for years as long as the drugs are used in conjunction with other interventions as part of a comprehensive weight control program. These other interventions include diet, exercise, and behavior modification.

The supposed short-lived effectiveness of diet drugs is something I learned in my pharmacology course at medical school. I had to *unlearn* it when new data were released. Many doctors still hold on to the earlier information and resist acceptance of the latest findings.

Many doctors, by nature, are conservative. I'll agree that, in many instances, this is an appropriate approach. However, when conclusive scientific data are systematically ignored for years, that's not being "conservative," that's being out of touch—which is not in the patient's best interest. With the help of this book, both you and your doctor can be up-to-date on the latest information about treating your weight problem with drug therapy.

Myth 3: Diet drugs don't work very well. Once you stop taking them, you will regain the weight.

Reality: Part of this statement is true. If you stop taking diet medication, you may start regaining weight. This does *not* mean that drugs don't work. It actually means the drugs *do* work. Let me explain. There are several ways to determine drug effectiveness. In the case of diet drugs, the drug may cause more weight loss over time than a placebo. Another way to determine a drug's effectiveness is to demonstrate that the effect of the drug disappears after it has been discontinued. Medication effectiveness is actually inferred from the rapid increase in weight in the majority of people who stop diet medication, even though they continue a low-calorie diet, exercise regimen, and behavior modification program.

In the late eighteenth century, German scientist and Nobel Prize winner Robert Koch developed postulates—basic principles—concerning drug effectiveness that are the most rigorous to date. To fulfill Koch's postulates one must demonstrate that:

- The treatment produces the desired effect.
- Withdrawal of the treatment reverses that effect.
- Reinstitution of the treatment realizes the effect once again.

The latest studies make it clear that diet drugs fulfill these criteria. This leads us to the conclusion that the drugs do indeed work. They work to control your weight problem.

Diet drugs don't *cure* obesity. If diet drugs did cure the disease, we could take them for a time, stop taking them, and then be thin forever! Wouldn't that be great? It just doesn't work that way. Although some drugs cure diseases (for example, antibiotics can cure bacterial infections), most drugs only *control* disease. It's unfortunate, but diet drugs are frequently held to a higher standard than other drugs. No one would dispute the effectiveness of insulin in the treatment of diabetes, nor would they scoff at the treatment of high blood pressure with antihypertensive medication. Both of these medications are effective in treating their respective diseases. But what happens when these medications are discontinued? With diabetes, the blood sugar rises immediately. The same is true with high blood pressure. Both of these diseases are lifelong metabolic diseases that must be treated on a continuous basis, and in most cases, forever. It is commonly accepted that the drugs used to treat these diseases merely control, not cure, the disease. Ironically, the only way some people can stop taking these medications and control their problems is by losing weight!

Not everyone gains weight after discontinuing diet medication. Some people have a long-term benefit from their diet medication and are able to maintain their weight without the drugs. If you do experience weight gain after stopping the medication, Chapter 11 will guide you toward maintaining your goal weight forever.

Myth 4: Most diet drugs are still dangerous. They significantly increase your risk of high blood pressure, stroke, heart attack, and sudden death from irregular heartbeats.

Reality: Any drug, including diet drugs, can cause a host of side effects. However, diet drugs cause no more side effects than many other prescription medications. If you are currently taking a medication (any medication), go to the library and look it up in the *Physician's Desk Reference* (PDR). The PDR lists information about all drugs currently available in the United States. I guarantee you will find your drug has side effects ranging from diarrhea to hepatitis, seizures to difficulty breathing, hair loss to acne. While diet drugs do have the potential to cause side effects, serious side effects are rare, most are mild, and they often eventually improve even when you continue to take the medication. Side effects are of two types: *idiosyncratic*, which means they occur in a small percentage of users at low doses and often for unexplained reasons; and *dose-dependent*, which means they predictably occur in many people when the drug is given in a high enough dosage. All drugs also have a *therapeutic index*. This is a dosage range below which the drug is ineffective, and above which the drug is toxic. Some drugs have a therapeutic index that is so narrow, patients must have their blood tested regularly to be sure the levels of the drug are not too high (e.g., digoxin for heart failure, lithium for manic-depression, and theophylline for asthma). Most diet drugs have a wide therapeutic index and none require blood level monitoring.

Dose-dependent side effects can usually be controlled by keeping the dose of the drug within the therapeutic index. This means that as long as you take no more than the prescribed amount of the drug, any dose-dependent side effects will be minimized. Serious, idiosyncratic side effects are extremely rare. Bear in mind, when you take *any* drug for the first time, there is the potential, however slight, for a serious side effect. In Chapter 4, we'll assess your personal risk: benefit ratio for diet drugs.

A comprehensive list of side effects associated with diet medication is provided in Chapter 7 and/or Appendix I. The most common complaint from people taking phentermine is a dry mouth. Some people will also experience body stimulation. Meridia™ can elevate blood pressure but usually only to a small extent. Xenical™ prevents the absorption of dietary fat and can therefore make your stool (bowel movements) somewhat oily. Most of these diet drug side effects do not require you to stop taking the medication.

The "bad rap" label for diet drugs probably started with amphetamines. While they curbed appetite, they also raised blood pressure and pulse, and were extremely addictive. Let me be perfectly clear: None of the current diet medications are as dangerous as amphetamines. Phentermine and Meridia™ have minimal or no potential for addiction and Xenical™ absolutely none.

Myth 5: We would have heard a lot more about these diet drugs if they were so effective.

Reality: From the late 1980s to the mid-1990s we heard very little about diet drugs. Most of their use was in weight loss "mills" and there were little, if any, found in mainstream family practitioners' offices. So why weren't the drug manufacturers touting their wares in the doctors' offices? Surely there was money to be made by extolling the virtues of these drugs. Why were consumers kept in the dark for so long?

The answer lies in simple economics. Drugs such as phentermine have been on the market for so long their patent rights have expired. When drugs go "off patent," dozens of generic drugs flood the market, causing the price and profit margins of the brand name drugs to fall. The profit on these drugs falls so low that it doesn't pay to advertise them. This means that drug sales representatives will spend the few minutes they have telling doctors about the newest patent-protected drugs they represent, and not bother to mention those off patent. It may surprise you to learn that many physicians get the latest drug information directly from the sales representative of the drug. In other words, they're only hearing about new drug therapies through those who represent a particular drug.

Phen/fen and Redux caused a renewed interest in drug treatment of obesity, but that was soon extinguished when evidence of their toxicity was published. Now that two patent-protected diet drugs (Meridia™ and Xenical™) are available, doctors are being reacquainted with the benefits of diet drugs. This should result in a renewal of interest in treating the obese with drugs. Even though the new drugs are terrific, keep in mind that the older, generic drugs—Ionomin™, Adipex-P™, or Fastin™ (phentermine)—and over-the-counter medications such as Dexatrim™ or Acutrim™ (phenylpropanolamine) still work well.

Myth 6: Diet drugs are only for seriously obese people.

Reality: Studies clearly demonstrate that even mildly overweight people (BMI>25) carry an increased risk of heart disease and death. Therefore, even moderate degrees of obesity need treatment. If diet, exercise, and behavioral modification alone have not worked for you, you should consider taking diet drugs. You are a candidate for diet drugs if your BMI is greater than 30, or if it's 27 and you have an obesity-related disease such as diabetes, hypertension, or hyperlipidemia. Remember, remaining obese at any level is dangerous to your health.

Myth 7: Obese people don't need to take drugs. They just need to exercise more self-control.

Reality: This simplistic view of obesity is outdated and erroneous. Everything doctors now know about obesity—the genetic link, defective satiety perception, and multiple metabolic disturbances—demonstrates that obesity should be treated as a disease. Standard diet therapy often isn't enough. By understanding the true causes of obesity, the drug therapy approach becomes a more rational treatment for many individuals.

Myth 8: Obesity isn't a serious medical problem.

Reality: Next to smoking three packs of cigarettes a day, remaining obese is probably the best way to get heart disease, stroke, and cancer. Mortality rates increase as your body weight increases from 20 percent above ideal weight (IBW) to 40 percent above IBW. Cancer of the colon, breast, uterus, and prostate are more common in the obese. While a "risk-benefit ratio" should be considered when using any drug, the risk of using antiobesity drugs in most individuals is less than the risk of remaining obese.

There are other barriers that have undermined the advance of drug treatments for obesity. Some doctors worry unnecessarily that they risk reprimand by their licensing boards or even the Drug Enforcement Administration (DEA) if they "overprescribe" diet drugs. Insurance companies often will not pay doctors to treat obesity unless a patient already has diabetes or high blood pressure. Insurance companies often do not reimburse their clients for diet drugs.

Although obesity is one of the most costly and widespread diseases in America, traditionally it has been "put on the back burner" in terms of research funding. For years the National Institutes of Health (NIH) heavily funded research to fight or cure diseases associated with obesity, such as cancer and heart disease. Yet money for obesity research was less available. Fortunately, the NIH has recently started an initiative to "wage war" on obesity. It is also fortunate that the private sector, namely drug companies, remains heavily involved in antiobesity research.

Now that I've dispelled some myths surrounding the drug treatment of obesity and identified a few of the barriers to that treatment, let's find out if you are a candidate for diet drugs.

4

Who Is a Candidate for Diet Drugs?

Some people assume incorrectly that diet drugs are used only to treat people who are "really, really fat." Others inappropriately use nonprescription diet drugs (e.g., Dexatrim™, generic name: phenylpropanolamine) when they are just slightly overweight. From what you've read so far in *The Complete Book of Diet Drugs*, you may be wondering if diet medication is right for you.

Let's review some facts about obesity and diet drugs:

- Many studies demonstrate that even mild to moderate obesity is associated with a significantly increased risk of cardiovascular disease and early death. For example, if your BMI increases from 26 to 32, your mortality increases 90 percent. Based on this fact, it is estimated that every year, nearly 1,000 out of every 1 million people die an obesity-related death.
- The diet drugs that are currently available control appetite and lower body weight. This is true with both long- and short-term use.
- Most people tolerate diet drugs well. Side effects are usu-

ally minimal. For most people, the benefits of diet drugs far outweigh their side effects.

- Serious side effects are extremely rare now that fenfluramine is no longer available.

Are you a candidate for diet drugs?
As shown in Table 4.1, you are a potential candidate for diet drugs if:

- Your BMI is >30
- Your BMI is >27 and you have an obesity-related health problem (e.g., diabetes, hypertension, hyperlipidemia, coronary artery disease)*

*Some experts require two or more risk factors to be present if the BMI is greater than 27 and less than 30.

Table 4.1   Who Is a Candidate for Drug Therapy?

Body Mass Index

Height (feet/inches)

Weight (lbs)	5'0"	5'3"	5'6"	5'9"	6'0"	6'3"
140	27	26	23	21	19	18
150	29	27	24	22	20	19
160	31	28	26	24	22	20
170	33	30	28	25	23	21
180	35	32	29	27	25	23
190	37	34	31	28	26	24
200	39	36	32	30	27	25
210	41	37	34	31	29	26
220	43	39	36	33	30	28
230	45	41	37	34	31	29
240	47	43	39	36	33	30
250	49	44	40	37	34	31

Source: F. Xavier Pi-Sunyer, M.D.: *Current Approaches to the Management of Obesity*, 1996. Drug therapy may be used for those in the lightly shaded areas (BMI of 30 or higher) or those in the darkly shaded areas (BMI of 27 or higher) who have one or more obesity-related health problem.

If you fulfill the above criteria, you should definitely consider diet medication if one of the following scenarios also describes you:

You haven't been able to lose a significant amount of weight in the past, even with a low-calorie diet, exercise, and a behavior modification program.

Chances are, if dieting hasn't worked before, it isn't going to work this time. Even the latest fad diets aren't likely to shed your pounds permanently. TV personality Oprah Winfrey succeeded in losing weight with one-on-one dietary counseling from a registered dietitian, a personal trainer, and a personal chef. This kind of constant, personalized attention can help you succeed at weight loss, but it comes with a price tag very few can afford. And then, of course, Ms. Winfrey put her weight back on anyway.

After losing weight, you can't maintain your new, lower weight.

Maintaining weight loss is, without a doubt, the biggest obstacle dieters face. It is the most common cause of failure of any given diet program. Statistics show that within 2 years (3 to 5 years if you exercise and use behavior modification techniques), close to 95 percent of all dieters regain any weight they have lost. In many cases, people gain back even more weight than they lost. Most diet drugs are effective in helping people maintain their new, lower weight as long as the medication is taken. The one exception appears to be Prozac™. The antiobesity effect of the drug tends to wear off after 6 months of treatment.

The issue of using diet drugs to maintain weight loss brings up some important and somewhat controversial questions. In order for previously obese people to maintain their goal weight, should diet drugs be given to them if their BMI is less than 27 if they begin to regain weight? Should diet drugs be continued at least intermittently indefinitely? I'll discuss these issues in the upcoming chapter on weight maintenance.

You have a weight-related disease such as hypertension, hyper-lipidemia, or diabetes.

If you have one or more of these diseases, successful weight loss and maintenance is critical for your health. By losing just a portion of your excess weight, you can improve or possibly even eliminate your health problem. In this situation, many physicians prescribe diet medications even if the BMI is only greater than 27. Of course, the decision whether or not to start any treatment depends on the "risk-to-benefit ratio," a careful analysis of the expected benefits of therapy weighed against the potential risks of that therapy.

Whenever faced with a decision, your brain automatically considers the options available and searches for the one with the most benefit and the least risk. Perhaps when you're faced with a big decision, you make a list of the benefits and risks involved in order to clarify the process. If the good outweighs the bad, you may proceed with a particular plan. If the reverse is true and the bad outweighs the good, you may scratch the idea. This process is essentially how doctors decide the risk-to-benefit ratio of any given treatment. Keeping this in mind, I have presented in Table 4.2 a partial list of the risks associated with remaining obese, versus the risks of losing weight with diet drugs. This may help you decide whether diet drugs are a good choice for you (see Chapter 7 for more information on drug side effects).

Table 4.2
Assessing the Risk/Benefit Ratio of Diet Drugs

Risk of Remaining Obese	Risk of Diet Drugs†
Early death	Dry mouth*
Diabetes	Sleep disturbance**

Risk of Remaining Obese	Risk of Diet Drugs†
High triglycerides	Drowsiness**
High total cholesterol	Constipation**
Low HDL (good) cholesterol	Hair loss (reversible)
Hypertension	Central nervous system stimulation
Coronary artery disease	Restlessness
Congestive heart failure	Inability to concentrate
Blood clots	Headache
Gout	Tremor
Fatty liver	Decreased sex drive
Gallstones	Blurred vision
Sleep apnea	Depression
Breast cancer	Palpitations
Prostate cancer	High blood pressure
Colon cancer	Nausea
Uterine cancer	Diarrhea
Arthritis	Stroke***
Menstrual irregularity	
Infertility	
Psychological dysfunction	

† These are potential risks found with phentermine, Meridia™ and other sympathomimetic drugs (see Chapter 5). Xenical™ does not cause these side effects but can make stools greasy.
* Most common side effect (occurs in about 23% of patients).
** Common side effect (occurs in 5% or more of patients).
*** Extremely rare side effect.

Table 4.3 uses another technique to determine if diet drugs are the right choice for you.

Table 4.3

If Weight (BMI) Is:	And Weight-Related Health Risk Factor(s) Are:	Importance of Diet Drugs Is:
Under 27	None	0
27–30	1 or more	2+
Over 30	None	2+
Over 30	1 or more	3+

*Scale of 1–3. 1 is not as important, 3 is very important.

Contraindications to Diet Drugs

There are few instances where diet medication is either absolutely contraindicated (should never be given), or at least relatively contraindicated (be given only if the risk of remaining obese is very high). Table 4.4 indicates those conditions.

Table 4.4   Absolute Contraindications to Diet Drugs

Pregnancy	Concurrent use of MAO inhibitors or lithium*
Lactation (nursing mothers)	Known allergy to specific diet drug
Severe psychosis	Severe uncontrolled hypertension*
Anorexia nervosa	Heart, kidney, or liver failure
Alcoholism	Concurrent use of migraine medication (sumatriptan,
Drug abuse	dehydroergotamine)*

Relative Contraindications to Diet Drugs

Poorly controlled hypertension*	Cardiac arrhythmia*
Glaucoma*	Symptomatic coronary artery disease*
Depression*	Concurrent use of serotonin selective reuptake
Anticipated surgery*	inhibitors (Prozac™, Effexor™, Paxil™)*

* Only contraindicated for use of Meridia™, phentermine, and related sympathomimetic drugs (see Chapter 5). Xenical™ can still be used.

Let's take a look at a case history to see how this all works out: Joan was a 56-year-old woman who was 5 feet 3 inches tall and weighed 220 pounds. She had severe lumbar disk disease with sciatica. She needed an operation known as a "laminectomy." Her back was so bad that she had a hard time getting out of bed. Since she was so incapacitated, she was unable to exercise. Consequently, Joan began gaining even more weight. She wanted to schedule the operation but her orthopedic surgeon said she would have to lose 40 pounds first. When Joan came to my office, she was nearly in tears. She was totally defeated because she needed to lose the weight, yet because of her immobility, kept gaining instead. She also cited that the stress of this situation made her a "nervous eater." Joan was caught up in a vicious cycle.

In part because of her weight, Joan's blood pressure was around 180/110 even though she took her beta-blocker (high blood pressure medicine). Her family doctor said "no" to diet drugs because of hypertension. It was clear to me, however, that her hypertension was going to climb along with her weight.

Although in the past doctors have had to deny diet drugs to those with poorly controlled hypertension, we now have a drug that does not raise blood pressure. I prescribed Xenical™ and additional medication for her blood pressure. Over a period of 4 months, Joan's weight and blood pressure dropped and she was able to schedule the surgery. Joan came through the surgery with flying colors and remains on Xenical™.

At this point, you should have a good idea whether or not you are a candidate for diet drugs. If you are a candidate, you may still not be sure that the drug option is for you. The next chapter will help you with your decision. It includes information about each of the diet drugs currently available.

5

The Diet Drug Options

For the first time ever, doctors and patients now have access to a wide array of FDA-approved pharmaceuticals that are effective for weight control. Although the number of these drugs is still small compared to the number of drugs available to treat other diseases (e.g., medications for high blood pressure), physicians can now find a drug that can cause significant weight loss for most people.

The drugs currently available for weight loss and control are very effective. They all have been shown to cause significant weight loss in scientific studies and their side effects are considered acceptable. Pharmaceutical manufacturers see the demand for such drugs. The weight loss market is very attractive to them. Therefore, they are putting time and money into researching new drugs that will improve treatment of obesity even further. As a result, the search continues for the *ideal* diet drug. Short of a drug that would simply cure obesity or burn calories despite the amount of food we eat, what are the qualities of an ideal diet drug?

An ideal diet drug would:

- Cause a dramatic decrease in body weight, approaching, but not going below, ideal body weight.
- Be effective in maintaining body weight for as long as the drug is taken, without having to increase the dose.
- Be proven safe for long-term use (at least two years, but preferably safe indefinitely).
- Cause a reduction in body fat while sparing body protein.
- Have minimal side effects and no potential for addiction.

Although we have not yet reached "diet drug nirvana," there are many drug options today that, when used appropriately, will help you lose your excess weight and keep it off. What's really exciting is that these drugs also work in individuals who have tried, but have never had success with, permanent weight loss. And these drugs can usually accomplish this without causing significant side effects.

Next is an outline of the drugs your doctor can prescribe, and the over-the-counter drugs you can take yourself. You will probably recognize some, such as Meridia™, Xenical™, phentermine, and Dexatrim™. I will introduce others not so familiar, such as Mazinor™ (maxindol) and Tenuate™ (diethylproprion).

Don't be concerned if, after reading this chapter, you find yourself in a quandary facing a plethora of diet drug options. The next chapter helps sort out these options and, along with advice from your physician, helps you select a drug regimen that will suit you.

How Do Diet Drugs Work?

There are several different ways a drug can help you shed pounds. One way is to reduce appetite by blocking the part of the brain that makes you want to eat, or "the feeding center" of the brain. This center is located in the hypothalamus (the part of the brain that controls body functions such as temperature and weight). Other drugs can stimulate the part of the brain that makes you feel full or satiated. This brain center, which is located in a separate area of the hypothalamus, causes you to stop eating sooner than you normally would. Some drugs slow down stomach emptying, which makes you feel fuller with less food. Other drugs stimulate your expenditure of energy, or burn fat even when you are sleeping. Finally, there is a new class of drugs that interferes with the absorption of a nutrient such as fat.

Most of the drugs currently available work by reducing appetite and, to a lesser extent, by burning fat. Xenical™ (orlistat) is the exception. It works by interfering with the absorption of dietary fat. Many drugs that are not yet available also have novel ways of working. (See Chapter 6 for information on drugs in development.)

Diet drugs that work by reducing appetite generally do so by increasing brain levels of norepinephrine (NE) or serotonin. Let me explain. The brain's nerve cells communicate with each other by sending signals. These signals are in the form of chemicals called "neurotransmitters." Two of these neurotransmitters are called "norepinephrine," also known as "noradrenalin," and "serotonin." Neurotransmitters are released from one nerve cell and then stick to the next nerve cell. This alters the function of that neighboring cell. The neurotransmitter is then usually taken back up by the original cell (reuptake) to prevent overstimulation of the neighboring nerves. Diet drugs act by either releasing one of the neurotransmitters (NE) or by preventing the reuptake of the neurotransmitters (NE or serotonin).

NE is used by nerve cells in the sympathetic nervous system, and causes a wide range of actions. These actions affect heart rate, breathing, and eating behavior. In some parts of the brain, NE reduces appetite, while in other areas, it actually causes an increase. However, when you take a **sympathomimetic** drug, that is, a drug that either stimulates release of NE (e.g., phentermine, diethylpropion, mazindol) or prevents the reuptake of NE (sibutramine), the net effect, in almost all cases, is a reduction in appetite.

Serotonin is another important neurotransmitter with wide-ranging effects on behavior. Drugs that cause release of serotonin from the nerve ending (fenfluramine compounds — Pondomin, Redux) were associated with pulmonary hypertension and valvular heart disease and are no longer available. In contrast, drugs that work by preventing the reuptake of serotonin by the nerve ending (Meridia™, Prozac™, Effexor™) are not associated with severe heart and lung problems.

Carbohydrates (e.g., potatoes, pasta) can be converted to, and cause release of, serotonin in the brain. Serotonin has been shown to improve mood, increase feelings of fullness by slowing down stomach emptying, increase the burning of fat, and decrease appetite by turning off the craving for carbohydrates. (See Figure 5.1.)

Is this scenario familiar? It is 4:00 P.M., and you are feeling a

Figure 5.1

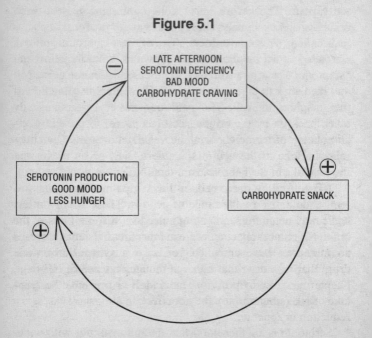

bit blah. You are hungry and crave the chocolate cake that's calling your name on the countertop. You know you should probably have a healthier snack, but the cake seems irresistible, not to mention—*it's there!* You rationalize eating just a sliver. Well, maybe just a second sliver won't hurt. The next thing you know, you've inhaled a quarter of the cake.

The theory expounded by Dr. Judy Wurtman is that obese individuals treat their "blah" feelings with carbohydrate-rich food in order to increase brain serotonin and improve their mood. However, a drug that increases brain serotonin can improve mood without the need for snacking.

You may now be asking yourself, "Why do I need to know how diet drugs work? Does it really matter?" The answer is, "yes." Drugs that work by releasing NE have different side effects from drugs that work by preventing the reuptake of serotonin, which are still different from drugs that block fat absorption. Read on to find out more about each of the available diet drugs.

The three prescription sympathomimetics listed in Table 5.1 are approved by the FDA for three months. You may have already tried one or more of these in the past. If you took the drug for just three months, chances are you haven't solved your weight loss problem. That's because, for most people, the drugs work only while you are taking them. Because the FDA approves certain drugs for only three months, it doesn't mean they aren't safe beyond that time period. It also doesn't limit the amount of time a doctor can continue to prescribe them. Although the FDA does regulate the manner in which drugs are advertised and promoted to doctors, FDA regulations do not prevent a doctor from prescribing drugs at different doses, for different lengths of treatment, or even for different purposes than the drug was originally intended (e.g., some doctors use Prozac™ for weight control, even though it is approved by the FDA as an antidepressant). These so-called "off label" uses of drugs by doctors are extremely common.

Prescription Norepinephrine-like Drugs

Table 5.1 Prescription Sympathomimetic Diet Drugs*

Brand Name	Generic Name	Tablet Dose (mg)	Dose Range (mg)	Dose Instructions	Usual Dose
Adipex-P™	Phentermine	37.5		Start with	30 mg or
Fastin™		15 or 30	15–37.5	15 mg/day (or 1/2 37.5 mg)	37.5 mg Adipex-P
Ionomin™		15 or 30		before breakfast. Increase to 30 mg/ day or 37.5 mg if needed and well tolerated.	tablet before breakfast.
Mazinor™	Mazindol	1		1 mg tablet/day. Depending on	1 mg, twice a
			1–3	effectiveness	day with
Sanorex™		1 or 2		and side effects, up to three 1 mg tablets/day with meals.	meals.
Tenuate™	Diethylpropion	75	75	1 tablet a day.	1 tablet
Tepanil™					a day.

*All prescription sympathomimetics listed are considered schedule IV drugs (limited potential for abuse) by the DEA. Direx™ (benzphetamine) and Anorex™, Wehless™, and Obalan™ (phendimetrazine) are schedule III drugs with greater potential for abuse and are therefore not recommended for *The Complete Book of Diet Drugs* program.

Physicians have a great deal of knowledge regarding obesity, its causes, and treatments. It makes no sense to limit sympathomimetic drugs to three months. Of course, it would be reassuring if more studies showed long-term safety. But such studies may never be completed. Because none of these drugs is patent protected now, the pharmaceutical industry has little motivation to pursue these studies. Only the federal government research arm, the National Institutes of Health (NIH), would be in a position to fund long-term safety studies for phentermine-like drugs. Until that time, it is up to individuals and doctors to decide on the length of each treatment.

Are you ready to get started on a drug-assisted weight control program? Some of you may feel like giving diet and exercise alone one last try. Others may be saying "Show me hard data," before deciding whether or not to use diet drugs. As a scientist as well as a physician, I believe the more informed you are, the better. Therefore, I am going to provide you with information generated by selected scientific studies proving the effectiveness of each drug mentioned in this book. Some of this information is technical. But by reviewing the outcomes of the studies, you can get a feel for the amount of weight loss you can expect from a given drug regimen and how long it takes to get there.

Adipex-P™, Fastin™, and Ionomin™ (Phentermine)

Phentermine is derived from amphetamine, but has fewer side effects and little of the addictive properties of amphetamine. It stimulates the release of NE and dopamine in the central nervous system. Many studies demonstrate the ability of phentermine to cause weight loss. In one study lasting 24 weeks, phentermine users (30 mg a day) lost 10 kilograms (22 pounds) compared to placebo users, who lost only 4.4 kilograms (about 10 pounds). All participants in the study were given an individualized diet, which explains why the placebo users still lost some weight (remember that drugs are always given with diet, exercise, and behavior modification for full effect).

In another study lasting 36 weeks, subjects were offered a 1,000-calorie diet. Those given 30 mg of phentermine a day were more successful with sticking to the diet and lost an average of 13 kilograms (29 pounds) compared to the 4.8 kilograms (10.5 pounds) lost by subjects given a placebo.

In a double-blind (neither the doctor nor the patient knew

what treatment the patient was taking), placebo-controlled study, phentermine given on an intermittent basis was just as effective as when it was given daily. Both methods of administration worked better than the placebo.

Mazinor™ (Mazindol)

Mazinor™ is a sympathomimetic-like drug that reduces appetite by directly blocking the feeding center (located in the hypothalamus) of the brain. Mazinor™ is the only antiobesity drug licensed in Japan. In a Japanese study published in the *American Journal for Clinical Nutrition,* 388 obese patients were given 0.5 mg to 3 mg of mazindol a day for 14 weeks. Patients who completed the study lost an average of 4.6 kilograms (about 10 pounds). Mazinor™ suppressed appetite in 71 percent of the people, which was similar to the percentage of people who actually lost weight (79 percent). In another study, Mazinor™ was given to people who had lost weight using a very low-calorie diet (VLCD). These diets (e.g., Optifast, Medifast, NutriSource) used to be extremely popular in the 1980s. (Remember when Oprah Winfrey lost a lot of weight on Optifast? Everyone flocked to Optifast centers. Remember when Oprah regained all of the weight and then some after stopping Optifast?) Half the subjects were given a placebo and half were given Mazinor™ 1.5 mg per day. Fifty-three percent of those given Mazinor™ maintained their decreased body weight for at least 1 year, whereas only 20 percent of the people taking a placebo were able to stay at their reduced weight.

Mazinor™ or a placebo was also given to 228 obese patients for 12 weeks. Mazinor™-treated patients had more significant appetite and weight reduction than placebo-treated patients. In studies performed outside Japan, Mazinor™ also fared well. Patients in one study lost an average of 8.4 kilograms (18.5 pounds) in 14 weeks at the 3-mg-per-day dose.

Side effects experienced during these studies included dry mouth (25% of patients), constipation (22%), stomach discomfort (12%), nausea (10%), sleep disturbance (9%), and dizziness (6%). However, most of the side effects were mild and disappeared even though the drug was continued. No one had changes in blood tests.

Tenuate™ (Diethylproprion)

Tenuate™ works by stimulating the sympathetic nervous system. In one study lasting 25 weeks, Tenuate™ (75 mg per day) decreased weight by 11.7 kilograms (26 pounds) compared to a loss of 1.6 kilograms (3.5 pounds) in placebo users on a "strict" diet. In another study (lasting only 12 weeks) Tenuate™ users lost 9.1 kilograms (20 pounds) and placebo users 4.5 kilograms (10 pounds) while on a 1,000-calorie diet.

Overview of the Effectiveness of Prescription Sympathomimetic Diet Drugs

In 1973, the FDA reviewed 105 double-blind, placebo-controlled studies of sympathomimetic, appetite-suppressing medications to ensure the drugs were effective. An active drug was given to 3,182 patients, while 4,543 patients took placebo medication. The FDA concluded that people following a low-calorie diet lost 0.25 kilogram (0.5 pound) per week more when taking diet drugs than when taking a placebo. While a half pound a week may not seem like a lot, over a 6-month period it translates into an additional 12 pounds lost over and above whatever weight you would lose by dieting without drugs. On the basis of their study, the FDA determined that appetite suppressants were definitely effective.

Nonprescription Sympathomimetic Diet Drugs

Dexatrim™ and Acutrim™ (Phenylpropanolamine)

These over-the-counter products are appetite suppressants that work in a way similar to phentermine and Mazinor™. Although phenylpropanolamine (PPA) is a sympathomimetic chemical related to amphetamine-like drugs, it has a better safety profile and is not subject to abuse. It is also one of the few diet drugs approved by the FDA for over-the-counter (OTC) use. PPA is also approved by the FDA as a decongestant. In fact, more PPA is purchased by consumers as a cold medicine than for weight control.

One might think that PPA is less effective than prescription sympathomimetic drugs because OTC drugs often have weaker effects than their prescription counterparts. In some studies, however, PPA appears to be just as effective as phentermine in causing weight loss. Dr. Michael Weintraub reviewed scientific literature dealing with PPA and weight control. He found several double-blind studies completed before 1982 and grouped the results together. Today we call this a "meta-analysis." Weintraub found 1,098 patients who received PPA with or without caffeine and 784 who received a placebo. The PPA users lost 0.27 kilogram (0.6 pound) more per week than placebo users. Remember, the FDA study showed that prescription sympathomimetic diet drugs cause a 0.25 kilogram per week greater weight loss than placebo. Thus, it seems that PPA may be equally effective as prescription drugs such as phentermine.

Some scientists may criticize the above conclusion because the Weintraub results are being compared to the FDA study reported years earlier in a different patient population. Yet, other studies have also found no difference in the magnitude of weight loss when the effects of PPA, Mazindol™, and Tenuate™ were compared. For instance, in one study Mazinor users lost 0.64 kilogram per week, Tenuate users 0.84 kilogram per week, and PPA users 0.64 kilogram per week.

Some of the newer PPA studies have demonstrated results similar to prescription diet drugs for the first month of treatment, but by the end of the studies the prescription drugs outperformed PPA. The FDA has approved the use of PPA for up to 3 months. For longer periods of time, a doctor should be consulted.

Side effects were monitored in most of these studies. Nineteen percent of PPA users experienced side effects compared to 14 percent of placebo users. The PPA side effects were mild and usually transient. There have been rare reports of stroke and death in patients receiving PPA. It has not been conclusively proven, however, that PPA was the cause of these catastrophic events.

PPA is given as a 75 mg sustained release capsule to be taken once a day, usually before breakfast. Since it is OTC, it can be taken without a doctor's supervision. However, being a sympathomimetic, it can raise blood pressure and should not be used in people with poorly controlled blood pressure. It should also be used with a doctor's supervision if you have diabetes, thyroid disease, heart disease, or depression. As with many medications, it is always a good idea to let your doctor know that you want to take PPA before starting the drug.

Other OTC Options

Benzocaine

Benzocaine, an anesthetic, is the only other drug besides PPA that is approved by the FDA as an over-the-counter product for weight control. It likely works by numbing one's sense of taste or smell, and preventing the hunger signals from the stomach to reach the brain.

The actual data supporting benzocaine are scant. Only one study has been published demonstrating that benzocaine causes a robust 0.32 kilogram per week weight loss greater than placebo (remember prescription drugs, such as phentermine, caused a 0.25 kilogram per week weight loss greater than placebo). In another study comparing benzocaine to PPA, however, benzocaine (12 mg in chewing gum) caused no weight loss at all, while PPA users lost 0.23 kilogram per week and placebo users lost 0.11 kilogram per week. By combining PPA and benzocaine, people lost only 0.12 kilogram per week. Due to the lack of information on benzocaine, I do not recommend using it for weight control.

Caffeine

Caffeine is not approved by the FDA for weight control; however, several studies demonstrate that at the 200-mg dose available OTC for drowsiness (e.g., NoDoz™), caffeine has an effect on appetite. It is not clear how caffeine exerts this effect on appetite, but it is thought to prevent the breakdown of NE (the neurotransmitter whose release is stimulated by phentermine). Caffeine is rarely used alone for weight control. In Europe, it is often combined with ephedrine with excellent results. In the United States, caffeine has been paired with PPA, but this combination is no longer used.

Ephedrine

Ephedrine is the active ingredient in the herb Ma Huang, which is made from dried young branches of *Ephedra sinca* and other related plants. Ma Huang is sold in health food stores. Ephedrine has an adrenaline-like effect on the body. The drug causes weight loss by increasing metabolic rate as well as appetite suppression. Ephedrine is an OTC drug used to treat asthma but all asthma preparations containing ephedrine also contain theophylline. It's not a good idea to use asthma medicine for weight control. Ephedrine is most effective when combined with caffeine but this combination should be given only with a doctor's supervision. Later in this chapter, when I talk about combining drugs, I will give you more information on this extremely effective OTC drug regimen.

Prescription Serotonin-like Drugs

Table 5.2
Serotonergic Diet Drugs

Brand Name	Generic Name	Tablet Dose (mg)	Dose Range (mg)	Dosing Instructions	Usual Dose
Prozac™	Fluoxetine*	10–20	20–80	Start with 20 mg in the A.M. If there is no response in a few weeks, double the dose (20 mg twice a day). The dose should never exceed 80 mg per day.	20 mg per day in the morning.

*Not FDA approved for weight loss.

Prozac™ (Fluoxetine)

Prozac™ increases brain serotonin by preventing the reuptake of serotonin at the nerve endings in the brain. It is approved by the FDA for the treatment of depression, not for weight control.

Nevertheless, several studies have shown that SSRI (specific serotonin reuptake inhibitor) antidepressants often cause weight loss. The problem with SSRIs such as Prozac™ is that the weight loss is usually not sustained, even when the person continues to take the medication.

In one study, people given 60 mg a day of Prozac™ in divided doses lost an average of 5 kilograms (11 pounds) within 10 weeks of treatment compared to just 2 kilograms (4.4

pounds) in the placebo group. However, by 60 weeks, Prozac™ users had lost only 2 kilograms (they regained 3 kilograms between weeks 10 and 60).

Older people seem to lose more weight in the long term than younger patients and smokers lose less (probably because smoking itself tends to keep off weight). If users of Prozac™ didn't lose significant weight in the first month of treatment, there was only a 17 percent chance they would lose weight in the long term. Some of the more common side effects of Prozac™ are tiredness, tremors ("the shakes"), and sweating.

The SSRIs are not a first choice drug for most people with weight problems. In selected patients, however (especially those obese individuals where depression is a significant problem), a trial of Prozac™ or Effexor™ may be very useful. Some clinicians feel Effexor™ works better than Prozac™ for weight control. See Table 5.3.

Table 5.3
Combined Sympathomimetic/Serotonergic Diet Drugs

Brand Name	Generic Name	Tablet Dose (mg)	Dose Range (mg per day)	Dose Instructions	Usual Dose
Effexor™	Venlafaxine*	25 37.5 50 100	75–225	Start at 25 mg 3 times a day with meals. Depending on results, you can double the dose to 50 mg 3 times a day. The maximum dose is 75 mg 3 times a day.	25 mg 3 times a day with meals.
Meridia™	Sibutramine	10	10–15	Start at 10 mg per day. Can increase by 5 mg to a maximum dose of 15 mg per day.	10–15 mg per day

*Not approved by FDA for weight loss.

Effexor™ (Venlafaxine)

There is a paucity of information about the ability of Effexor™ to cause weight loss. I sometimes will use it for less than 6 months in patients who need to lose weight and are clinically depressed. If patients do not lose more than 4 pounds in the first month, I usually stop the drug.

Meridia™ (Sibutramine)

Meridia™ is in a class of its own. It works by preventing the reuptake of both serotonin and NE by the nerve terminal. Thus, it has both serotonergic and sympathomimetic properties, and is the first effective SNRI (serotonin-noradrenaline reuptake inhibitor). The antidepressant drug Effexor™ was actually the first SNRI but has a very limited ability to block the reuptake of NE. Originally developed as an antidepressant, Meridia™ was soon found to have a strong effect on weight. In contrast to the antidepressant Prozac™, Meridia™ causes long-lasting weight reduction in overweight patients. The drug not only suppresses appetite and stimulates a sense of fullness, but also burns fat. The drug does not appear to be an effective antidepressant.

In one study, 1,047 obese patients were given a placebo or Meridia™ in a dose of either 1 mg, 5 mg, 10 mg, 15 mg, or 30 mg once daily in combination with diet and exercise for 24 weeks. The higher the dose of Meridia™, the more weight was lost. The placebo group lost less than 2 kilograms (4.4 pounds) while those on the 30-mg-a-day dose of Meridia™ lost about 8.5 kilograms (18.7 pounds). Weight loss was still continuing at the end of 24 weeks in those patients receiving 15 mg or more of Meridia™.

When people were given 15 mg of Meridia™ once a day for 24 weeks, 56 percent lost at least 5 percent and 34 percent lost at least 10 percent of their starting weight. The success rate with Meridia™ is much higher if you are able to lose at least 4 pounds in the first month. On the basis of this and other studies, the FDA has approved Meridia™ for long-term use (1 year).

Patients receiving Meridia™ may experience dry mouth, insomnia, and fatigue, but as with other diet drugs, these symptoms are usually mild and transient. A slight increase in systolic blood pressure may occur, but is not felt to be a significant problem for people with normal blood pressure. The effect on blood pressure usually happens within the first 2 months. The drug is not recommended for people with uncontrolled hypertension and heart disease. Meridia™ has not been associated with primary pulmonary hypertension (PPH) and valvular heart disease. PPH is more likely to occur with drugs that release serotonin (Pondomin, Redux) rather than drugs that work mainly by preventing the reuptake of neurotransmitters (Meridia™, Prozac™, and Effexor™).

Table 5.4
Lipase Inhibitor

Brand Name	Generic Name	Dose Range	Usual Dose	Instructions
Xenical™	Tetrahydrolipstatin (orlistat)	240–360 mg per day	360 mg per day	Take a 120 mg tablet with each fat-containing meal.

Xenical™ (Orlistat, Tetrahydrolipostatin)

There is little debate that excessive intake of dietary fat is a major factor in causing and perpetuating obesity. We are all told to cut way back on fat. But just how far should we go? The problem with lowering fat intake is that much of the flavor and texture of food comes from its fat content. The lower you go, the harder it is to stay on your diet. Fake fats, like Olean™ or Olestra™ (see Chapter 8) help to an extent. They taste and feel like fat, but some people can detect a slight difference in taste and there are only a few products available with fake fats. Xenical™, a drug recently released by the Roche drug company, permits you to eat regular fat but then prevents its digestion and absorption so the fat stays in your intestines and never reaches your hips. Xenical™ sticks to and blocks an enzyme called "lipase." Lipase is responsible for digesting dietary fat, or triglycerides, into smaller molecules (glycerol and fatty acids), which can then be absorbed by the small intestines. By blocking lipase, Xenical™ cuts down on the fat calories your body receives. Xenical™ blocks the absorption of approximately one-third of dietary fat.

In a study published by Dr. M. L. Drent in 1995, 360 mg a day of Xenical™ caused about a 4.5-kilograms (10-pound) weight loss over 12 weeks. This was 2 kilograms (4.4 pounds) more weight loss than that seen in the placebo group. These investigators also found that Xenical™ decreased serum cholesterol levels.

In a study published in 1998 by the European Multicenter Orlistat Study Group, 688 patients from 15 European centers were studied to determine the effect of Xenical™ (120 mg 3 times a day) on weight loss. Subjects received a placebo or Xenical™ for 1 year. In the second year, subjects were reassigned either Xenical™ or a placebo to determine the effect of Xenical™ on weight maintenance. Xenical™ users lost 10.2 percent of their body weight (22.7 pounds) in the first year compared to a 6.1 percent loss of body weight (13.4 pounds) in the placebo group. Patients who switched from the placebo to Xenical™ lost an additional 2 pounds in the second year. Subjects who used Xenical™ in the first year and who stayed on Xenical™ in the second year regained only half as much weight as those patients who were switched to a placebo in the second year. Total cholesterol, LDL cholesterol, and blood sugar decreased more in the Xenical™ group than with a placebo.

In a large multicenter United States study of 391 obese diabetic men and women, Xenical™ (120 mg 3 times a day) for 1 year caused a 6.2 percent loss of initial body weight, compared to 4.3 percent in the placebo group. Xenical™ users had better control of blood sugar as evidenced by a lower hemoglobin A_{1C} and fasting blood sugar and lower cholesterol and triglyceride levels. Scientific studies indicate it is safe to use Xenical™ for at least 2 years.

Some patients using Xenical™ may notice a change in their bowel habits. Stools may be greasier and may be associated with mild abdominal bloating and discomfort (similar symptoms to those experienced with Olean™ or Olestra™). Very few people find these side effects (which are not dangerous) significant enough to stop taking Xenical™. You may want to consider these digestive side effects as positive since they may cause an aversion to fatty foods, thereby limiting their appeal.

Xenical™ should be used only in fat-containing meals. For best results you should use a diet which contains about 30 percent of daily calories from fat and divide the fat evenly among the three meals. It is recommended to take a vitamin supplement while on Xenical™ because the medication may partially block the absorption of some vitamins. Take the vitamin at least 2 hours before or after using Xenical™. For most people, bedtime works best.

Combination Drug Treatment

Many diseases, such as hypertension, are often treated with a combination of drugs, rather than a single drug. This is because either the single drug is not effective by itself, or because it requires such a high dose to be effective that side effects can be a problem. By combining drugs that produce the same end result, but do so by different means, one can often achieve better results: an improved desired outcome with fewer side effects.

Ephedrine plus Caffeine

Although caffeine and ephedrine are rarely used for weight control, a large study from Denmark showed that combining 20 mg of ephedrine with 200 mg of caffeine three times a day caused significant weight loss. In one study, the combination of ephedrine and caffeine was even more effective than prescription diet drugs. In another study of 180 obese patients, the combination of ephedrine and caffeine given over 24 weeks resulted in a 13-kilogram (28.6 pound) loss of weight, 3.4 kilograms more than the placebo group. The study was continued for a year (without placebo), and as long as ephedrine was given, the weight loss was maintained. The authors concluded that 75 percent of the weight loss was caused by appetite suppression and 25 percent by the ability of ephedrine to burn fat. Because ephedrine has an adrenaline-like effect and caffeine is a stimulant, it was not surprising that 60 percent of the patients had some side effects. These side effects included tremors, fast heart rate, and rise in blood pressure. However, most people were able to tolerate the side effects and they tended to disappear within a few weeks. Although each of these drugs are OTC, I believe this combination of drugs should always be given under doctor's supervision and never used in patients with high blood pressure or heart disease. If you use Ma Huang as a source of ephedrine, be sure to use the standardized preparation containing 6 percent ephedrine.

Phentermine plus Prozac (Phen/Pro)

When Pondomin (fenfluramine) was withdrawn from the market in 1997 because of the potential for heart and lung toxicity, some physicians substituted Prozac™ (fluoxetine) for the "fen" (fenfluramine) of the widely used phen/fen regimen. Since both Pondomin and Prozac™ are serotonergic drugs, they felt Phen/Pro may work as well as Phen/fen without the potential to cause valvular heart disease and pulmonary hypertension. A few preliminary studies did show the combination was effective in enhancing weight loss but there have not been any long-term safety and efficacy studies to date. Eli Lilly & Company, the makers of Prozac™, does not recommend using phentermine and Prozac™ together (although this statement was not based on any specific data).

Since Prozac™ seems to work for only the first 6 months (see above), theoretically Phen/Pro should not be any better than phentermine alone beyond the first 6 months of treatment. Although Phen/Pro seems to be a potentially promising combination to treat obesity, I cannot recommend its use until more reliable information about its safety and effectiveness is available.

Herbal Phen/Fen (Ephedrine plus St. John's Wort)

St. John's wort contains hypericin extracted from the leaves and flowers of a perennial shrub native to both Europe and the United States. Hypericin is felt to be a mood enhancer similar to the specific serotonin reuptake inhibitors such as Prozac™. Ephedrine, extracted from the herb Ma Huang, has a stimulant, sympathomimetic effect like phentermine. Thus, the combination of a serotonergic-like substance (St. John's wort) with a sympathomimetic-like substance (ephedrine) might produce a phen/fen-like effect on weight loss. Although this combination has been used on a fairly large scale, currently there is no definitive documentation of its safety and effectiveness.

Other Theoretical Drug Combinations

It is tempting to combine Xenical™, a drug which blocks fat absorption, with any of the other diet drugs, for example, Meridia™ or phentermine (Xen/phen). One would anticipate a synergistic effect on weight loss. That is, the person would lose more weight than if he used either drug alone. Studies are actually in progress examining these potential drug combinations, but until the results roll in, I would not recommend unproven combination drug regimens.

Putting It All Together

We now have several drug options to aid the overweight in their quest to lose weight and keep it off. None of the drugs actually cures obesity — however, each drug is effective in controlling the disease.

As well as the drugs work, some of you may be disappointed if you don't actually reach your "ideal" body weight. As you'll see in Chapter 9, there are many different types of goals when it comes to losing weight. The most important goal is to reduce health risks. Drug therapy can often help you to accomplish that goal.

Many of you will have excellent results with drug-assisted weight loss, but studies show that a certain percentage of people have little or no benefit from a single drug or a combination of drugs. I believe we are just "getting our feet wet" when it comes to treating obesity with drugs. I predict a much more aggressive approach to treating obesity in the future. Multiple drug regimens will be the rule, not the exception. We may see people taking phentermine and Xenical™ or a selective thermogenic drug that burns fat (see Chapter 6) along with Meridia™ and Xenical™. These multiple drug combinations may allow those apparent "nonresponders" to respond to treatment, and the "responders" who lose between 5–10 percent of their weight to lose up to 20–25 percent of their body weight over time.

The key is having several classes of drugs (i.e., SSRIs, sympathomimetics, SNRIs, selective thermogenics, enzyme blockers) and several choices of drugs in each category. If you don't respond to one drug regimen within 4 weeks, you try another or add another from a different class. This is the same aggressive approach that has improved the management of inflammatory bowel disease (some of my patients are on prednisone, azothiaprine, sulfasalazine, and mesalamine enemas all at the same time) and hypertension (some patients require a combination of Calan SR, Analopril, hydrochlorthiazide, and propranolol). Combination drug therapy will be key for people who want to reach their ideal body weight.

In the next chapter, we will look at future treatments of obesity.

6

Diet Drugs in the Pipeline

The pharmaceutical industry refers to drugs that are still in development (not yet approved by the FDA) as drugs "in the pipeline." How are new drugs developed? Some chemicals are accidentally found to possess a certain property or drug effect. For instance, while Prozac™ and Meridia™ were being developed for the treatment of depression, they were incidentally found to cause weight loss. Other chemicals are specifically designed to fit like a key in a lock into a specific receptor on a cell that then activates a desired body function. These are sometimes called "designer drugs" and their chemical structure is often computer generated.

Once a chemical either is found to possess a desired action (for instance, weight loss) or, by virtue of its structure, is thought likely to possess that effect, it becomes a candidate drug and is placed "in the pipeline" for development. Initially, animal studies are performed to make sure the drug is not toxic. Then an IND (investigational new drug) application is filed with the FDA so human studies can be performed. The drug must then pass three phases of development before an NDA (new drug application) can be submitted to the FDA for final drug approval.

Before the 1990s there were very few diet drugs in the pipeline. Obesity wasn't considered a real disease. Patients, doctors, drug companies, and the FDA didn't consider diet medication to be an important part of obesity treatment; now all of that is changing. If you are impressed with the results of the diet drugs already on the market, wait until you see what's coming up in the next few years such as hormone look-alikes that signal your brain to stop eating, and drugs that actually burn fat. Let's preview the exciting new advances that may soon make the treatment of your weight problem even more effective.

Satiety Peptides

Cholecystokinin (CCK)

The perception of satiety or fullness is controlled by the "satiety center" of the brain, which is located in the hypothalamus. The hypothalamus controls unconscious body functions such as blood pressure, body temperature, and breathing. Chemical and nerve input from the body influence the satiety center. When food and drink distend the stomach, they activate nerves that travel to the spinal cord and then connect to the hypothalamus. This signals the brain that a meal has begun. When food (especially fat and protein) reaches the small intestine, a specific hormone called "cholecystokinin" (CCK) is released into the bloodstream. CCK works to increase satiety in several ways. It delays emptying of the stomach, which magnifies the feeling of fullness. The hormone can also directly activate the same stomach nerves that respond to stomach distention. CCK may also directly reach the central nervous system to signal fullness. Once food is digested and absorbed, nutrients like glucose and amino acids may also signal the satiety center of the brain. Thus, stomach, intestinal, and postabsorption signals all work in concert to let us know when enough is enough.

Several pharmaceutical companies are trying to develop a CCK-like drug. Dr. Gerald Smith from Cornell reviewed 14 studies demonstrating that CCK can reduce the intake of food in humans. CCK injected intravenously caused an average 27 percent reduction in food intake in lean subjects and a 21 percent reduction in food intake in obese individuals with very few side effects.

This is all well and good, but there is one problem with CCK: it is a peptide (a small protein). When peptides are taken by mouth, digestive enzymes break down and inactivate them. Even if peptides could be protected from digestion, they would still be too large for the small intestine to absorb them. The Fisons pharmaceutical company has had some success (in animal studies) with CCK taken intranasally by spray. The mucous membranes inside the nose are able to absorb some peptides. For example, calcitonin, a hormone used to treat osteoporosis, and vasopressin, a drug for diabetes insipitus, are two peptides that are given intranasally. They are already approved by the FDA and are on the market.

The strategy employed by other companies, including Eli Lilly, Glaxo, and Hoffman La Roche, is to create a peptoid. A peptoid is a chemical that has a three-dimensional shape similar to a particular peptide, but much smaller. The hope is that a peptoid will retain all or much of the biologic activity of the original peptide with the added benefits of being indigestible and easily absorbable. To date, the CCK peptoids that retain biologic activity (that is, the ability to delay stomach emptying) cannot be absorbed, and the ones that can be absorbed have lost their biologic activity. With computer modeling, ingenuity, and more money, an effective CCK peptoid may soon be a reality. Other strategies to stimulate satiety involve the use of a special dietary supplement (Satietrol—see Chapter 8) and a digestion-resistant CCK-Releasing Peptide (CCK-RP) to trigger release of CCK from the small intestine.

Enterostatin

Enterostatin is an exciting, newly discovered peptide that selectively blocks the desire to eat fat. Enterostatin is made in the pancreas and initially is part of a larger molecule called "procolipase." After a meal, procolipase is secreted into the small intestines. There it is split by the pancreatic enzyme trypsin. One half of procolipase ends up as "colipase," a substance needed for fat digestion, and the other part becomes enterostatin. Enterostatin, in some unknown way, decreases our desire to eat fatty foods.

Several animal studies have demonstrated the ability of enterostatin to selectively prevent fat intake without effects on carbohydrate or protein ingestion. What is even more unique is that enterostatin works whether it is given by mouth or injected. The animals don't seem to compensate for reduced fat calories by increasing intake of carbohydrates or protein.

If taking enterostatin by mouth turns out to decrease the intake of dietary fat in humans, we may truly have another exciting drug—one that keeps us satisfied without overeating those rich, calorie-laden, flavorful fatty foods. If you already adhere to a strict low-fat diet, enterostatin will probably not be for you. The peptide has no effect on reducing fat ingestion in laboratory animals already on a low-fat diet.

Amylin

Amylin, another peptide that can slow the emptying of the stomach, can also have a strong effect on the intake of food. Whenever special endocrine cells in your pancreas release insulin, they release amylin as well. When amylin is injected under the skin of rats, it causes their stomachs to slow emptying almost by half.

When combining amylin and CCK, each appears to enhance the effect of the other. In one revealing study, researchers found that the combined injection of amylin and CCK was *20 times* more potent in suppressing food intake than either peptide given by itself. In design now are human studies to examine the effect of amylin on food intake. The need to inject the peptide will probably decrease its marketability except for people with diabetes. Yet, a spray of a CCK/amylin combo into each nostril (unobtrusively performed behind a napkin, of course) just before a meal could become commonplace in the twenty-first century.

Glucagon-like Peptide-1 (GLP-1)

Glucagon is a hormone released from special endocrine cells in the pancreas. Glucagon starts as a larger molecule called "proglucagon." While proglucagon is converted to glucagon in the pancreas, something else happens in the central nervous system (CNS). In the CNS, proglucagon is converted to a peptide that looks and acts very much like glucagon itself. We call this glucagon-like peptide "GLP-1." Known to powerfully decrease the intake of food, GLP-1 has raised hopes regarding its possible future designation as a magic bullet for treating obesity. Unfortunately, as currently used, GLP-1 must be injected directly into the brain to inhibit the intake of food. I only mention GLP-1 because it has received a good deal of attention in the professional literature. Clearly, though, unless researchers find a way of getting GLP-1 into the brain without injection, this peptide will remain where it is today — on the drawing board!

Neuropeptide Y (NPY) and Galanin

NPY and galanin are peptides that strongly *stimulate* food intake when injected into the brain. So why do we need to discuss these peptides? The answer is quite simple. If you know how to make someone eat, you can block that effect and make him or her eat less. There are probably more drugs on the market that block the effect of a body chemical than drugs that mimic the action of a particular body chemical. For instance, one of the best-selling class of drugs is the H_2 blockers (Tagamet™, Zantac™, Pepcid™, and Axid™). They treat heartburn and ulcers by blocking the effect of histamine, a body chemical that stimulates acid secretion in the stomach. By developing NPY and galanin blockers, we could have two new classes of drugs to treat obesity. Even as you read, drug companies, using computer modeling, are creating chemicals that can prevent NPY or galanin from sticking to their respective receptors in the brain. If they are designed so they can withstand digestive enzymes, are absorbable and cross from the bloodstream to the brain, these, too, could be new blockbuster drugs to treat obesity.

Leptin

Of all the candidate drugs to treat obesity, leptin has received the most attention. Perhaps the $20 million price tag Amgen paid to Rockefeller University for the rights to develop and market leptin accounts for its notoriety. The story behind leptin is quite intriguing. For years, we've known there had to be a protein that was either missing or malfunctioning in genetically obese mice and rats (so-called "OB/OB mice" or "FA/FA rats" inherit a double dose of a defective gene that results in their being obese). Recently, new techniques in molecular biology allowed scientists to unravel the obesity gene in rodents and discover the actual genetic defect. It turns out the OB gene causes the creation of a protein called "leptin," which is made exclusively by fat cells. Leptin, which blocks production of NPY in the brain, appears to have at least two major functions. One is to increase body metabolism; another is to inhibit food intake.

OB/OB mice are unable to make leptin. Therefore, they overeat and have a slow metabolism. This inevitably results in obesity. When researchers inject leptin into obese mice, however, the mice decrease their eating and, in time, lose weight.

It didn't take long to discover that while obese rodents lacked leptin, obese humans actually made too much of the protein. Dr. Jose Caro and coworkers at Jefferson Medical College of Thomas Jefferson University in Philadelphia, for example, found high levels of leptin in most obese individuals. Not only do obese people have higher levels, but it appears that the heavier you are, the more leptin is found in your bloodstream.

Based on those results, we must conclude that, unlike mice, most human obesity is probably not due to a deficiency of the OB protein leptin. Just because there is no leptin deficiency, however, doesn't mean that obese humans have no leptin abnormality. In juvenile-onset diabetes, high blood sugar is caused by a deficiency of insulin. In adult-onset diabetes, there are high insulin levels, which indicate the body is resistant or poorly responsive to that hormone. Similarly, obese humans may have high leptin levels because their bodies are *resistant* to this important regulator of body weight. This doesn't necessarily mean leptin can't be used to treat obesity. By giving extra leptin, the body's resistance to the hormone may be overcome and weight loss may result. Human studies will soon tell us if leptin will be useful in treating obesity.

Selective Thermogenic Drugs

Our body weight is finely balanced by the number of calories we consume in the form of food and by the number of calories we expend in the form of energy. When calories "in" equals calories "out," our weight stays the same. We can lose weight either by eating less (no fun), or by exercising (apparently not fun for everyone), or by a combination of both. It would be great if there were a third option: a drug that would speed body metabolism and burn body fat without relying exclusively on exercise. If such a drug really worked, you could maintain your body weight no matter what you ate! You could even lose weight while you sleep.

It might surprise you that doctors have known for decades

that two different body chemicals can do just that. Yet when used at doses effective for weight loss, these body chemicals each exhibit significant side effects. One of the chemicals is thyroxin. Released by the thyroid gland in your neck, thyroxin has major effects on body metabolism. When given in doses high enough to achieve weight loss, however, the hormone can cause the symptoms of thyrotoxicosis (sweating, tremors, anxiety, palpitations, fast heart rate, and inability to sleep).

The other chemical is adrenaline. When released by the adrenal glands, which sit on top of your kidneys, adrenaline directs your "fight or flight" response to a situation that you perceive as dangerous. When you're frightened, it is an adrenaline surge that causes alertness, sweating, goose bumps, and dilation of your pupils. Unfortunately, the negatives outnumber the positives here. Adrenaline side effects are just too uncomfortable to bear even if the chemical is able to burn fat.

Nonetheless, researchers are now on the trail to develop selective thermogenic drugs that can burn fat without causing adrenaline-like effects. How are they doing this? They're studying the surface of the cell and how adrenaline interacts with fat and heart muscle cells. For example, researchers know that adrenaline fits like a key into a lock called a "receptor" on the outside surface of fat and heart muscle cells. As it turns out, the shape of the adrenaline receptor (adrenoreceptor) on the fat cell is slightly different from that of the heart adrenoreceptor. While adrenaline can stick to any adrenoreceptor, the new selective thermogenic drugs are designed to stick or bind only to the fat cell adrenoreceptor (also called the beta-3 adrenoreceptor). Drugs that activate the beta-3-adrenoreceptor have little or no ability to stick to the adrenoreceptors on heart muscle, thereby causing fewer unwanted side effects such as an activation of the "fight or flight" response.

In this regard, recent studies using selective thermogenic drugs have proven quite successful, especially in rats whose fat cells contain many beta-3-adrenoreceptors. Obese rats not only lose weight, but also have better control of blood sugar when taking these drugs. On the other hand, preliminary studies in humans have not been as promising. It turns out that humans don't have as many beta-3-adrenoreceptors on their fat cells as rats. In a recent study involving obese women, for example, a selective beta-3-adrenoreceptor stimulant given for two weeks did not increase resting metabolic rate. In another study involving obese individuals with and without diabetes, however, a selective beta-3-adrenoreceptor stimulant did produce a small increase in body metabolic rate with a corresponding small but significant loss of weight. Although more work is needed on selective thermogenic drugs, they remain an exciting area of antiobesity drug research.

There Is No Going Back

Drug treatment of obesity is here to stay. While a host of drugs that are proven effective in weight management are already available for your use, we know that even more drugs are on the way. There is no going back to the Dark Ages where a few "nifty" diet and exercise tips were the only advice you could get from the medical establishment. Be assured that:

1. Drug companies and the FDA are finally serious about finding new and better drugs for weight control.
2. We will never again have to wait 20 years before a new prescription diet drug comes on the market.
3. Diet drugs are and will continue to be an accepted and important part of treatment programs for obesity.

In the next chapter, I will help you and your doctor choose a diet drug regimen that will fit your needs

7

The Best Regimen for You

Over-the-Counter or Prescription Diet Drugs?

If you have already decided to:

- attempt to lose weight and keep it off *and*
- give diet drugs a try

then the next step is to decide if you want to go it alone with an over-the-counter (OTC) drug like phenylpropanolamine, or consult your physician regarding the use of prescription diet medication. Even if you think you qualify for the OTC drug version of my program (see below), it is always a good idea to keep your doctor informed about your intentions. It is imperative that you consult your physician before starting diet medication if one or more of the items listed in Table 7.1 apply to you.

Table 7.1
Conditions Requiring Physician-Supervised Weight Control

Current Weight *less than* 30 percent of ideal body weight or BMI< 30 (if not obese but still want to lose weight)	Heart disease
	Gallbladder disease
Age < 18 years	Use of certain drugs
Eating disorder (anorexia nervosa, bulimia)	Lithium
Lactating woman	Antidepressants
Pregnant	Decongestants
High blood pressure	Glaucoma
Diabetes	Enlarged prostate

If you do not satisfy any of the conditions listed in Table 7.1, then you may qualify for self-medication. If so, I usually recommend starting with Dexatrim™ or Acutrim™ (e.g., phenylpropanolamine).

Table 7.2
Available Preparations of Phenylpropanolamine

Brand	Formula	Dose (mg)	Dose Form	How to Take
Dexatrim™	Maximum strength plus vitamin C (180 mg)	75	Capsule Caplet	One at midmorning (10 A.M.) with a full glass of water.
	Maximum strength extended duration	75	Tablet	Same as above.
Acutrim™	Complete (contains fiber, vitamin B$_{12}$ chromium picolinate)	75	Caplet	One tablet midmorning with a full glass of water.
	Diet gum	7.5	Gum	Chew one or two pieces before meals or whenever you feel the urge to snack. Do not take

Brand	Formula	Dose (mg)	Dose Form	How to Take
Acutrim™ (cont'd.)	Diet gum	7.5	Gum	more than 6 pieces per day or more than 2 pieces in a 4-hour period.

Table 7.2 outlines the wide range of pheylpropanolamine preparations available. I usually recommend starting with either Dexatrim™ Maximum Strength Extended Duration or Acutrim™ Complete. Both of these preparations deliver phenylpropanolamine to the bloodstream gradually over the day, so whenever you eat, there is always some drug in your system. Furthermore, because the drug is gradually absorbed, peak blood levels may not be too high, and the potential for side effects such as nervousness, dizziness, or sleeplessness may be lessened.

If you find you are having a particular problem controlling your appetite at lunch time, Dexatrim™ Maximum Strength Plus Vitamin C capsules or caplets, when taken in the morning, may deliver higher blood levels of phenylpropanolamine at lunch time. With the exception of Acutrim™ Diet Gum, never take more than one dose of any preparation in a single day. Generic formulations of phenylpropanolamine are available and generally cost less than half the price of the name brands.

Even though some of the preparations tout their formulas as caffeine-free, the truth is that *all* of the current phenylpropanolamine products are caffeine-free. Some preparations contain vitamin C, but the addition of the vitamin does not affect appetite control. In my view, the vitamin C formula offers little advantage because, while dieting, you need more than just vitamin C supplementation. Acutrim™ Complete contains fiber (Garcinia Cambogia, 200 mg) and chromium picolinate (50 mg—see Chapter 8). I recommend taking a high-potency vitamin whenever you are dieting. Minerals, including calcium and iron, must also be replaced, especially if you are eating fewer than 1,500 calories per day.

Working with Your Doctor to Choose the Right Diet Drug for You

You know there are several prescription drug options from which your doctor can choose. But some doctors are familiar with just one drug or combination of drugs and use those for all their patients. I believe drug-assisted weight loss is best accomplished if the choice of drug(s) is tailored to the individual. Some people don't respond to one drug, yet do respond to another. If patients don't lose at least 4 pounds after 4 weeks, they should be switched to another drug. The more drugs in a doctor's "little black bag," and the more the doctor understands how and why they work, the better the chances for success in your effort to lose weight.

There are several issues that doctors examine before choosing a particular drug to treat patients. These are:

- Effectiveness
- Side effects
- Cost

Naturally, your doctor wants to prescribe a medication that will really work, won't make you sick, and won't cost a fortune. In Table 7.3, I have attempted to rate the diet drugs, taking into consideration their effectiveness, side effects, and cost.

Table 7.3
Rating the Diet Drugs

Brand Name	Generic Name	Effectiveness	Side Effects	Cost
Adipex-P™	Phentermine	***	***	$
Fastin™				
Ionomin™				
Effexor™	Venlafaxine	**	**	$$$
Mazinor™	Mazindol	***	***	$
Meridia™	Sibutramine	***	**	$$$
Prozac™	Fluoxetine	*	**	$$$
Tenuate™	Diethylproprion	***	***	$
Xenical™	Orlistat	***	*	$$$

***is the most, * is the least.
$$$ is the most expensive, $ is the least expensive.

Although rating the effectiveness and side effect profiles of drugs is a fairly subjective exercise, I have done so based on my personal clinical experience and the experiences of other physicians who treat patients with weight problems. Identifying which drugs are better than others can be difficult. Many doctors try to sidestep the issue, but patients always ask the question: "Which is the best diet drug on the market?" or "Which one do you use for your patients?" To such patients and to my readers, I will offer my preferences with the understanding that these are my views and not necessarily those of other experts.

I generally use Adipex-P™, Fastin™, or Ionomin™ (one of the phentermine preparations); Meridia™; or Xenical™. If a patient does not have an insurance prescription plan, the cheapest treatment is phentermine. I usually start with 15 mg a day and, if necessary, raise the dose to 30 (Ionomin™, Fastin™) or 37.5 (Adipex-P™) mg per day if no undesirable side effects are experienced. If phentermine is not effective (less than 4 pounds of weight loss in 4 weeks) or if there are disturbing side effects at the 30 mg dose, I would stop the phentermine and give the patient Xenical™ or Meridia™. Xenical™ (120 mg) is given three times a day. It is usually well tolerated. A few people using Xenical™ experience fecal leakage and find an "oil slick" on their underwear if they are eating too much fat. Despite the potential for some gastrointestinal side effects (see Table 7.4), Xenical™ is probably the safest diet drug on the market. For those individuals who have bowel problems, Meridia™ may be useful.

Meridia™ (10 mg) is given once a day in the morning. If necessary, the dose can be increased to 15 mg a day, but higher doses are not recommended due to an increased risk of side effects (high blood pressure, etc.).

I usually select Xenical™ for my hypertensive patients since it does not raise blood pressure (phentermine and Meridia™ may cause an increase in blood pressure).

If depression is a large component of the problem—especially if depression may be causing my patient to overeat—I may prescribe an antidepressant. The SSRI antidepressants, while not approved by the FDA for the treatment of obesity, nevertheless are often effective, not only in improving spirits, but in lowering weight. In my experience, Effexor™ works a little better than Prozac™. Prozac™ is effective only for approximately 6 months. After 6 months, your weight may again increase despite continuing on the drug. Effexor™ is usually started by taking 25 mg with breakfast, lunch, and dinner. If necessary, the dose can be doubled or even tripled to achieve control of depression and (we hope) weight as well. Don't be fooled, though, because not all antidepressants cause weight loss. Elavil™ (amitriptyline), for example, often causes weight gain.

Side effects are an important factor in selecting a drug. All drugs have side effects and diet drugs are no exceptions to the rule. In Table 7.4, I have listed some of the more common diet drug side effects. Most people will not experience any significant side effect(s) that would cause them to stop taking the drug, so don't be frightened away by this laundry list of items that sound like cruel and unusual punishment. If you look in the PDR (*Physician's Desk Reference*), just about any drug you have ever taken also has a long list of potential side effects.

Table 7.4
Potential Diet Drug Side Effects*

Body System	Sympathomimetics (phentermine, Mazinor™, Tenuate™, phenylpropanolamine)	SSRI/SNRI (Prozac™, Effexor™, Meridia™)	Lipase Inhibitor (Xenical™)
Neurologic	Stimulation	Insomnia	
	Restlessness	Nervousness	
	Sleep disturbance	Fatigue	
	Headache	Headache	
	Fatigue, drowsiness	Anxiety	
	Blurred vision	Tremor	
	Tremor	Dizziness	
Heart/Lung	Palpitations (fluttering feeling in chest)	Fast heart rate	
	Fast heart rate	High blood pressure	
	High blood pressure		
Digestive	Dry mouth	Dry mouth	Oily spotting
	Nausea	Nausea	Flatus with discharge
	Constipation	Constipation	Fatty/oily stool
	Diarrhea		Increased defecation

*Partial list.

Let's Start

After analyzing the pros and cons of each drug, you and your doctor can now chose a particular drug regimen. Your chances for losing significant weight and keeping it off are excellent. More important, your risk of developing diabetes, high blood pressure, arthritis, etc., is about to be greatly reduced. Don't despair if, after you start your medication, things don't go well at first. Your doctor may need to adjust the dose of the drug you are taking or switch you to an entirely different type of drug. Remember the general rule: If you don't lose 4 pounds in the first month, you need to change the drug regimen. You also need to remember the admonition that diet drugs are not a free ride. Your diet program must also include good dietary advice, an exercise program, and behavior modification. So don't start your medication until you have read the upcoming chapters on these subjects.

You may have tried or at least heard of several dietary supplements touted to be useful for weight loss. In the next chapter we take a look at some of them.

8

Nondrug Weight Loss Products

Because such a generous, multimillion-dollar price tag is attached to the research and development required to patent, and then market, a new drug, only the largest pharmaceutical companies can afford the effort. Under normal circumstances, smaller companies are simply shut out. Still, because the antiobesity market is so vast and holds great promise for financial reward, smaller companies definitely want a part of the action, especially in terms of nutritional supplements, where they seem to operate best. Regulation of nutritional products for use in a particular disease, however, is not as nearly as severe as those regulations applied to drug use. This laxity in regulation is both good and bad. It is good for the company marketing a nutritional product; the cost of bringing the product to market is just a fraction of the cost for drug approval. On the other hand, lack of sufficient regulation may prove to be a bad thing for those people who take the product. Many companies—some reputable, others not so reputable—have gotten on the "nutraceutical" bandwagon with an ever-increasing array of weight control products appearing in your local pharmacy or health food store.

"But what are nutraceuticals?" you may ask. Nutraceuticals are foods or nutritional products given for a desired therapeutic effect. How are they different from drugs? I'll illustrate the difference between a nutraceutical and a drug by the following example: Dietary fiber—in the form of wheat bran—increases stool bulk and can be useful in alleviating constipation. The product Colace is a pill, and since its manufacturer claims it treats constipation, Colace is regulated as a drug. Some people may find wheat bran as effective as Colace. Yet as long as wheat bran is tasted and consumed as a food, and as long as the people marketing wheat bran don't make any claims that it treats constipation, the product is not considered a drug and does not have the regulations associated with a drug. Even a ham sandwich would be considered a drug if you put it in a capsule and claimed it could treat malnutrition. So most manufacturers of nutritional products never come out and say: "Our product will treat obesity," or "Our product will suppress your appetite and cause significant weight loss." The FDA considers these statements as claims that only drugs can make and satisfy. As a result, manufacturers of nutritional weight-loss products restrict the claims they make. In effect, they consider their products as useful adjuncts to a weight-loss program by way of four criteria: (1) They add a sense of fullness while one is on a low-calorie diet (e.g., fiber products, Satietrol); (2) they improve lean body mass (e.g., chromium picolinate); (3) they prevent the absorption of dietary fat (e.g., chitin); or (4) they prevent fat production (e.g., thermogenic tea).

Food additives, on the other hand, are nutritional products added to regular food, which in some way change the properties of the original food. Food additives used for weight control are sometimes called "dietary diluents" in that they dilute the number of calories you consume when they are substituted for calorie-laden food. Fake fats (e.g., Olestra™ and Simplesse™) and artificial sweeteners (e.g., aspartame, saccharine) are common examples of dietary diluents used for weight control.

It would be impractical to discuss every nutritional product now marketed and used for weight control. Frankly, there are just too many of them. So I have chosen to review a few of the more popular dietary supplements, diluents, and other nondrug products. Some may be helpful, others are a waste of money, and some we do not possess enough information to make an informed decision.

Fiber Products

Fiber is a nondigestible carbohydrate found in fruits, vegetables, and grains. We now recognize fiber to be an essential part of our diet, reducing the risk of some cancers, heart disease, and many gastrointestinal disorders. Because fiber resists digestion, it increases the bulk in the stool and causes it to pass through the bowel more quickly. The bulking effect of fiber also takes place in the stomach, where fiber can promote a sense of satiety or fullness. Fiber can delay emptying of the stomach, which again results in a full feeling. To a small extent, fiber also can prevent the absorption of food. By preventing even 40 calories a day from being absorbed, a 4-pound weight loss can result in 1 year.

Unfortunately, in order to feel full enough to eat less, you really have to consume a lot of fiber. Professor John Blundell from the University of Leeds in the United Kingdom found it takes as much as 30 grams of fiber consumed in a beverage to substantially reduce the intake of food in a subsequent meal. Although 30 grams of fiber a day is recommended for optimal health, most people consume far less. Furthermore, most people consuming 30 grams of fiber at one sitting would feel extremely bloated and uncomfortable.

Some types of fiber appear to be more effective than others. For instance, guar gum, oat bran, glucomannan, and to a lesser extent psyllium, seem to be more effective than other fibers such as cellulose or wheat bran in causing weight loss. By taking supplements enriched with guar gum or glucomannan, you may be able to reduce food intake and your weight with lower amounts of fiber. Guar gum is obtained from the Indian cluster bean, while glucomannan comes from the Japanese kinjac root. Both can be purchased in health food stores. In one study, 10 grams of guar gum twice a day for one year caused an average weight loss of 49.5 pounds. In another study, 15 grams of guar gum a day for 4 months caused a weight loss of 5.5 pounds compared to 0.9 pound in the placebo group. In yet another study, obese women taking 10 grams of guar gum before lunch and dinner lost an average of 9.4 pounds after 2 months, even though they had received no diet instructions.

Another source of fiber, glucomannan, was also found to reduce weight gain. At a dose of 1 gram taken an hour before each meal for 2 months, glucomannan caused a 5.5-pound weight loss, compared to a 1.5-pound weight gain in those people ingesting a placebo. In a further study researchers found that people consuming oat bran biscuits before meals (8 grams of fiber per day) lost an extra 12.8 pounds of weight over a year than people just adhering to a 1,000 calorie diet without added fiber (36.1 vs. 23.3 pounds lost). Researchers found similar results with people consuming citrus fiber, high fiber bread, and a mixture of vegetable grain and fruit fiber.

Certainly, fiber is good for you and does seem to aid in weight loss. Gradually incorporating fiber into your diet is an excellent way to go. You should also know that, when fiber reaches the colon, bacteria ferment it and hydrogen gas is released. Thus, if you use too much fiber right away, you may experience bloating, flatulence, and cramps. Start by taking about 3 grams of guar gum or 1 gram of glucomannan or 2.5 grams of oat fiber wafers (approximately six wafers) a day. Gradually increase the dose, so by the end of 3 months you are taking 15 grams of guar gum or 6 grams of glucomannan or 7.5 grams of oat fiber a day consumed in divided doses before each meal.

Chromium Picolinate

Chromium is an essential mineral needed by the body to maintain a normal blood sugar level. Chromium increases the body's sensitivity to insulin, the hormone responsible for regulating blood sugar. Chromium may also have other actions. It may lower LDL (bad) cholesterol while increasing HDL (good) cholesterol, and it may reduce body fat while increasing muscle mass. When chromium is combined with picolinic acid, the result is chromium picolinate — a form of chromium that the body is better able to absorb. The body needs about 200 mcg (micrograms) of chromium a day; this is easily achieved in a normal diet. Many scientists see a role for chromium supplements only to treat chromium deficiency, a rare clinical situation. There are a few human studies, however, which demonstrate a positive effect of chromium picolinate on weight loss. In one such study, patients taking chromium picolinate lost an average of 4.2 pounds over a 2.5-month period compared to 0.4 pound in the placebo group; Chromium picolinate was far more effective in men than women (men lost 7.7 pounds compared to 0.1 pound in the placebo group; women lost 3.2 pounds compared to 0.2 pound in the placebo group). In another study, chromium picolinate, at a dose of 400 mcg a day for 2.5 months, resulted in a 3.5-pound weight loss. When taking body composition into account, researchers found that there actually was a loss of 4.6 pounds of fat and a gain of 1.1 pounds of muscle.

In a more recent study, 122 moderately overweight individuals who took chromium picolinate (400 mcg) lost an average of 6.2 pounds of body fat as opposed to only 3.4 pounds in those individuals in the placebo group.

While the theory behind chromium picolinate and the initial results seem promising, more human data is needed. Nevertheless, chromium picolinate is readily available in health food stores and pharmacies, and scores of overweight people are giving it a try.

Chitosan

Chitosan is made from chitin, the hard substance found in shellfish and insect shells. Chitosan may cause some weight loss by binding to dietary fat and preventing its absorption. Unlike Xenical™, which binds to the pancreatic enzyme that digests fat, chitin binds to fat itself. You are unlikely to get as much weight loss with Chitosan as with Xenical™. As with Xenical™, you should take a vitamin supplement at bedtime.

Hydroxycitrate (Citrimax™ and Citrin™)

Hydroxycitrate is the principle acid extracted from the rind of a fruit called Garcinia Cambogia. It is reported to be beneficial for weight control because it allegedly prevents the conversion of carbohydrates to body fat. Like chromium picolinate, most of the data supporting the role of hydroxycitrate for weight loss come from animal studies, with only a few preliminary human studies performed. Nonetheless, in one human study, Thom and coworkers studied 60 patients (44 women and 16 men). They gave hydroxycitrate (440 mg before meals) to 30 patients and gave a placebo to the other 30 patients. They then put the patients on a 1,200-calorie diet and told them to exercise 3 times a week. The patients receiving hydroxycitrate lost an average of 6.4 kilograms (14 pounds) in 8 weeks while the placebo group lost only 3.8 kilograms (8.4 pounds).

In another human study, researchers gave a combination of hydroxycitrate (500 mg) and chromium picolinate (100 mcg) three times a day before meals to obese patients for 8 weeks. The study was "open label," which means the researchers knew the participants were taking the product and there was no placebo control group (this study design makes the interpretation of results difficult). Weight dropped in men from an average of 210.7 pounds before starting the study to 204.6 pounds at 4 weeks and remained at 204.6 pounds at 8 weeks. In women, weight declined from 183.8 pounds to 179.4 pounds by 4 weeks and to 174.3 pounds in 8 weeks.

Satietrol

Satietrol is a dietary supplement that stimulates a feeling of fullness or satiety and helps the weight loss process. Satietrol contains potato fiber, oleic acid, casein macropeptide and other nutrients and fibers designed to stimulate and sustain release of the satiety hormone CCK. (See Chapter 6.) CCK slows down stomach emptying, leading to early satiety and a decrease in food intake. Sateitrol is a high-protein beverage consumed before a low-calorie meal. Satietrol does satisfy the claims made on its behalf: in scientific studies it enhances satiety and decreases hunger. Obese subjects were less hungry for up to 3.5 hours after eating if they took Satietrol 15 minutes before a meal compared to a placebo beverage of equal volume and calories. (For more information, check out www.Satietrol.com.)

Food Additives

Fake Fats

Just about every health-conscious diet, whether designed for heart disease, digestive problems, or weight control, advocates the lowering of fat calories. Many try to restrict the fat in our diet to 30 percent of total calories. But to reduce fat intake below 30 percent of our total caloric intake can be difficult, since much of the flavor, aroma, and texture of food comes from its fat content. While most of us are consuming less whole milk, eggs, and red meat, we are still eating too much cheese, oils, and ice cream. For some people, a "sweet tooth" is not the problem; it's the "fat tooth" that gives them trouble. Fake fats are designed to help us solve this dilemma. They taste and feel like fat on the way down, but because they are not absorbed, they are calorie-free.

Olestra™

Olestra™ is the end result of some chemical tinkering. Regular fat consists of a glycerol molecule attached to 3 fatty acid molecules. By substituting a long string of sugar molecules (sucrose polyester) for glycerol and by adding 6 to 8 fatty acids instead of 3, Procter & Gamble produced Olestra™, a nondigestible, nonabsorbable "fake fat." Another name for Olestra™ is Olean™. Although Olestra™, for all practical purposes, tastes, feels and behaves like a fat, it contributes no calories, cholesterol, or fat to the diet. Many people can't tell the difference between foods made with, or fried in, oil containing Olestra™ and those containing regular dietary fat. Olestra™ has been approved by the FDA for replacement of up to 35 percent of the fat used in shortenings and oils for home use, and up to 75 percent of the fat used in fried snacks such as potato chips. Olestra™ also causes positive effects on blood cholesterol by decreasing saturated fats in the diet.

There are a few negatives regarding Olestra™. Because Olestra™ is not absorbed, it continues to travel through the gastrointestinal tract. If eaten in large enough quantities, Olestra™ can cause loose, oily stools and abdominal cramps. Furthermore, Olestra™ may stick to fat-soluble vitamins (D, E, K, and A) and also prevent their absorption. We have not, however, seen clinically significant vitamin deficiencies in users of Olestra™.

One might think that substituting Olestra™ for dietary fat would, by itself, result in weight loss over time. But studies by John Blundell in Leeds, England, demonstrate you can fool your taste buds but you can't fool your brain. He found that people who were given Olestra™ in a meal made up for the fewer calories taken in by eating more later in the day. By the next day, the people who ate the Olestra™ meal had eaten the same number of calories as those who had eaten a meal containing regular dietary fat. Although the Olestra™ users eventually made up for the lost calories, they did it by increasing carbohydrate consumption, not fat. It's good news that Olestra™ should be able to help us lower the fat content of our diets, but to achieve weight loss, the fake fat must be used in conjunction with standard approaches to weight management, including a low-calorie diet and regular exercise.

Simplesse™

Although Simplesse™, like Olestra™, has the taste and texture of fat, it in no way chemically resembles fat. It is made from egg white and milk protein that is mixed and heated by a process called "microparticulation." This fake fat is actually a protein that has been beaten and shaped into round particles that roll over each other easily, thus giving it a creamy texture.

The FDA considers Simplesse™ to be "generally recognized as safe" (GRAS) for use in frozen desserts. The Nutrasweet Company markets Simplesse™ under the brand name Simple Pleasures™. Kraft is marketing an egg and milk protein product that is very similar to Simplesse™ called Trailblazer™. While Simplesse™ can be present in mayonnaise, salad dressing, sour cream, and yogurt, it cannot be used in cooking because heating causes it to lose its texture. It may be applied to warm foods, however, such as Simplesse™-containing butter on warm toast or Simplesse™-containing sour cream on a baked potato.

Artificial Sweeteners

The Surgeon General's report has stated loud and clear that Americans need to reduce sugar intake. Although many nutritionists have preached the evils of sweets, the primary repercussions of excess dietary sugar are the promotion of obesity and tooth decay. Just as fake fats dilute calories by replacing dietary fat, artificial sweeteners dilute calories by substituting for dietary sugars. More Americans are switching to low-calorie foods and beverages, most of them containing artificial sweeteners.

Table 8.1
Artificial Sweeteners

Saccharin (Sweet 'n Low)	Alitame
Aspartame (Nutrasweet™)*	Sucralose
Acesulfame-k (Sweet One™)	

*In Diet Coke, Diet Pepsi, and most other diet soft drinks.

Saccharin

Saccharin, the oldest sugar substitute, was discovered in 1879. Saccharin is derived from a petroleum product and gram for gram is more than 300 times sweeter than sugar. There was some concern back in the 1970s that, like cyclamate (the first artificial sweetener), saccharin may cause bladder cancer. Congress prevented the FDA from banning the sweetener, and to date there is no evidence that saccharin causes bladder cancer in humans.

How can artificial sweeteners help you lose weight? At first glance it seems a "no-brainer." Just use nonnutritive sweeteners (zero calories) instead of sugar (about 1,800 calories per pound). You will lose weight and the food will still taste great. As usual, however, things are not that easy. It turns out a sweet taste actually makes you feel hungry.

When you consume sugar, the sweetness of the sugar stimulates hunger. However, this feeling is overcome by the sugar's calories, which when absorbed by the body, suppress hunger and stimulate fullness. By contrast, hunger caused by saccharin's sweet taste may actually make you overeat. One study revealed that when freely feeding rats were offered saccharin-sweetened water to drink, they ate 10–15 percent more food than when only given unsweetened water to drink. In another landmark experiment, a tube (gastric cannula) was placed into the stomach of rats and the rats were allowed to "sham drink" (the beverage is tasted but not absorbed by the body). The rats drank a concentrated calorie-laden solution, which drained out through the stomach tube before it could be absorbed by the small intestine. The tube was then clamped after the drink drained out and the rats were offered food. The rats that sham drank the concentrated sugar solution ate 30–40 percent more in the following hour than when they sham drank water. Thus, it appears that sweetness in general drives hunger and that nonnutritive sweetness may actually work against you when it comes to weight control. The one exception seems to be aspartame.

Aspartame

Aspartame was discovered by accident in 1965. Because it is derived from protein and consists of 2 amino acids (dipeptide), it is considered a nutritive sweetener (calorie-containing) as opposed to a nonnutritive sweetener such as saccharin. Since aspartame on a gram-per-gram basis is greater than 200 times sweeter than sugar, it doesn't take much aspartame to sweeten food. For instance, less than 1 calorie of aspartame can sweeten a 12 ounce can of Diet Coke. Aspartame loses its sweetness when heated for long periods of time and is not used in baked products.

Aspartame contains the amino acid phenylalanine and therefore should not be taken by people who have phenylketonuria (the disease they test for when they prick a newborn's heel to get a blood sample). Although anecdotal reports have linked aspartame-containing products to headaches, seizures, gastrointestinal distress, and other disturbing symptoms, most scientific studies demonstrate the product to be extremely safe even for children and pregnant women. Of course, as with all products, there may be rare aspartame intolerance in certain people.

For some reason, aspartame seems to inhibit rather than stimulate eating behavior. Although aspartame is sweet and contains only trivial calories, something about its chemical structure reduces the drive to eat. Dr. John Blundell from Leeds, England, found that when aspartame (at a dose equivalent to that found in one or two cans of Diet Coke) was placed in gelatin capsules (to hide its sweet taste) and then consumed, subjects ate on average 138 fewer calories in a meal consumed 1 hour later. The results are more variable when aspartame can be tasted. In general, the results demonstrate that aspartame-containing beverages either do not change or slightly suppress eating behavior.

Other studies confirm Dr. Blundell's results. They show that long-term use of aspartame may result in weight loss. Dr. George Blackburn of the New England Deaconess Hospital showed that the addition of aspartame-containing foods to a low-fat, low-calorie diet enhanced compliance and resulted in more weight loss. Women aspartame users lost 16.5 pounds in 12 weeks compared to the control group, who lost 12.8 pounds. Aspartame, however, did not appear to benefit the men. When the same research group followed patients during the maintenance phase after initial weight loss, low aspartame use was associated with a higher weight gain.

To my knowledge, the other artificial sweeteners now available—acesulfame-k, sucralose, and altitame—either do not have the appetite-suppressing effects of aspartame or have not been tested. For those of you who like diet beverages and are trying to lose weight, aspartame appears to be the sweetener of choice.

Meal Substitutes

Meal substitutes are a popular and convenient way to lose weight, especially in individuals who tend to overeat at mealtime. For example, a person can substitute a can of Slimfast or Sweet Success™, which contain a low-calorie tasty liquid, for a meal or meals, preferably breakfast and lunch. For dinner, that person would then eat a low-calorie meal consisting of regular food. Physician supervision is not necessary as long as the person consumes one regular meal per day and total daily food intake is at least 1,000 calories.

Some liquid meal replacements are extremely low in fat and calories and high in protein. These so-called "liquid protein diets" (e.g., Optifast, Medifast) usually contain fewer than 750 calories per day and offer only 1–2 grams of fat per day. During active weight loss with these products, the dieter usually avoids regular food. With such a restrictive daily intake of calories, weight loss can occur rapidly. In fact, the average patient can lose 20–25 pounds in the first month. Only significantly obese people, however, should follow this type of diet with supervision by their physician.

Not surprisingly, many people experience a significant weight gain after they stop using meal substitutes. As a result, diet medication may be useful for weight maintenance while you are gradually switching from meal replacement to regular food.

Dermatological Products

Thigh Cream

Thigh creams that claim to get rid of cellulite contain varying amounts of the asthma drug aminophylline. Nobody knows how thigh cream works (or for that matter if it does work). There are scientific theories involving aminophylline working its way through the skin to fat cells, where the drug causes the cell to burn fat. Some people think the product causes skin

Table 8.2

Rating Nondrug Weight Control Products

Product	Recommended	Probably Effective But Need More Information	Comments
Fiber	X		Need very large amounts to control appetite.
Chromium picolinate		X	Also useful in diabetes to control blood glucose.
Chitosan		X	Can make stools greasy. Need vitamin supplement.
Hydroxycitrate		X	Probably safe but questionable effectiveness.
Satietrol		X	May help control blood sugar in diabetics. Decreases hunger while dieting.
Olestra	X		Helps lower dietary fat intake. Possibility of digestive symptoms.
Simplesse™	X		Helps lower dietary fat intake. Can't use in heat.
Aspartame	X		Helps lower dietary sugar intake.
Meal replacements	X		Convenient low-calorie meals.
Liquid protein diet	X		Only with physician supervision.
Thigh cream		X	Cosmetic only.

lumpiness/cellulite to smooth over due to fluid shifts in the skin. A few years ago at the North American Association for the Study of Obesity (NAASO), a study by the distinguished scientist George Bray showed that a thigh cream containing aminophylline actually caused a decrease in thigh circumference. As far as I know, actual fat loss has not been confirmed by more sophisticated tests such as computerized tomography (CT scan). What is quite clear is that the effect quickly wears off when you stop applying the cream.

Now that you or your physician have selected your diet drug regimen, let's learn more about the wonderful reduced-calorie meal plans I recommend to maximize your satisfaction while safely losing weight.

9

The Complete Book of Diet Drugs Diet Plan

Ready, Set, *Go!* You now have the latest information on the diet drugs you can use to achieve your weight loss goals. You and your doctor have tailored a drug regimen that is suited to you. You are ready to start losing weight today! So how do you do it? Do you just cut back on your food portions and hope for the best? Do you give up desserts and hope the medication will eliminate your sweet tooth? Do you scan the fashion mags for the latest fad diet? After all, you're about to take diet drugs. Your appetite is about to be controlled — so anything goes, right? Not quite. Let's take a closer look at the best way to lose weight while taking these drugs. You are about to learn how to eat well, enjoy your food, satisfy your particular cravings, and lose weight, too. With the diet drugs, you will have control over *how much* you eat. After reading this chapter, you will know *what* to eat to lose weight and feel completely satisfied at the end of the day.

The details of the diet plan can be found later in this chapter. But before starting the diet, you should set some goals for yourself. When you think of goals, I know what goal comes to mind first: your goal weight. We'll get to that soon, but first let's examine some other goals that are universal to all dieters.

Goals for Dieting

Goal 1: Enjoy My Diet

Now you are saying, "That goal is unrealistic." Many of you will agree when I say that most dieters assume they will *not* enjoy their diet. In fact, you may feel that the phrase "enjoying a diet" is an oxymoron! Yet if you don't enjoy your diet or feel you are constantly sacrificing, there is little or no chance that you will be able to maintain the diet and achieve your weight loss goal. It is imperative, therefore, that you find a diet plan that affords pleasure as well as results. So how do you do that? Two ways: One way is to incorporate delicious, yet lower-calorie recipes into your meal plan; another is to develop good eating habits that will intensify your eating pleasure.

You can lighten your caloric load by three different routes: (1) reducing the number of calories in your current recipes (we'll show you how); (2) trying new low-fat recipes from this book; and (3) buying low-fat commercial food products. For example: Let's say you are used to eating dessert every day. Many of us have a sweet tooth and have a hard time resisting sweets, especially after a meal. Instead of eating a rich fatty dessert such as apple pie, which contains 280 calories, try a Cranberry Baked Apple, which has only 97 calories (see recipe in Chapter 19), or a fresh apple dipped in 1 tablespoon of hot, fat-free caramel sauce (110 calories). Factor this amount of caloric savings (170 calories) into many other foods in the day's meal plan, and you have major caloric savings. Major caloric savings means major weight loss! Experiment with these recipes and the lower-fat products in your supermarket and you will discover that low-calorie eating can be extremely satisfying. The more recipes and low-fat methods of food preparation you learn and use, the more likely that you will achieve long-term success.

Developing good eating habits is essential for losing weight and maintaining your goal weight. In addition, good eating habits can actually intensify your eating pleasure. Be aware of the food you eat and savor each bite. It is important to eat slowly. It takes 20 minutes for our brains to recognize we have eaten something and to send out the signal that we are full. If your meal is completely *over* in less than 20 minutes, you run a significant risk of eating too much. When you eat quickly until your stomach feels distended, 20 minutes later your brain doesn't just say "full," it says "stuffed"! Try this experiment the next time you sit down to a meal. Set the timer for 5 minutes and begin eating your meal. When the timer goes off, stop eating and observe. Did you eat more than one-quarter of your meal? If the answer is yes, then it is time to slow down. By slowing down, you will get the feeling of fullness (satiety) before you have overeaten as well as get more satisfaction out of eating. You can find many more eating tips in this chapter and also in Chapter 11 on weight maintenance.

Goal 2: Feel Good

Getting Your Essential Nutrients (Vitamins and Minerals)

The Complete Book of Diet Drugs diet plan is nutritionally balanced. You can't find a healthier diet! Approximately 25 percent or less calories are from dietary fat, 12–15 percent from dietary protein, and 55–63 percent from carbohydrates. We stress eating vegetables and fruit and limiting intake of saturated or animal fats. We also encourage you to work your way up to eating at least 15–20 grams of fiber on the weight loss plans and 25–30 grams of fiber per day by the time you are on the maintenance plan.

In order to feel good both physically and mentally, it is important to eat all the essential nutrients. Depriving yourself of the essentials will lead to nutritional deficiencies and ill health. Weakness and depression can result from an overly restricted diet. Essential nutrients are supplied in so many different foods that, when eating an unrestricted diet, a deficiency is unlikely. When restricting calories becomes necessary in order to lose weight, however, it is possible to get short-changed on a few vitamins and minerals. Remember to take a high-potency vitamin and mineral supplement while dieting (this is especially important if you are restricting calories to 1,200 or fewer per day). In addition, check with your physician to see if you are on any medications or supplements that may interfere with the absorption of a nutrient or its function in the body (e.g., Xenical™, Olestra™).

Fluid

Think of water as your zero-calorie friend. Water is an important part of the metabolic process and should be included daily in your meal plan. Eight or more cups of fluid per day are recommended for the average person. If you are very active or perspire a lot during hot weather, your need for fluid will increase. Dehydration sets in before you even begin to feel thirsty, so it's important to drink plenty of water with exercise or extreme heat. Begin your meals with a cup or two of water to increase the volume in your stomach; this will contribute to a feeling of fullness and decrease your risk of overeating at that meal.

Fiber

Although fiber is not considered an essential nutrient, it does contribute to good health. Insoluble fiber—as found in wheat bran, fruit, and vegetables—prevents constipation and may be associated with a decreased risk of colon cancer. Soluble fiber—as found in fruits, vegetables, and oats—has been shown to be beneficial in lowering blood glucose and blood cholesterol. For an individual on a weight reduction regimen, fiber-containing foods promote satiety. Therefore, I highly recommended that you include raw vegetables at the beginning of a meal to help make you feel full and to add to your chewing enjoyment. Convenience is always a motivating factor, so be sure to have plenty of raw snap peas, cherry tomatoes, sliced cucumbers, baby carrots, sliced red peppers, and celery sticks ready to eat in your refrigerator.

Goal 3: Be Successful

A positive attitude is a necessary component to achieving weight loss. Many of you have experienced pitfalls with previous diets. Long-term success depends on your ability to overcome any eating problems or obstacles that have prevented you from losing weight in the past. This requires recognizing your eating problems and working to change your behavior to overcome them. It may help you to make a list of potential solutions to your eating problems so you can use it when the problem arises. In a moment of weakness, a list of ideas for coping may mean the difference between diet success and diet failure.

Below is an example of an eating problem and a list of potential behavior changes you can make to overcome the problem:

Possible Solutions/Behavior Changes:
1. Have a pot of herbal tea, decaffeinated diet soda, or delicious spring water to fill me up.
2. Have raw carrots, cucumbers, and salad with diet dressing available if I need chewing satisfaction.
3. Save unbuttered popcorn or another fat-free snack for the evening. Turn off the TV when it is time to eat the snack. I want to be totally aware of what I am eating.
4. Do activities other than eating, i.e., reading, sewing, calling a friend, walking, going out to the library, etc.

My Eating Problem: Overeating at night—even when I'm not hungry!

Many overweight people eat even when they are not hungry. The diet drugs will help here, especially in eliminating overeating and reducing hunger-induced eating. Be that as it may, you must change your behavior if you still eat even when you are not hungry. Each time you feel that urge to overeat at night, try a solution and see which one works for you. During your diet plan, write down all the eating problems that occur and any possible solutions that help you resolve the problem. If you have difficulty coming up with solutions, refer to Chapter 11, where I identify obstacles to dieting success and their solutions.

How to Select Your Goal Weight

Now it is time to determine your goal weight. How successful you feel about your diet often depends on your ability to achieve this goal weight. First, let's look at what would happen (and for many of you has already happened) if you didn't do anything about your weight problem. The dotted line in Figure 9.1 describes what happens to patients with untreated or poorly treated obesity.

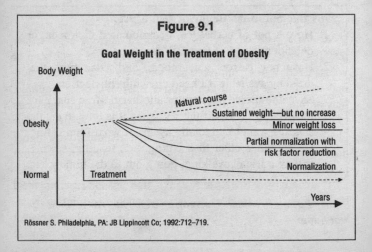

Figure 9.1

Goal Weight in the Treatment of Obesity

Rössner S. Philadelphia, PA: JB Lippincott Co; 1992:712–719.

When doctors study the course of a disease left untreated, they call it the *natural history* of that disease. The results of a treatment program for a disease can be compared to the course of the natural history of the disease to see if the treatment works. When obesity is not treated, weight tends to creep up even further over time. Therefore, any treatment that prevents further weight gain over time would be considered an effective treatment.

For most of you, a goal of just maintaining your weight at its current level would be too modest unless you have already lost weight on a diet. As you can see in Figure 9.1, however, a treatment that results in maintaining your present weight is still an accomplishment.

Unfortunately, staying at your current weight will probably not reduce your risk of developing high blood pressure, diabetes, high cholesterol, certain cancers, and other disease. On the other hand, you now know that by losing 10 percent of your body weight, you can reduce or eliminate these health risks. For instance, a woman who is 5 feet 4 inches and weighs 200 pounds can reduce health risks just by losing 20 pounds. At 180 pounds she still isn't close to her ideal body weight of 146 (BMI=25), but she has attained a significant goal; and arguably the most important goal: she has lost weight.

Many of you would like to attain a normal weight. Depending on your starting weight, how long you have been at your current weight, and your age when you were last at a normal weight, the goal of achieving a BMI of 25, for example, may or may not be practical. As we have seen, weight loss tends to level off after 6 months, often before you have achieved your ideal body weight. Of course, aggressive treatment with higher doses of diet drugs and multiple drug regimens may permit more people to reach their ideal body weight.

If your starting BMI is between 27 and 30, and reaching ideal body weight, or a BMI of 25, is a reasonable and definitely attainable goal. If your BMI is above 30, and especially if it is over 35, a more rational approach would be to set goals in a stepwise fashion. Your first milestone should be to lose 10 percent of your starting weight.

After achieving your initial goal, you should try to maintain this sensible goal weight for at least a month (use the maintenance plan, Chapter 11), before pursuing a lower weight. This will allow your body to get used to your new weight. Then you will be ready to plan new goals closer to your desirable weight.

Achieving a Safe Rate of Weight Loss

Most experts are generally conservative regarding how fast you should lose weight. Sure, you would love to lose 10 pounds in 10 days (the fashion magazines tell you it can be done), but there are reasons why that may not be such a great idea. Most physicians in the field of bariatric medicine recommend losing no more than 1 percent of your body weight per week. For most dieters, that translates to 1.5–3 pounds per week.

When we go on a diet, we tend to focus on the amount of weight we are losing. What is just as important as the amount of weight we lose, however, is the quality of weight that is lost. Losing weight too fast can cause your body to burn too much muscle (lean body mass), rather than fat. And this is something you don't want to happen.

Any time you lose weight, the weight that is lost is never 100 percent from your excess body fat. Ideally, we prefer that at least 75 percent of the weight that is lost comes from fat stores. Studies by Trevor Silverstone in London show you can lose only about a third of a pound a day before you start losing a disproportionate amount from your lean body mass. So by keeping your rate of weight loss to less than one-third of a pound per day (about 2.3 pounds a week), and by exercising (see Chapter 10), you can maximize the quality of the weight lost and preserve your lean body mass.

Don't be too concerned if you lose more than 2–3 pounds in

the first week or two. When you start dieting, initially you tend to lose a lot of water from your body. Just keep well hydrated by drinking several glasses of water a day. On the other hand, don't be discouraged when weight loss inevitably slows or temporarily plateaus after a few weeks. Cheer up, because any weight lost during this period is mostly fat.

If you are very overweight (BMI>35), it's okay to lose weight a little faster—perhaps 3 to 5 pounds per week. Studies have shown that seriously obese individuals can maintain a good quality of weight loss (i.e., > 75 percent of weight loss from fat stores) even when they lose over 3 pounds a week. But even it you are seriously obese, as your weight approaches a BMI of 30, you should definitely slow down to a weight loss of about 2 pounds per week.

A pound of weight is made up of about 3,500 calories. In order to lose a pound of weight, you have to purge those 3,500 calories from your diet. Therefore you need to eat 500 calories per day less than you usually do (i.e., a calorie deficit of 500 calories) to lose 1 pound in a week, or restrict 1,000 calories per day to lose 2 pounds in a week. The meal plans offered in this chapter range from 1,200 to 1,500 calories per day. I will help you select a meal plan that should give you a calorie deficit of about 500–1,000 calories per day.

A simple formula follows to give you a rough estimate of how many calories you should eat per day in order to lose weight: Multiply your current weight in pounds by 13. From that sum, subtract the number 500 if you want to lose one pound per week, 1,000 if you want to lose 2 pounds per week, or 1,500 if you want to lose 3 pounds per week. The result will be the number of calories to eat each day. For example: A 180-pound woman can lose 2 pounds per week by consuming 1,340 calories per day.

$$180 \times 13 = 2,340$$
$$2340 - 1000 = 1,340 \text{ calories per day}$$

If you lose more than 3 pounds per week two weeks in a row, you need to add calories to your diet. If you are not losing weight, you need to restrict calories further. In addition, your doctor may consider changing the type or dose of your diet medication(s). Always remember that adding additional exercise to your routine burns extra calories and can help you get back on track (see Chapter 10).

Selecting Your Meal Plan

To simplify matters, you can choose from one of two meal plans, depending on your sex and height. If you are a woman less than 5 feet 7 inches tall, then a 1,200-calorie meal plan is appropriate for you. It provides adequate protein and nutrients during the weight loss phase. If you are a man or woman taller than 5 feet 7 inches, then a 1,500-calorie meal plan is suggested. This will allow a slightly greater protein intake for a taller person. If you are losing weight too rapidly, consult Appendix II to find meal plans with higher calories.

The Meal Plans

The meal plans in this book are based on the American Dietetic Association and American Diabetes Association's Exchange Lists found in Appendix II. Exchange lists are foods listed together because they are alike. Each serving of food has about the same amount of carbohydrate, protein, fat, and calories as the other foods on that list. That is why any food on a list can be "exchanged" or traded for any other food on the same list. For example, you can trade the slice of bread you might eat for breakfast for ½ cup of cooked cereal. Each of these foods equals one starch choice.

There are three main groups of exchanges: the Carbohydrate group, which includes starches, fruit, milk, and vegetables; the

Meat and Meat Substitute group (protein); and the Fat group. The Meat and Meat Substitute group is divided into very lean, lean, medium-fat, and high-fat foods.

Both the 1,200-calorie and 1,500-calorie meal plans allow you choices from all the exchange groups found in Appendix II, with the exception of the higher fat meats and dairy products. Because fat is hidden in the medium- and high-fat meat groups as well as in whole milk products, caloric intake will increase with the use of these foods. To illustrate, lean meat contains 55 calories per ounce while high-fat meat contains 100 calories per ounce. Skim and very low-fat milk contain 90 calories per cup, whereas whole milk has 150 calories per cup. Thus, you should choose mainly from the very lean and lean meat exchanges and the skim and very low-fat milk list until you are on the maintenance plan.

Since fat is concentrated in calories and must be eaten sparingly, you are allowed only two fat exchanges for the whole day. But don't deny yourself fat-free condiments, such as mustard and salsa. You can also use fat-free salad dressings on salads, pasta, and as a meat marinade. The exchange lists will give you more information on "free" foods and beverages.

Foods are listed in the exchanges with their serving sizes, which are usually measured after cooking. When you begin, you should measure the size of each serving. This may help you learn to "eyeball" correct serving sizes.

The following chart shows the amount of nutrients in one serving from each exchange list.

Table 9.1
Exchange Lists for Meal Planning

Group/Lists	Carbohydrates (grams)	Protein (grams)	Fat (grams)	Calories
Carbohydrate Group				
Starch	15	3	1 or less	80
Fruit	15	—	—	60
Vegetable	5	2	—	25
Milk				
Skim	12	8	0–3	90
Low-fat	12	8	5	120
Whole	12	8	8	150
Other Carbohydrates	15	Varies	Varies	Varies
Meat and Meat Substitutes				
Very lean	—	7	0–1	35
Lean	—	7	3	55
Medium fat	—	7	5	75
High fat	—	7	8	100
Fat Group	—		5	45

The meal plans are divided into three meals with a snack at night. This type of meal plan promotes satiety and lessens the risk of bingeing. People who skip meals are more likely to overeat later in the day. In addition, by eating more frequently, you will feel more energetic throughout the day.

Below is the breakdown of food exchanges allotted for each meal. Examples of food selections within each exchange group are next to each exchange. You will be able to make your own menus from the exchange lists in Appendix II, choosing foods that *you* want to eat. Simply select foods that you like from the exchange lists, and plug them into the meal plans. When two or more choices are allowed within an exchange group, you have the option of selecting two different choices or doubling the portion size of one choice. A more elaborate explanation of how to use the exchange groups and the foods available within each group can be found in Appendix II.

1,200-Calorie Sample Meal Plan

(For women less than 5 feet 7 inches)

EXCHANGE	EXAMPLE

Breakfast

1 fruit	1 small banana
1 starch	½ cup Shredded Wheat
1 skim milk	1 cup skim milk

Lunch

2 meats	½ cup tuna
2 starches	2 slices bread*
1 vegetable	Sliced tomato, lettuce
1 fat	1 tbsp reduced-fat mayo
Free food	Iced tea

Dinner

3 meats	3 oz turkey
2 starches	½ cup sweet potato*
	1 plain roll
2 vegetables	1 cup green beans*
1 fat	1 tsp margarine

Night Snack

1 starch	Pudding*
1 fruit	(made with low-fat milk)
1 milk	1 cup skim milk

*Portion size has been doubled.

1,500-Calorie Sample Meal Plan

(For men and women 5 feet 7 inches and taller)

EXCHANGE	EXAMPLE
Breakfast	
1 fruit	½ cup orange juice
2 starches	1 English muffin*
Free food	2 tsp low-sugar jelly
1 milk	1 cup skim milk
Free food	Coffee
Lunch	
3 meats	3 oz chicken breast
2 starches	2 slices whole-wheat bread*
1 vegetable	Sliced carrots, cucumbers
1 fat	2 tbsp reduced-fat salad dressing
Free food	Iced tea
Dinner	
3 meats	3 oz salmon fillet
2 starches	⅔ cup brown rice*
2 vegetables	1 cup broccoli*
1 fat	1 tsp margarine
1 fruit	⅓ small cantaloupe/melon
Night Snack	
2 starches	1 bagel*
1 fruit	1¼ cup strawberries
1 milk	¾ cup low-fat yogurt

* Portion size has been doubled.

Using the above examples and the instructions in Appendix II, try to develop some menus for yourself. Next, make a shopping list and buy only those foods that are on your plan. Keep high-calorie foods out of the house to avoid temptation. If you see a special food item in the supermarket, check the calories on the food label and substitute the food for an exchange that has similar calories. For example, 4 ounces of frozen yogurt has 80 calories and a milk exchange has 90 calories. Instead of drinking a cup of skim milk, you can pick the frozen yogurt. If you cut back on your dairy products on a regular basis, make sure you add a calcium supplement to your plan.

Diet-Related Side Effects

While we have discussed potential *drug* side effects, there is also the potential for *diet-related* side effects whether you use drugs or not. Table 9.2 lists some of the more common side effects associated with a weight-loss diet. The faster you lose weight (that usually means the more calories you restrict), the more likely you are to experience one or more of these side effects. You can usually avoid these disturbing, diet-related symptoms, however, by sticking to the general rule of 1 percent loss of body weight per week.

Table 9.2
Diet-Related Side Effects*

Diarrhea	Depression
Constipation	Gallbladder attack
Muscle cramps	Menstrual irregularity
Fatigue	Headache
Hair loss	Palpitations (irregular heartbeat)

*Partial list.

Chapter 13 includes tips on shopping and cooking that you will find helpful. For your convenience, three weeks of pre-planned menus based on the above mentioned 1,200- and 1,500-calorie plans are also included in Chapter 13. The menus feature tasty recipes designed specifically for this program by a Registered Dietitian. The recipes are relatively quick and easy to prepare, and low in calories and fat.

Writing It Down

I highly recommend tracking your weight loss. Photocopy Table 9.3 and record your weight each week. Seeing your progress on paper can be very inspiring and rewarding. Weigh yourself first thing in the morning twice a week. Expect to see some fluctuation in your progress as the rate of weight loss can fluctuate—just drinking 2 cups of water will temporarily increase your weight by 1 pound. If you feel you are retaining fluid weight but have been adhering to your diet plan, don't get discouraged. Water weight comes and goes and the scale will eventually reward your efforts. Keep in mind the long-term goal and you are sure to see significant progress after 12 weeks. It is also a good idea to keep a food diary. Keeping track of what you eat is a good way to avoid overeating. A food diary form can be found in Chapter 11.

Table 9.3
Monitoring My Weight Loss

Week	1	2	3	4	5	6	7	8	9	10	11	12
+8												
+6												
+4												
+2												
Start Wt.												
−2												
−4												
−6												
−8												
−10												
−12												
−14												
−16												
−18												
−20												
−22												
−24												
−26												
−28												
−30												

Pounds

Starting Weight = _____   Reasonable Weight Goal = _____

Table 9.4
Example: Monitoring My Weight Loss

Week	1	2	3	4	5	6	7	8	9	10	11	12
+8												
+6												
+4												
+2												
Start Wt.	178											
−2		176										
−4												
−6			172									
−8				170	170							
−10						168						
−12							166	166				
−14									164			
−16										162	162	
−18												159
−20												
−22												
−24												
−26												
−28												
−30												

Starting Weight = 180 pounds   **Reasonable Weight Goal = 160 pounds**

10

Exercise for Faster, Easier Weight Loss

Years ago, many people felt that exercise was only for people who were "fitness freaks" or for those who were dieting. Now, nearly everyone knows that exercise is important to maintain a healthy body. Regular exercise affords a bounty of health benefits. It can help reduce stress, improve mood, increase energy, reduce sleeplessness, strengthen muscles, burn calories, and raise metabolism. It may also increase longevity. When you look at it that way, exercise is the best deal in town! So why do so many of us still avoid it? Why is America the home of the couch potato? I've heard all of the excuses: not enough time; too expensive for equipment or a health club; too hard; too boring, etc. Well, excuse time is over and exercise time is here. I am going to tell you how to incorporate exercise into your life, starting today!

Your Energy Balance

The key to weight loss is to burn more energy (calories) than you consume. If, on average, you eat fewer calories than you expend, you will lose weight. Of course, the converse is also true: If your average energy expenditure is less than your energy intake, you will gain weight. Any kind of exercise or physical activity contributes to weight loss by providing additional energy expenditure. It is important to note, however, that results of hundreds of weight loss studies have shown that exercise *alone* is often not an effective way for most people to lose weight. You must combine all three of the components discussed in *The Complete Book of Diet Drugs* to ensure long-term weight management: calorie restriction (with or without drug therapy), exercise, and behavior modification.

How Exercise Helps Weight Loss

Let's examine the role exercise plays in your goal to lose weight.

Burns Calories

When you expend energy, you burn calories (remember, calories are energy). To lose 1 pound, you must burn 3,500 calories. Later in this chapter, I'll tell you how many calories you can burn with various exercises.

Lowers Set Point

Your body has a mechanism called a "set point," which maintains your weight at a certain level despite external influences. In other words, when you overeat or undereat, your body internally adjusts by altering body metabolism to maintain your weight at its set point (obese people have a higher set point than normal-weight individuals). For example: If you are stranded on a desert island without food, your body tries its best to protect you from losing too much weight by maintaining your set point. Even though you are consuming less, your metabolism slows to prevent you from losing too much weight. This slowing is limited, and by restricting enough calories, you will lose weight. But your body is fighting against you because it doesn't know whether you are on a diet or you are stranded on a desert island. Exercise can prevent your set point from slowing down the weight loss process by raising body metabolism.

Raises Body Metabolism at Rest

Burn extra calories while you sleep? It sounds too good to be true! Well, while everyone knows that metabolism increases *during* exercise, what you may not know is that exercise can also raise your metabolic rate even when you are at rest (your basal metabolic rate). There appears to be a small but definite residual effect of exercise on metabolism that lasts hours after your exercise program has ended.

Preserves Body Muscle

Exercising during a weight loss program encourages the body to burn excess fat while building up muscle tissue. And since muscle is the most metabolically active tissue in your body, increasing muscle mass means increasing body metabolism.

Reduces Appetite

Most people experience a reduction in appetite after exercise. Why this happens is not entirely known, but it may be related to exercise-induced changes in glucose and insulin levels.

Not only does exercise assist you in losing weight, but it improves your overall health. In fact, some studies indicate that even if you can't lose weight, as long as you remain fit, you may avoid obesity-related diseases and have a normal lifespan.

Getting Started

Many times, getting started is the hardest part of any venture; this includes exercising. The most important thing to bear in mind is that exercise takes many forms and you can pick what is right for you. There is no one "right" exercise; variety and flexibility are the keys to a successful exercise program.

In our fast-paced world of modern conveniences, the need to exert ourselves shrinks daily. Contrary to societies of the past, fewer of us are laboring in the fields and in factories at jobs that require physical exertion. Homemakers aren't scrubbing clothes on a washboard or cleaning out the barn. Now many of us drive to work, take the elevator to our offices, sit at a desk most of the day, and then drive home to "veg" in front of the tube. We don't even need to leave the couch to flip the channels! But as dieters, we now have to adjust our thinking to deliberately incorporate physical activity into our lives.

Some exercise can be part of your daily routine. For example, make it a policy to walk everywhere say, less than a quarter-mile away. Next time you shop, resist taking the parking spot closest to the store. Park a bit farther away and get some exercise. Have you ever driven your car from the parking spot in front of one store to another space closer to a store farther down the shopping strip? If so, you've missed a perfect opportunity to exercise! Do you wait impatiently for the elevator to take you up one flight? Next time remember this: "Up one, down two." This simply means, make it a policy to take the stairs if you are only going up one or down two flights. You can increase the number of flights as your fitness improves. Many lawn and garden tools are available in manual and power versions. Opt for the manual ones, and you will do your body and the environment a favor. You can use this concept to think of more ways to increase your physical activity without even regarding it as exercise.

If you have tried to exercise before, but failed, here are some tips on how to get started.

- *Begin slowly.* If you are new to exercising, don't expect to compete in a marathon in a week.
- *Set realistic goals.* You know Rome wasn't built in a day. And you won't be fit after two aerobic sessions. But if you find a program you like, the process of getting fit should be as enjoyable as the result.
- *Choose activities you enjoy and vary your routine.* Let's face it, there is no way you will sustain any workout program that you dread. There are so many options, you can pick several that suit you.
- *Have a plan, but be flexible.* A regular exercise schedule is ideal. This eliminates the many excuses that tend to cut down our time for workouts. What happens when you do have a legitimate conflict? Try to reschedule that lost workout for another time the same week. Maintain a schedule of exercising 3 to 5 times per week. Avoid scheduling your workout time immediately after meals or just before bed. Exercising on a full stomach can result in cramps and heartburn. And because exercise can stimulate your body, plan to finish your routine at least one and a half hours before bedtime.
- *Keep records.* Most activities can be charted (see Table 10.6 at end of chapter) to show how much progress you have made. Actually seeing the results on paper can be very heartening!

Note: Before starting any exercise program, check with your physician. This is especially important if:

- You are over 45 years old.
- You or anyone in your immediate family has experienced a heart attack or stroke.
- You have experienced chest pains, shortness of breath, loss of balance, or dizziness.
- You are seriously obese.
- You are a heavy smoker.

- You have a preexisting medical condition such as diabetes, hypertension, or hyperlipidemia (increased triglycerides or cholesterol).

Warm-Up and Stretching

No matter what type of exercise you plan to do, allow a few minutes to warm up before you begin. A good way to do this is to walk or move in place for a minute or two. Warming up will increase the circulation to your leg muscles, so when you start your exercise, the muscles will respond to the added energy demand with less fatigue. Warming up also raises the temperature of your muscles, which in turn, increases their elasticity. This reduces the chance of muscle injury and makes stretching your muscles easier and safer.

When you have warmed up, spend a few more minutes stretching. Stretching helps prevent injury during exercise. It also increases flexibility, allowing your joints to maintain a good range of motion. Remember, it is dangerous to stretch muscles that are cold; injury could result.

Stretching Principles

- Sustain a stretch. Move slowly into a stretched position and hold this position for 15–20 seconds.
- Never bounce while stretching. Rapid bouncing actually works against muscle flexibility by causing muscles to contract, rather than relax.
- Never stretch to the point of pain. Stretch only as far as you can without feeling pain.
- Never hyperextend (lock) knee or elbow joints during a stretch.
- Breathe while stretching. A slow, rhythmic breathing pattern will help you reach a full range of motion with your

muscles. Slowly exhale as you move into a full stretch. Slowly inhale as you release the stretch.

- Repeat the stretch for each muscle group 3–5 times.

Cooling Down

Once you are finished exercising, take a few minutes to cool down. As with the warm-up, you can cool down by walking at a comfortable pace. The cool-down allows your heart to slow down gradually, and you will be less likely to feel light-headed or dizzy from a lack of blood to your brain. After the cool-down, do some additional stretches of those muscles you were working during the exercise.

Aerobic and Nonaerobic Exercise

Of course, you have heard of aerobics, but just what are they? Aerobic exercises are those that use a large number of your muscles at a reasonably low level of intensity and can be maintained over a long period of time. Nonaerobic exercises are also called "muscle-strengthening exercises." Nonaerobic exercises use only a small number of muscles or a single muscle group. These muscles are exercised at a high intensity and each exercise can be sustained only for a short period of time. Table 10.1 lists some examples of aerobic and nonaerobic exercises.

Table 10.1

Aerobic Exercises	Nonaerobic Exercises
Brisk walking	Sit-ups
Dicycling	Leg lifts
Jogging	Bench press
Swimming	Leg curls
Roller-skating	Arm curls

Aerobic exercise is recognized for its importance in helping to prevent the number one cause of death in the United States: cardiovascular disease (heart disease and hypertension). It has also been noted to lower the risk for, and severity of, diabetes and certain types of cancer. These health benefits are due to the improved functioning of your heart, lungs, circulatory, and metabolic systems, as well as the lowering of your body fat.

Nonaerobic exercise (muscle strengthening) is known to aid in preventing osteoporosis ("brittle-bone disease"). Nonaerobic exercises that are done with isolated muscle groups and at high levels of muscle tension are also valuable in your quest to lose weight. By strengthening your muscles, you can expect:

- Increased muscle strength.
- Increased muscle endurance.
- Decreased muscle fatigue.
- Increased bone strength in your arms and legs.
- Increase in your basal metabolic rate.

Remember, when you increase your metabolic rate, you increase your energy expenditure even while you sleep!

Burning Fat

The muscles you use when you exercise require additional fuel in order to support your body's movement. During the initial phase of any exercise, metabolism (the burning of body fuels) occurs without adequate oxygen. This is known as "anaerobic metabolism." Carbohydrates, rather than fat are usually burned during this phase. After 2–3 minutes into the exercise session, your increased breathing rate and depth, heart rate, and blood flow to exercising muscles start to deliver additional oxygen to your cells. Now your exercising muscles can meet some of their energy demands with "aerobic metabolism." Both fat and carbohydrates are used to fuel aerobic metabolism. The amount of time you spend exercising and the intensity of the exercise affect how much fat and how much carbohydrate you burn during your workout.

During an aerobic workout, the more intense the exercise, the lower the contribution of your fat stores to meet your energy demands. Conversely, the more moderate the intensity of the exercise, the more fat fuels will be burned to support your energy demand. Experts feel that exercising at 60–80 percent of maximum heart rate is sufficient for maximum fat-burning effect. The amount of time you exercise also affects what fuels will be used to provide the added energy required by the activity. After the first few minutes of exercise, you start to use fat as fuel, but carbohydrates remain the primary long-term energy provider. Studies have shown that you must exercise more than 20 minutes to get a substantial contribution from fat stores to fuel your movements. Since we know that sustained exercise expends more energy and burns more fat, aerobic exercise appears to be the best choice for people interested in losing weight.

Heart Rate

Your heart rate is an accurate indication of how hard you are exercising. Any movement you make from a resting position increases your heart rate in order to circulate more blood to the muscles you are using. The more movement you make, the higher the heart rate. To use heart rate as an indicator of exercise intensity, however, you need to know your maximum heart rate. To determine your maximum heart rate in beats per minute (bpm), simply subtract your age from 220 (see Table 10.2)

Table 10.2
Age-Predicted Maximum Heart Rate Levels

220 - Age	Maximum Heart Rate (bpm)
220 - 20	200
220 - 25	195
220 - 30	190
220 - 35	185
220 - 40	180
220 - 45	175
220 - 50	170
220 - 55	165
220 - 60	160

In general, experts advise gradually exercising up to, but never exceeding, your maximum heart rate.

In order to determine how intensely you are exercising, take your pulse* immediately after you stop exercising. Count how many beats in 30 seconds, starting with 0, and multiply this number by 2. This total is your exercise heart rate. Calculate your Percent Exercise Intensity with the following equation:

(Exercise Heart Rate ÷ Maximum Heart Rate) x 100 = Percent
Exercise Intensity

For example: After a brisk walk, a 35-year-old woman has an exercise heart rate of 125 bpm. Her maximum heart rate is 220 − 35 = 185 bpm.

*To take your pulse: Place your first two fingers (never the thumb) on the pulse site. The preferred location is the radial artery, which is located under your wrist. Another choice is the carotid artery, which is the large artery on the side of your neck. Apply only a small amount of pressure and move your fingers over the area until you locate the strongest pulse. *Never apply strong pressure, especially on the carotid artery. Too much pressure can slow your heart rate and possibly interfere with the blood supply to your brain.* If you can't find your pulse, ask your doctor or nurse to assist you in learning the technique.

Percent Exercise Intensity

$(125 \div 185) \times 100 = 68\%$
of Maximum Heart Rate

Table 10.3
Level of Exercise Intensity

45–55% of maximum heart rate	Low-intensity exercise
56–75% of maximum heart rate	Moderate-intensity exercise
76–90% of maximum heart rate	High-intensity exercise

Your heart is like all the other muscles in your body. The more you work out, the stronger your heart will be. The stronger your heart, the greater the amount of blood it can circulate with fewer beats per minute. Track your heart rate response to your exercise program every 2–3 weeks. You will notice that as you become more fit, you will be able to do the same amount of exercise, but your exercise heart rate will decrease (you may choose to increase the intensity of your exercise at this point). In fact, as you improve your fitness, even your resting heart rate will decrease. The fittest athletes have the slowest resting heart rates.

The Fitness Test

Before starting an aerobic exercise program, I recommend that you perform a test to determine your current level of fitness. By knowing your present fitness level, you will be able to measure your progress as your fitness improves. This test was developed by Staywell Health Management Systems and has been shown to be an effective test of aerobic fitness for the general adult population.

The fitness test entails walking 1 mile as fast as you can without stopping. Your fitness level will fall into one of five classifications: excellent, good, average, below average, and low. The classifications are based on your age and the amount of time it takes you to complete the mile walk.

The first thing you need to do is to map out a flat walking route exactly 1 mile in length. There are many possibilities for walking sites. You can walk on a street or sidewalk (use your car odometer to verify the distance), or you may use a running track. Outdoor tracks are ¼ mile in length: walk around 4 times from the inside lane. If you choose an indoor track, make sure you know how long the track is before you begin since indoor tracks vary in length. Some malls and local parks have walking/jogging trails with mileposts for tracking your distance. One thing to consider if you are on a path or street is to walk ½ mile one way, and then turn around and walk the other ½ mile back to the starting point. If you are tired at the end of the mile, you will be near your home or car.

Step two is to walk the mile as fast as possible without stopping, timing yourself with a stopwatch. Table 10.4 indicates your current fitness status.

Table 10.4
Aerobic Walk Fitness Test

Aerobic Fitness Classification	Time Measured in Minutes:Seconds			
	Women Under 40 years old	Women 40 and Older	Men Under 40 Years Old	Men 40 and Older
Low	20:01 or more	22:01 or more	19:31 or more	21:31 or more
Below Average	18:30–20:00	19:31–22:00	18:01–19:30	19:01–21:30
Average	16:01–18:30	17:01–19:30	15:31–18:00	16:31–19:00
Good	13:31–16:00	14:31–17:00	13:01–15:30	14:01–16:30
Excellent	13:30 or less	14:30 or less	13:00 or less	14:00 or less

Aerobic Fitness Test, developed by Staywell Health Management Systems, Minneapolis, Minnesota.

The Exercise Options

Table 10.5 is a list of physical activities and their corresponding energy expenditures. These caloric values are an approximation of how much energy you will burn with each activity. Note the description of the pace of each activity and remember that you must sustain the activity for 1 hour at that pace to burn the stated number of calories.

Table 10.5
Energy Expenditure of Aerobic Activity per Hour

Calories per Hour Expended at Given Body Weight

Activity	Description	125 lbs	150 lbs	175 lbs	200 lbs	225 lbs
Walking	2.0 mph	143	170	200	228	255
	3.0 mph	200	238	280	319	357
	4.0 mph	257	306	360	410	459
Jogging	5.2 mph	513	612	720	819	918
Running	7.0 mph	656	782	920	1047	1,173
Bicycling	14–15.9 mph	570	680	800	910	1,020
Bicycling,	Moderate effort	399	476	456	637	714
stationary	Vigorous effort	599	714	840	956	1,071
Aerobics	Low impact	285	340	400	455	510
	High Impact	399	476	560	637	714
Stair climbing	Moderate effort	342	408	480	546	612
Ski machine	Moderate effort	542	646	760	865	969
Baseball	Recreational game	285	340	400	455	510
Bowling	Recreational game	171	204	240	273	306
Dancing	Ballroom, disco	314	374	440	501	561
Golf	Power cart	200	238	280	319	357
	Carrying clubs	314	374	440	501	561
Racquetball	Recreational game	399	476	560	637	714
Tennis	Doubles	342	408	480	546	612
	Singles	456	544	640	728	816

Based on Ainsworth, B. E. et al. Compendium of Physical Activities: Classification of energy costs of human physical activities. *Medicine and Science in Sports and Exercise*, 25(1): 71–80, 1995.

Exercise Options

I cannot overstress this point: You must pick the exercises that you enjoy. And since variety is the spice of life, be sure to vary your exercise routine enough to keep it interesting and keep you motivated to do more. Since some exercises will be limited to appropriate weather conditions or access to certain facilities, you may find these limitations force you to vary your routine accordingly. So walk one day, play tennis another, and try to incorporate exercise 3–5 times during the week. Below is a list of a few of the popular exercise options you may want to consider.

Walking

The advantages to walking are many. Walking involves a skill you already have and it is suitable to people of all fitness levels. Walking can be a light stroll or the pace can be increased to provide a thorough aerobic and fat-burning workout. No special equipment is required, except for a decent pair of shoes. Your neighborhood is an obvious choice for setting up a walking route, but you should also consider other options. Many community parks have walking trails, and local malls are usually open early to accommodate indoor walkers. Walking "travels" well too. You can do it at home, while on vacation, or on a business trip.

Jogging

Jogging improves the performance of your cardiovascular system. This improvement not only directly benefits your health, but can also improve your performance in other sports such as swimming, basketball, and tennis. Jogging or running can be added to your walking routine as your fitness increases. Consider adding a jogging segment to your regular walking route and increase the number of segments as your stamina allows. Remember, in order to burn significant fat, you must sustain your exercise for at least 20 minutes or more, so it is important to add jogging or running to your program gradually for the greatest fat-burning effect.

Aerobics

"Aerobics" is commonly used as a catchall word to include all types of exercise routines. These exercises can be done at home or at an organized facility. Home options include follow-along televised exercise shows and home exercise videotapes and audiotapes. The equipment involved is usually minimal but may require a mat and some hand weights. Some routines also require a "step" for step aerobics. If you are using tapes, I suggest you vary them often for a more well-rounded, less-repetitive routine. I would also like to offer a word of caution. Many celebrities are touting themselves as exercise authorities and offer their own exercise videos. Some of these videos are worthwhile; others are strictly self-promotions. Look for routines that are well rounded and aren't selling expensive equipment as part of the package. Be sure to keep safety in mind and never attempt to do any exercises that hurt.

If you are looking to get out of the house, all health clubs offer aerobic classes. There are also many independent instructors that lease spaces in churches or schools and offer regular classes. Some classes may even offer dance routines as part of their program. The instructors and the music are often the biggest variables in aerobic classes. Try a few to see which ones you like the best.

Tennis

The way I like to exercise is while playing a sport. You can get an effective workout with many sports while you focus on the game instead of the exercise. One of my favorite sports is tennis. Tennis is a sport for all fitness levels and abilities that you can play throughout your entire life. And while you can spend a lot of money to play tennis—fancy clothes and expensive equipment—you can also play it at a reasonable price. Most townships or public schools offer courts free of charge; all you need is a racquet (it can be bought secondhand), athletic shoes, and a can of balls.

Tennis is a great sport for aerobic conditioning and fat-burning, but you have to keep moving! While the pros work up a sweat playing doubles tennis, the average "club" tennis player finds it easier to keep moving in a game of singles. Another option is to sign up for a tennis clinic or tennis aerobics. These clinics typically consist of an hour and a half of tennis drills that are orchestrated by an instructor. Class sizes vary between four and eight people and you can improve your stroke as you work out. Be sure to find an instructor who will give you the right workout to enhance your current fitness level. You can sign up for clinics at tennis clubs, schools, and Ys.

Swimming and Aqua Jogging

Swimming is another wonderful exercise that provides many health benefits. Swimming exercises the entire body, yet places less stress on the joints than "high-impact" exercises.

Aqua jogging, a more recent development, is just like walking or jogging, but while suspended in the water. There are different types of equipment necessary for aqua jogging: One type involves wearing a foam belt around your waist to keep you afloat (aqua jogging requires water deep enough to avoid touching the bottom as you jog). Special weblike gloves can also be worn to propel you as you jog. Another option is to purchase large plastic perforated "moon boots" and barbells for this exercise. The boots and barbells increase resistance in the water, thus increasing the difficulty of your workout.

Both swimming and aqua jogging provide a good, low-impact, cardiovascular workout. And you can perform both year-round. For access to indoor pools, check with your local health clubs, Ys, community centers, and public and independent schools. Always observe water safety rules when engaging in any water activity.

Monitoring Your Progress

Once you have started an exercise program, make it a habit to track your progress. Use a log to record your activity. You can customize this sample log to suit your needs and particular exercise activity.

Table 10.6
Sample Exercise Log
Aerobic Activity
Resting Heart Rate: _____ (bpm)

Day	Activity	Distance (miles)	Duration (minutes)	Speed (mph)	Calories Burned	Exercise Heart Rate

Total Calories Burned/Week: _____

Exercise Summary

- Any type of exercise or physical activity will contribute to creating an energy deficit.
- Moderate-intensity aerobic exercise that can be sustained for 20 or more minutes burns more body fat than a high-intensity exercise that can be maintained for only a short period of time.
- Nonaerobic exercise (muscle-strengthening exercise) promotes increases in your basal metabolic rate by building muscle mass.
- Creating an energy deficit through calorie restriction alone (dieting without exercise) will reduce your basal metabolic rate, making it more difficult to lose weight.

11

Weight Maintenance
(After Weight Loss)

Congratulations! Most of you have reached your goal weight. You feel great and look fabulous. Some of you may have lost 5 percent of your initial weight and would like to maintain that weight before losing more weight. Or you may have lost 10 percent of your initial body weight and reduced your risk for obesity-related diseases. While a few of you may have struggled to get here, many of my patients have told me how easy it was to lose weight with *The Complete Book of Diet Drugs*.

Now, how do you keep the weight off? Most of you want to be at this new weight (or an even lower weight) 5 to 10 years from now. Yet statistics tell us that only about 5 percent of dieters can achieve that ultimate goal without diet medication. Even though *The Complete Book of Diet Drugs* offers a state-of-the-art weight maintenance program, it is likely that many of you will start to regain the weight you lost unless you continue to take—at least intermittently—weight loss medication. Those of you who incorporate exercise in your life in a big way may be able to keep weight off without continuing on medication. As strongly as I recommended exercise during weight loss, it is *more* important during weight maintenance.

Figure 11.1

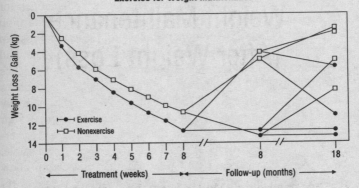

Exercise for Weight Maintenance

Modified from Pavlou KN, et al. *Am J Clin Nutr.* 1989;49:1115–1123.

To illustrate the importance of exercise, Figure 11.1 shows how exercisers are able to maintain their weight loss while those who shun exercise are not. If the nonexercisers begin exercising, they are able to lose weight again. If the exercisers stop exercising, they regain their weight. If you want to avoid taking medication—or take a reduced dose—during weight maintenance, *exercise is the key to preventing weight gain.*

Some of you may even be willing to accept the possibility of regaining a small portion of your lost weight. But I think we can all agree that regaining the entire amount of weight is unacceptable. Most studies indicate that the body's set point is fixed and doesn't change when a person loses weight, even if the lower weight is maintained for years. That means you have to be diligent in keeping up with proper eating habits and exercise or you will eventually regain your weight. Let me show you how to maintain your new weight forever.

Eating Well

One of the mainstays of eating properly is to adhere to a low-fat diet. Research backs this up: The Dietary Guidelines for Americans (1990), the Surgeon General's Report on Nutrition and Health (1988), the National Cholesterol Education Program (1993), the National Research Cancer Committee on Diet and Health (1988), and National Institutes of Health Evidence Report (1998) all agree that maintaining a healthy diet includes limiting your fat intake to 30 percent or less of your total daily calories. Limiting fat in your diet will not only decrease your risk of chronic diseases, such as coronary artery disease and certain types of cancer, but will also help keep your weight stable.

In order to maintain your new weight, you need to know how much food you can eat without losing more weight or regaining any pounds. Your daily activity level will also influence your caloric requirements. The greater your activity level, the more calories you need to maintain your body weight. Most people can describe their activity level as either "sedentary" or "moderately active." You are sedentary if you spend a large portion of the day sitting, driving, playing a musical instrument, doing school or office work, or participating in an activity that does not result in sweating. You are moderately active if you spend a large portion of the day walking, stair climbing, mowing the lawn, gardening, or participating in vigorous exercise at least three times a week.

How to Determine Your Caloric Needs to Maintain Your Weight

Table 11.1 lists the estimated number of calories needed to maintain your current weight based on your sex. Determine your activity level before consulting the table and round your age to the nearest number listed (e.g., age 32, use the age 30 column; age 58, use the age 60 column).

Table 11.1

Men's Caloric Needs*

Height	20-year-old Mild Activity	20-year-old Moderate Activity	30-year-old Mild Activity	30-year-old Moderate Activity	40-year-old Mild Activity	40-year-old Moderate Activity	50-year-old Mild Activity	50-year-old Moderate Activity	60-year-old Mild Activity	60-year-old Moderate Activity
5'4"	1,969	2,120	1,881	2,024	1,795	1,933	1,704	1,834	1,616	1,740
5'5"	2,083	2,243	1,994	2,148	1,905	2,052	1,817	1,957	1,729	1,862
5'6"	2,189	2,357	2,056	2,215	1,968	2,120	1,880	2,024	1,791	1,929
5'7"	2,213	2,382	2,124	2,287	2,036	2,193	1,947	2,097	1,860	2,003
5'8"	2,278	2,453	2,199	2,358	2,101	2,263	2,013	2,168	1,925	2,072
5'9"	2,343	2,522	2,254	2,427	2,166	2,332	2,077	2,237	1,989	2,142
5'10"	2,407	2,599	2,272	2,497	2,230	2,402	2,142	2,307	2,084	2,212
5'11"	2,473	2,664	2,385	2,569	2,217	2,474	2,209	2,379	2,130	2,295
6'	2,539	2,734	2,450	2,639	2,364	2,543	2,273	2,449	2,185	2,353
6'1"	2,603	2,803	2,514	2,710	2,426	2,612	2,337	2,517	2,249	2,422
6'2"	2,667	2,873	2,579	2,778	2,491	2,682	2,402	2,587	2,314	2,492
6'3"	2,731	2,941	2,643	2,846	2,555	2,751	2,466	2,656	2,378	2,561
6'4"	2,799	3,014	2,710	2,919	2,622	2,824	2,534	2,729	2,445	2,633

Women's Caloric Needs*

Height	20-year-old Mild Activity	20-year-old Moderate Activity	30-year-old Mild Activity	30-year-old Moderate Activity	40-year-old Mild Activity	40-year-old Moderate Activity	50-year-old Mild Activity	50-year-old Moderate Activity	60-year-old Mild Activity	60-year-old Moderate Activity
5'	1,654	1,780	1,591	1,714	1,530	1,648	1,469	1,582	1,408	1,516
5'1"	1,687	1,817	1,626	1,751	1,565	1,686	1,504	1,620	1,443	1,554
5'2"	1,715	1,847	1,654	1,781	1,592	1,715	1,531	1,649	1,470	1,583
5'3"	1,756	1,891	1,695	1,826	1,634	1,760	1,573	1,694	1,512	1,628
5'4"	1,794	1,932	1,729	1,862	1,668	1,796	1,607	1,730	1,546	1,665
5'5"	1,824	1,964	1,763	1,898	1,702	1,833	1,641	1,767	1,579	1,701
5'6"	1,858	2,001	1,797	1,935	1,735	1,869	1,674	1,803	1,613	1,737
5'7"	1,893	2,038	1,832	1,973	1,771	1,907	1,709	1,841	1,648	1,775
5'8"	1,928	2,076	1,867	2,010	1,806	1,945	1,745	1,879	1,683	1,813
5'9"	1,962	2,113	1,901	2,047	1,840	1,981	1,778	1,915	1,717	1,849
5'10"	1,996	2,150	1,935	2,083	1,873	2,018	1,812	1,952	1,751	1,886
5'11"	2,031	2,187	1,969	2,121	1,908	2,055	1,847	1,989	1,786	1,924
6'	2,064	2,223	2,003	2,157	1,942	2,092	1,881	2,026	1,820	1,960

*Caloric needs are based on the Harris-Benedict Equation and multiplying activity factors of 1.3–1.4 for mild and moderate activity level respectively.

Sample meal plans that range from 1,200 calories to 3,000 calories per day can be found in Appendix II. Choose a meal plan close to your maintenance calorie needs. Like the weight loss diet plans, each meal is broken down into food exchange groups (also found in Appendix II). All of the plans are well balanced, low in fat, and high in fiber. Refer back to the section in Chapter 9 on meal plans and the instructions in Appendix II if you still need help using the exchange lists and meal plans.

Substituting Foods

When the foods you want to eat don't quite match your exchanges, you need an alternative. The calories of each exchange are listed in the meal plans so you can substitute convenience foods or recipes of the equivalent calories into your menus (assuming they also contain less than 30 percent fat). To make comparisons, refer to the Nutrition Facts Label of prepared foods. Use the measurement conversions listed in Table 11.2 to assist you.

Table 11.2
Measurement Conversions

3 teaspoons (tsp)	=	1 tablespoon (tbsp)
2 tablespoons (tbsp)	=	1 fluid ounce (oz)
4 fluid ounces (oz)	=	½ cup
8 fluid ounces (oz)	=	1 cup
12 fluid ounces (oz)	=	1½ cups

Table 11.3 is a list of low-fat, low-calorie frozen entrées that you can use in your diet. Determine the number of calories in the frozen entrée and subtract them from the calories allowed for that meal. The difference in calories between your meal and the entrée can be made up in vegetables, starches, fruits, or milk. You may find other convenience items not on the list on Table 11.3. For example: You want to eat Stouffer's Lean Cuisine Hearty Portions Oriental Glazed Chicken (14 oz) for lunch. The frozen entrée has 470 calories and you are allowed 560 calories on your 1,800-calorie meal plan.

$$560 \text{ calories} - 470 \text{ calories} = 90 \text{ calories}$$

Now you can eat an additional 90 calories of a food of your choice. You can choose an exchange that provides approximately 90 calories, such as a milk or bread exchange, or two exchanges that add up to 90 calories, such as a fruit exchange and a vegetable exchange.

Table 11.3
Calories of Frozen Convenience Meals

Healthy Choice		Weight Watchers/Smart Ones		Lean Cuisine/Café Classics (C.C.)	
Beef Macaroni	220	Bowtie Pasta and Mushrooms Marsala	280	Angel Hair Pasta	260
Beef Pepper Steak Oriental	250	Hunan Style Rice and Vegetables	250	Baked Chicken with Potatoes + Stuffing	250
Beef Tips Français	280	Kung Pao Noodles and Vegetables	260	Baked Fish with Cheddar Shells	260
Grilled Peppercorn Steak Patty	220	Paella Rice and Vegetables	280	Beef Pot Roast + Whipped Potatoes	210
Lasagna Roma	390	Parisian Style White Beans with Vegetables	220	C.C. Bow Tie Pasta + Chicken	270
Spaghetti + Sauce with Seasoned Beef	260	Pasta and Spinach Romano	240	C.C. Lasagna with Chicken Scallopini	290
Swedish Meatballs	280	Pasta with Tomato Basil Sauce	260	C.C. Chicken Breast in Wine Sauce	220
Chicken and Vegetables Marsala	230	Peking Style Rice and Vegetables	270	C.C. Calypso Chicken	280
Chicken Con Queso Burrito	350	Pilaf Florentine	290	C.C. Chicken Carbonara	280

Table 11.3
Calories of Frozen Convenience Meals

Healthy Choice		Weight Watchers/Smart Ones		Lean Cuisine/Café Classics (C.C.)	
Chicken Enchilada Suiza	270	Risotto with Cheese and Mushrooms	290	C.C. Chicken Mediterranean	230
Chicken Fettuccini Alfredo	260	Sante Fe Style Rice and Beans	290	C.C. Chicken Parmigiana	240
Chicken Imperial	230	Spicy Penne Pasta and Ricotta	280	C.C. Chicken Piccata	270
Country Glazed Chicken	220	Angel Hair Pasta	170	C.C. Chicken with Basil Cream Sauce	260
Fiesta Chicken Fajitas	260	Chicken Chow Mein	200	C.C. Glazed Turkey	250
Garlic Chicken Milano	240	Chicken Mirabella	170	C.C. Grilled Chicken Salsa	270
Grilled Chicken Sonoma	240	Fiesta Chicken	220	C.C. Grilled Fish and Vegetables	170
Grilled Chicken with Mashed Potatoes	170	Honey Mustard Chicken	200	C.C. Herb Roasted Chicken	210
Honey Mustard Chicken	260	Lasagna with Meat Sauce	240	C.C. Honey Mustard Chicken	270
Mandarin Chicken	280	Lacagna Florentine	200	C.C. Mesquite Beef with Rice	280
Sesame Chicken	240	Lemon Herb Chicken Piccata	200	C.C. Sirloin Beef with Peppercorn	220
Cheddar Broccoli Potatoes	310	Macaroni and Cheese	220	Cheddar Bake with Pasta	260
Cheese Ravioli Parmigiana	260	Ravioli Florentine	220	Cheese Cannelloni	230
Fettucini Alfredo	250	Creamy Rigatoni with Broccoli and Chicken	230	Cheese Ravioli	240
Garden Potato Casserole	210	Roast Turkey Medallions and Mushrooms	190	Cheese Stuffed Shells	210
Macaroni and Cheese	320	Shrimp Marinara	190	Chicken à l'Orange	250
Manicotti with Three Cheeses	260	Spicy Szechuan Style Vegetables + Chicken	220	Chicken and Vegetables	250
Vegetable Pasta Italiano	240	Broccoli and Cheese Baked Potato	250	Chicken Chow Mein with Rice	240
Zucchini Lasagne	330	Grilled Salisbury Steak	260	Chicken Enchilada Suiza with Rice	280
Penne Pasta with Tomato Sauce	230	Pepper Steak	240	Chicken Fettucini	300

Table 11.3
Calories of Frozen Convenience Meals

Healthy Choice		Weight Watchers/Smart Ones		Lean Cuisine/Café Classics (C.C.)	
Country Roast Turkey with Mushrooms	220	Swedish Meatballs	300	Chicken in Peanut Sauce	280
Beef and Peppers Cantonese	270	Chicken Enchiladas Suiza	270	Chicken Italiano with Fettucini + Vegetable	270
Beef Broccoli Beijing	300	Cheese Manicotti	260	Chicken Lasagna	290
Beef Stroganoff	310	Chicken Fettucini	290	Chicken Oriental with Vegetables	250
Charbroiled Steak Patty	280	Fettucini Alfredo with Broccoli	230	Chicken Pie	310
Mesquite Beef with Barbeque Sauce	310	Garden Lasagna	270	Classic Chicken Lasagna	290
Traditional Beef Tips	270	Italian Cheese Lasagna	300	Country Vegetables and Beef	220
Traditional Meatloaf	320	Lasagna with Meat Sauce	270	Deluxe Cheddar Potato	230
Traditional Salisbury Steak	330	Lasagne Alfredo	300	Fettucini Alfredo	300
Yankee Pot Roast	280	Lasagne Bolognese with Meat Sauce	300	Fettucini Primavera	280
Cacciatore Chicken	250	Penne Pasta with Sundried Tomatoes	290	Fiesta Chicken with Rice + Vegetables	250
Chicken Broccoli Alfredo	300	Spaghetti with Meat Sauce	290	Five Cheese Lasagna	230
Chicken Cantonese	280	Spaghetti Marinara	280	Glazed Chicken with Vegetable Rice	240
Chicken Dijon	270	Tuna Noodle Casserole	270	Homestyle Turkey	240
Chicken Enchilada Suprema	270	Ziti Mozzarella	280	Lasagna with Meat Sauce	290
Chicken Francesca	330	Chicken Cordon Bleu	230	Macaroni and Beef	280
Chicken Parmigiana	300	Penne Pollo	290	Macaroni and Cheese	290
Chicken Piquante	260	Stuffed Turkey Breast	230	Meatloaf and Whipped Potatoes	240
Chicken Teriyaki	230			Oriental Beef	240
Country Breaded Chicken	360			Oriental Style Dumplings	320
Country Herb Chicken	320			Penne Pasta Bolognese	270
Ginger Chicken Hunan	350			Roasted Turkey Breast and Stuffing	290

Table 11.3
Calories of Frozen Convenience Meals

Healthy Choice		Weight Watchers/Smart Ones	Lean Cuisine/Café Classics (C.C.)	
Mesquite Chicken Barbeque	310		Salisbury Steak with Macaroni + Cheese	290
Roasted Chicken	220		Spaghetti with Meat Sauce	300
Sesame Chicken Shanghai	310		Spaghetti with Meatballs	280
Southwestern Grilled Chicken	200		Stuffed Cabbage with Potatoes	180
Sweet and Sour Chicken	360		Swedish Meatballs with Pasta	280
Pasta Shells Marinara	380		Three Bean Chili with Rice	260
Grilled Glazed Pork Patty	280		Turkey and Country Vegetable Pie	320
Herb Baked Fish	340		Vegetable Eggroll	330
Shrimp and Vegetables Maria	270		Vegetable Lasagna	270
Shrimp Marinara	220		Mandarin Chicken	260
Country Inn Roast Chicken	250		Teriyaki Stir-Fry	270
Traditional Breast of Turkey	290		Chicken Marinara Rotini	260

There will likely be other times that you'll want to eat certain foods without sticking exactly to the exchange lists. In this case, you can simply count the calories for those foods and trade them for some calories in your plan. For instance, say your lunch meal plan calls for 3 lean meat ex-changes (55 calories each), 2 starches (80 calories each), 1 vegetable (25 calories), 1 fat exchange (45 calories), and no fruit or milk. This is a total of 395 calories. You're out and want to order a veggie stir-fry and some low-fat frozen yogurt topped with fruit. The restaurant provides nutrition information, so you know that the calories come close to your limit. What do you do? By all means, give your order to the waitress and enjoy!

Calorie counting gives you a lot of flexibility, but there is one important rule: It is fine to trade the calories of meats and fats for more starches, fruits, and skim milk, but the reverse is not recommended. Replacing starches, fruits, and skim milk with more meat and fat will significantly increase the fat content and alter the vitamin and mineral concentration of your diet. Therefore, changing your basic diet plan is good only as long as the fat content you consume stays the same or decreases. Continue to take a multivitamin mineral supplement to assure an adequate intake. If you have questions about your diet, consult a Registered Dietitian.

At the same time, it is important that you keep records during your diet. Recording what you eat will help you to understand your eating habits, which in turn will assist you in determining the proper solution to any problems. Make copies of Table 11.4 and write down any foods you eat, including the quantity and calories. You can determine calorie amounts by referring to the caloric level of that particular exchange group (see Appendix II) or by looking up the calories in Appendix III, which lists common foods and their nutritional values. At the bottom of the page, record any problems or obstacles that occurred throughout the day. Then record how you resolved the problem. This valuable information allows you to analyze ways to *improve* your diet. You can also use the information to plan ahead for special events. Read on.

Table 11.4
Food Diary

Food/Quantity	Calories

List Obstacles:

List Solutions

Table 11.5
Sample Food Diary

Food/Quantity	Calories
½ CUP ORANGE JUICE	60
1½ CUPS CORN FLAKES	160
8 OZ SKIM MILK	90
3 CUPS HERBAL TEA, 1 BAGEL + 2 TANGERINES*	160 + 60
TURKEY (3 OZ) SANDWICH (2 BREADS) WITH MUSTARD (FREE)	325
DIET SODA	
4 OZ SHRIMP (VERY LEAN MEAT), 2 TBSP GRATED PARMESAN	140 + 55
1 CUP SPAGHETTI	160
1 CUP GREEN BEANS	50
2 TSP OLIVE OIL (USED IN SHRIMP AND SPAGHETTI DISH)**	90
DIET SODA	
1¼ CUPS STRAWBERRIES	60
1 CUP PLAIN FAT-FREE YOGURT	90
TOTAL	1,500

List Obstacles

*Conference meeting—served cinnamon buns, pastries, bagels, cream cheese, and assorted cheeses.

**Shrimp recipe needed extra fat.

List Solutions

*Conference meeting—drank 3 cups of herbal tea to fill myself up and ate 1 bagel, 2 tangerines.

**Planned ahead with shrimp recipe—used mustard (fat free) on sandwich at lunch and saved extra calories.

The Path to Diet Success: It's Not Always a Straight Line

In the life of every dieter, there are potential roadblocks on the path to dieting success. These roadblocks may vary somewhat, but many of you will recognize the ones I examine here. Let's talk about some of the obstacles you might face in your quest to lose and maintain your weight, and also discuss the solutions these obstacles.

The "All You Can Eat" Buffet

You know the scenario: parties, weddings, smorgasbord buffets. The choices are vast, the food looks scrumptious, and it's free. In the past this has been an opportunity for you to indulge yourself *big time*. Now you are facing a crisis. Do you stick to your diet and go away feeling pretty deprived or do you throw caution to the wind, concoct every possible rationalization, and start pigging out?

First, plan ahead. Don't skip meals that day in anticipation of a food fest. Skipping meals will only make you ravenous and can lead to bingeing. But you can reduce the calories of a day's meal plan in order to allow yourself some extra flexibility at a special event. Refer to your eating diary so you know how many calories you have available. Make sure you are not starving when you arrive; take the edge off your appetite by having a small snack and drinking at least 12 oz of water before you arrive.

The next step is to enjoy yourself. Mingle, talk to people, walk around. When you are ready to eat, start with low-fat and low-calorie foods like raw vegetables (no dip). These offer chewing satisfaction and give your hands something to hold. Avoid drinking alcohol by sipping a seltzer with lime or a diet drink instead. Alcoholic beverages can wreak havoc on your diet since they decrease your control and add unwanted calories. If you feel you really want an alcoholic beverage, limit it to one and drink it as slowly as possible. When it is time for the main meal, look over all the foods and decide what you really want. Make up a platter and take your time enjoying every bite. Eat slowly so when other people are on their second and third helpings, you will still be enjoying your first.

Now what about those desserts? They look great, but maybe you decide you feel you can get by without one. If not, you may want to sample one small piece. If so, try sharing it with a friend and give them the larger piece. Again, take your time and enjoy every morsel.

After the meal is over, do something far away from the table and the food. Find some fun! Check out the dance floor; you'll get some exercise while you boogie!

What happens if you do go overboard? Let's say it's a big birthday bash for you and you just want to let loose. By the end of the evening you have really indulged yourself—lots of food, plenty of wine. What are you going to do tomorrow? Resist the urge to throw in the towel. It is not logical to think you have "blown it" now and are going off your diet forever. Remember that it takes 3,500 *extra* calories to gain even 1 pound. That's pretty hard to do in one meal. Accept the indulgence and get right back on the program. By the end of the week, you are unlikely to have gained any weight.

Let's Review

- Fill up on liquids and raw vegetables for a feeling of fullness and self-control.
- Choose seltzer with a twist or diet soft drinks rather than alcohol.
- If you do choose alcohol, make one drink last.
- Eat slowly, enjoy your food thoroughly.
- Share dessert with a friend; take the smaller portion.
- Move out of the eating area to discover other fun activities: dancing, good music, interesting conversations.
- If you do indulge, all is not lost—get right back on track with the next meal.

Diet Saboteurs

You know who I mean—there is always one in the crowd. It may be your spouse, your children, your friends, or your mother. Someone really doesn't want you to be thinner. Of course, there are different reasons for this, but much of the time that person's feelings stem from insecurity. After all, if you became thinner, you might look better than your friend. Or you might become more attractive to the other sex, which can create jealousy. Or your success might show just how determined and strong you are as a person. All of these can feel very threatening to those who are close to you. Picture this. You walk into your mother's house and the first thing she says is, "You look so skinny, you've lost so much weight, you're going to get sick." Then she starts offering you first helpings, then second helpings, then third helpings. You don't want to hurt her feelings, and it tastes so good. What can you do?

You can tell her how much better you feel on this new meal plan. In fact, even your doctor recommended weight loss. Anyone who truly has your best interests at heart can't argue when you explain how much better you feel on this new diet. Compliment your mother on her delicious food and let her know you manipulated your diet to fit in her wonderful meal. Tell her that now you are full, and would appreciate it if she didn't offer you more food. Learn how to say "No, thank you," and insist that others respect your wishes. Afterward you will feel good about yourself.

Let's Review

- Let a saboteur know that losing weight is important to your health.
- Let a saboteur know how much better you feel when you eat this way.
- Let "the cook" know you enjoyed her food—now she can feel good, too.

- Also let "the cook" know the effort you made to fit her delicious food into your meal plan—now she feels even better!
- Insist that others respect you when you say "No, thank you."

"I Must Have Chocolate!"

There may be times when you feel out of control. You start thinking about chocolate and want it right now. You can't get it out of your mind and won't feel satisfied until you eat it. The key here is to distract yourself as quickly as possible. If you train yourself to get involved quickly in another activity, this feeling may cease. The first step is to write down a minimum of 10 alternative activities that you find enjoyable or productive. Keep this list close by. When the thought of chocolate comes up, you will now take a large glass of ice water and refer to your list of alternative activities. You may decide to go for a walk, wash your car, do some gardening, finish the laundry, surf the Internet, read an article, go to a movie, or call a friend. Physical activity is always a good idea. Exercise can curb your appetite.

If the distractions aren't enough and you feel truly hungry, have low-calorie snacks around to satisfy your hunger. These may alleviate your desire for chocolate. If you have specific food cravings, try to keep those foods out of the house and workplace. Finally, if you decide to eat the chocolate, eat it very slowly so your enjoyment will last a long time, then return to your meal plan. Just as in the first scenario, one bar of chocolate will not outweigh all the progress you have made so far.

Let's Review

- Make a list of 10 alternative activities that you enjoy.
- Do a physical activity.
- Distract yourself by drinking a large glass of water.
- Substitute other low-calorie, low-fat foods if you are truly hungry.

- Keep the binge foods out of the house and workplace.
- If you go off your diet plan, quickly return to it. You have been too successful so far to give up.

What If I Start to Regain the Weight?

If you find that you are starting to regain weight during the maintenance phase, you can intensify your exercise and switch to a lower-calorie meal plan. If these measures are ineffective, discuss the possibility of restarting the diet medication with your doctor. I rarely allow my patients to regain more than 10 pounds before restarting diet medication. As I said, it doesn't make sense to allow someone to regain all of his or her weight before reinstituting the drug. There are several different ways diet medication can be used for weight maintenance.

- Take the same drug at the same dose you did on the weight-loss plan. Since the medication worked before, it will likely work again. This is the surest method to get back on track.
- Take the same drug you took for weight loss, only at a lower dose. If you continue to gain weight, you can increase the dose.
- Take the same drug at the same dose you did on the weight-loss plan, but take the drug every other day. If you continue to gain weight, increase the dose to every day.
- Take the same drug at the same dose you did on the weight-loss plan for three months. Stop taking the drug for three months and then start the process over. While this "holiday" approach may be the safest, it may not be the most pleasant. Your weight may fluctuate quite a bit and the side effects of sympathomimetic drugs (see Chapter 5) may be more noticeable.

You and you doctor will have to discuss how comfortable you both are using diet drugs longer than the FDA recommendation. Each reader must consider the individual risk-benefit ratio (see Chapter 4) before making the decision to continue medication. The newest drugs on the market appear to be safe for long-term use (especially Xenical™, which has excellent safety data for two years' use). I believe that lifelong drug treatment for obesity will eventually be a reality for many individuals.

PART II

The Complete Book of Diet Drugs
Meal Plan and Recipes

12

Introduction

Do you think that cooking and eating healthy requires more time and energy than you have to spare? When you are dieting, do you eventually fall back into old habits of eating high-fat, high-calorie convenience foods? Have you prepared "diet" meals and found them to be boring and tasteless? Well, you can learn the secrets of managing a healthy, tasty eating plan without spending hours in the kitchen. By adhering to the following six basic steps for meal planning, you will eat delicious, satisfying meals every day and eliminate the hassles you now associate with diet plans.

- Plan ahead.
- Organize yourself.
- Rely on shortcuts.
- Shop smart.
- Prepare on your own time.
- Know how to improvise.

Plan Ahead

Before the crunch is on and the urge to eat has hit, know what you're going to eat. If you wait until you're tired and hungry to choose your meals, chances are you won't make good decisions. Well-planned, appealing meals can help you avoid the trap of reaching for the quickest (and often high-calorie) food when your defenses are the lowest. You can rely on our meal plans to create your own. In either case, you should think ahead for a few days (or a week). Make a list of what you'll have for meals and stock up on items you will need. If you have what you need to make dinner, you'll be less likely to hit the speed dial on your phone for the local takeout restaurant! Being prepared with a plan and the ingredients to follow through on it are key to easy meal preparation.

We have worked out a three-week meal plan for weight loss with you in mind. It is based on the exchanges and calorie levels described in Chapter 9. You will notice that some desserts and even a pizza delivery are included to keep your selections interesting! You can follow the plans just the way they are, or make your own adjustments by substituting foods of equal calorie value. Each of the meals has the calorie value listed to make it easier for you to modify. For example, if our meal plan provides a 350-calorie lunch, you can substitute a 350-calorie frozen meal instead. If the frozen meal provides only 250 calories, you have 100 calories left over to fill in as you please. Look in Appendix III to determine the calorie value and portion size of the food you would like to add. If you like the meal plan overall but don't care for one item—for instance, the vegetable side serving—refer to the exchange lists and choose a different vegetable side serving. The point is: You can follow our meal plans or have the flexibility to make your own.

Organize Yourself

Before you get started in the kitchen, think about what you'll be doing and how you'll get it done. If you're using a recipe, read it ahead of time. Gather all the ingredients and equipment before beginning. Break down large jobs into small tasks and finish the small things ahead of time—even the night before. You can chop vegetables, brown meat, or steam rice before you really get started, which will speed up your finished products.

Rely on Shortcuts

Combine steps, when possible, to save time and dirty dishes. For instance, if you want to top some pasta with blanched fresh vegetables, toss the chopped veggies into the pasta water during the last minute of cooking. Served with a dash of olive oil or broth and a light sprinkling of grated Parmesan cheese, you wind up with a tasty dish and only one pan to clean.

Choose recipes that involve a minimum of labor. The recipes included here were all developed and tested by a registered dietitian with ease of preparation in mind. Although some are quicker to prepare than others, they are all relatively simple and are based on ingredients found in most grocery stores. The portion sizes are designed specifically for your weight-loss plan.

Every recipe includes a Nutrition Facts label so that you can work it into your meal plans based on its calories. Remember that the "% daily values" listed on all food labels are designed for the general public and are based on consumption of 2,000 calories per day, a typical weight maintenance calorie level. While you are actively losing weight, you will be eating between 1,200 and 1,500 calories per day, so the "% daily values" will not apply to you.

Let someone else do the work for you! Use precut vegetables from a package or salad bar, no-bake lasagna noodles, and premarinated chicken breasts. Try frozen, prechopped onions, bagged salad mixes, and canned beans. Fresh pasta cooks almost instantly, or for fast results use a very fine dried pasta such as angel hair. Freeze homemade tomato sauce (see our recipe in Chapter 17) or find a low-fat tomato sauce that you like and keep it on hand for a quick meal. You can even find precooked rice and pasta in the freezer section of your grocery store.

(Beware the fat-laden sauces that many of these mixes contain. Use your own sauce or half the amount that the package provides.) Pick up a package of veggie burgers for a low-fat meal already fully cooked which requires only reheating. There are many varieties in grocery stores; see which ones you like best.

Shop Smart

You can't fix and eat good foods unless you have them on hand, so a large part of cooking healthy is shopping right. And since shopping can lead to temptation, you need to be able to get out of the store with just the items you want, not a cart full of goodies. Make sure you've had something to eat before you shop so you'll be less prone to impulse-buying. The outer edges of the store are generally where the healthiest foods are found—fresh produce, low-fat and nonfat dairy products, whole grain breads, and lean meats. If possible, stay out of the snack food aisles. Learn to read labels and know what they mean so you won't be fooled by deceptive advertising. Become familiar with some of the terms used on labels:

Calorie-free: up to 5 calories per serving
Sugar-free: up to 0.5 gram of sugar per serving
Fat-free: up to 0.5 gram of fat per serving
Low-fat: up to 3 grams of fat per 100 grams of food
Light/Lite: $\frac{1}{3}$ fewer calories than the regular version of a
    food

Check the portion sizes listed on labels when fitting these foods into your diet. Before you go to the store, make a list that includes items from the meals that you've planned. You should also keep some healthy staples on hand. Helpful items to have in the house include the following:

Staples for a Healthy Pantry

Foods

Canned beans—garbanzo, kidney, black, cannellini, and fat-free refried

Canned tomatoes—stewed, diced, crushed or pureed

Canned water chestnuts

Cholesterol-free egg substitute

Dry cereals, cornflake crumbs

Evaporated skim milk, plain yogurt

Fresh or dry pasta

Frozen vegetables

Frozen veggie burgers and veggie crumbles

Fruit-based fat replacement for baking

Low-fat tomato sauce or homemade frozen sauce

Presliced mushrooms

Raw baby carrots, salad in a bag, prechopped salad bar toppings

Reduced-salt broth—chicken, beef, or vegetable

Rice—converted, brown, or basmati

Roasted peppers

Salsa

Water-packed tuna

Seasonings/Condiments

Cooking oil spray

Dijon mustard

Dried herbs including basil, oregano, thyme, rosemary, and sage

Garlic cloves, green onions

Ginger (preferably fresh)

Lemon juice or fresh lemons, lime juice

Olive oil, canola oil, sesame oil

Parmesan or Romano cheese—grated or by the piece if you

prefer to grate your own

Parsley (preferably fresh)

Soy or tamari sauce

Spices including chili powder, ground cumin, cinnamon, and nutmeg

Vinegar—wine, cider, balsamic, or fancy varieties

White wine (keep single-serving bottles for cooking)

Equipment

2-quart casserole dish, assorted baking pans

2-, 3-, 4-, and 8-quart saucepans

Crock pot and/or pressure cooker

Kitchen scale, measuring cups and spoons

Microwavable dishes

8- and 12-inch nonstick skillets, nonstick grilling pan

Sharp cooking knives

Refillable spritzer made for spraying cooking oil

Prepare on Your Own Time

No one wants to spend his or her whole life in the kitchen. Decide on a time that's convenient for you to cook, then make the most of it. Prepare extra when you have the chance, then simply reheat when you're busy. Soups, sauces, pastas, casseroles, and rice dishes lend themselves to this technique. Choose a "cooking day" to fix one or two double recipes to eat later in the week. Refrigerate unused food promptly and use within three days, or label and freeze for another time. Remember to consider these frozen meals "prearranged," not "leftovers"! If you are cooking for a family, let everyone eat the same foods that you eat. While other family members may want larger potions, they certainly will benefit from eating healthful meals, too! Don't get caught in the trap of fixing separate foods for yourself and your family, because you will eventually give up your healthier eating habits just to save time. Instead, let others add additional fats, choose different snacks and side servings, or fix their own "junk foods." Once in a while, prepare a higher-calorie treat and let yourself enjoy a small portion along with everyone else.

Know How to Improvise

You can lighten up your favorite dishes by cutting back on certain ingredients and making substitutions in your recipes. For instance, the recipe for a traditional family favorite—macaroni and cheese—has been revised to reduce calories, fat, cholesterol, and sodium. The instructions for "New Style Macaroni and Cheese" are in Chapter 14. By using the substitution list below (and a little ingenuity), the calories for a 1-cup serving of macaroni and cheese are reduced from 580 to 310. Fat is slashed from 34 grams to 9 grams, saturated fat trimmed 21 grams to 5 grams, cholesterol cut from 100 milligrams to 29 milligrams, and sodium reduced from 740 milligrams to 510 milligrams. The end result is a delicious and satisfying meal that will help whittle your waistline.

Recipe Revision

Traditional Macaroni and Cheese	New Style Macaroni and Cheese
8 oz elbow macaroni	8 oz elbow macaroni
½ cup soft breadcrumbs	2 tbsp cornflake crumbs
2 tbsp butter	
¼ cup butter	2 oz low-fat cream cheese
4 tbsp flour	2 tsp cornstarch
2 cups whole milk	2 cups skim milk
8 oz cheddar cheese	5 oz ⅓-less-fat extra-sharp cheddar
½ tsp salt	½ tsp salt
⅛ tsp paprika	¼ tsp paprika
½ tsp dry mustard	½ tsp dry mustard

Traditional Macaroni and Cheese	New Style Macaroni and Cheese
Yield:	Yield:
5 servings, 1 cup each	5 servings, 1 cup each
Calories: 580	Calories: 310
Fat: 34 grams	Fat: 9 grams
Saturated fat: 21 grams	Saturated fat: 5 grams
Cholesterol: 100 milligrams	Cholesterol: 29 milligrams
Sodium: 740 milligrams	Sodium: 510 milligrams

Some of our recipes call for fresh herbs and spices, which taste better than dried seasonings. You can keep most fresh herbs in a jar of water (with their stems in the water like cut flowers) or store them in a plastic bag, and keep either in your refrigerator. If you prefer to use dried seasonings, reduce the seasoning measurements by one-half. You can make other substitutions in your recipes to improve their nutritional content by referring to the following table for guidelines.

Substitutions

If a recipe calls for:	Use or substitute:
Bacon	Canadian bacon, chopped ham, or prosciutto.
Baking chocolate, 1 oz	3 tbsp cocoa powder + 1 tsp canola oil.
Butter, margarine, or shortening	Reduce amount by ⅓ to ½; use canola or olive oil; for baking, substitute applesauce or fruit-based fat replacer.
Buttered crumbs	Cornflake crumbs.
Cheese, regular	Low-fat or fat-free cheese; use a reduced amount of highly flavored cheese such as feta or sharp cheese.
Chocolate chips	Use minichips and cut amount by ⅓ to ½.
Cream cheese	Low-fat or nonfat cream cheese.
Cream	Evaporated skim milk.
Egg, 1	2 egg whites or ¼ cup egg substitute.
Egg noodles	Eggless noodles.
Fudge sauce	Chocolate syrup.
Mayonnaise	Use fat-free mayonnaise or ½ reduced-calorie mayonnaise and ½ fat-free plain yogurt.
Nuts	Reduce amount by ⅓ to ½; toast to enhance flavor.

If a recipe calls for:	Use or substitute:
Ricotta cheese	Part-skim or fat-free ricotta; fat-free cottage cheese.
Roux (butter or margarine and flour base)	Cornstarch or mashed potato granules for thickening.
Salt	Reduce by ⅓ to ½.
Sautéing in butter or oil	Nonstick cooking spray, broth, or wine.
Sour cream	Nonfat sour cream or nonfat plain yogurt; for heated dishes add 1 tbsp flour per cup of yogurt.
Sugar	Reduce amount by ⅓ to ½.
Vegetable oil	Canola oil or olive oil.
Whole or 2% milk	1% or skim milk; evaporated skim milk.

Putting the Six Basic Steps into Practice

Developing healthy cooking and eating habits does not have to be time-consuming or boring. Our meal plans can be a quick-and-easy guide for you, and you have the option of tailoring them to your likes. Use them as a guide for your meals so that you're never caught wondering what to eat when you're hungry, tired, stressed out, or otherwise prone to making poor decisions. Get organized before you cook or shop. Be on the lookout for easy ways to save time without sacrificing nutrition. Try the recipes provided for you here, and scan other low-fat cookbooks or magazines for new ideas. Don't be afraid to tinker with your own favorite dishes to make them healthier. Keep in mind that every new meal, shortcut, or recipe remake may not be an instant success, so be prepared to be flexible when trying new ways of doing things. Most important, make healthy eating a priority in your life. Even with the assistance of diet drugs, permanent healthy habits are essential for healthy living and long-term weight control!

13

The Complete Book of Diet Drugs Three-Week Menu Plan

The three-week menu for weight loss is based on the meal plans given in Chapter 9 and incorporates the recipes from Chapters 14–19. As previously mentioned, men should follow the 1,500-calorie plan and women should follow the 1,200-calorie plan. If a woman is over 5 feet 7 inches tall, then she should choose the 1,500-calorie plan for weight loss. You will notice that each day's menu includes at least two or three of our recipes. If you are unable to prepare these many foods each day, you will want to modify the menus. Each meal lists the calorie and fat content, so you can make substitutions as needed. We suggest that you read the cooking tips in Chapter 12 and take advantage of our time-saving methods for fixing healthful foods.

Table 13.1
Average Daily Nutrient Content of Three-Week Menus

	1,200 Calories	1,500 Calories
Calories	1,215	1,510
Protein, grams	74	82
Carbohydrate, grams	185	240
Fat, grams	23	28
Saturated fat, grams	7	8
Cholesterol, milligrams	125	140
Sodium, milligrams	2,200	2,600
Iron, milligrams	12	15
Calcium, milligrams	1,000	1,100
Fiber, grams	16	20

Our suggested meals are low in fat, saturated fat, cholesterol, and sodium. Although the vitamin and mineral content of the menus is generally adequate, we recommend a multivitamin supplement during weight loss. Menstruating women may wish to choose a multivitamin with iron, since the 1,200-calorie plan provides about two-thirds of the USRDA for iron. The average nutrient content of the menus is listed in Table 13.1.

Beverages are not included in the menus, but are a very important part of your daily intake. You should add at least 8 cups of calorie-free fluids to your dietary intake every day. This includes water, mineral water or seltzer, coffee, tea, diet soda and other diet drinks, unsweetened or artificially sweetened iced tea, herbal teas, and club soda. Limit your caffeine-containing beverages such as coffee, tea, iced teas, and caffeinated sodas to one or two servings per day.

Dairy products should be skim or very low fat. For milk, skim is your best choice. Try a brand that has milk solids added for best flavor. If you really don't like skim milk, settle for 1 percent fat instead. If milk gives you indigestion, gas, or diarrhea, try lactose-reduced milk instead. When it comes to cheese, part-skim cheeses that contain 5–6 grams of fat per ounce are a reasonable choice and provide better flavor and texture than fat-free cheeses.

Choose lean meats and trim all visible fat from your meat. Select grades of meat that are lower in fat than prime cuts. For poultry, choose white meat over dark and remove the skin.

Fresh fruit is most nutritious and flavorful in season. If you use canned fruit, choose one that is packed in juice or light syrup. Frozen fruits that are unsweetened are convenient and can add variety to your meals when the fresh fruit selection is limited. For juices, you can make your own or buy 100 percent unsweetened juice, with orange or grapefruit juice suggested for many of the breakfasts. You can also substitute another unsweetened juice such as apple if you prefer a noncitrus juice. Serve juice over ice or mixed with seltzer if you want a larger portion.

With vegetables, fresh is best but frozen is fine, too. Enjoy your vegetables steamed, microwaved, or boiled in a small amount of water and served plain unless otherwise specified. You may add lemon juice, vinegar, broth, or herbs to your vegetables for flavor, but avoid adding extra fats and sauces excluded from your meal plans. If you're still hungry after eating a meal, try eating more vegetables. There's nothing wrong with increasing your serving sizes of vegetables, since they are low in calories, high in fiber, and packed with nutrients.

For breads, it's best to use those made of whole grains. Look for bread that lists whole-wheat flour as its first ingredient rather than just wheat flour. Try brown rice for a change from white—it takes longer to cook but provides more fiber and a delicious, nutty flavor. Choose cereals that are unsweetened or provide no more than 4 grams (1 teaspoon) of sugar per serving.

As far as fats are concerned, your best bets are olive, canola, safflower, and corn oils; margarines made with liquid forms of these oils as the first ingredient; and reduced-fat dressings made from these oils. Avoid solid shortenings and products listing hydrogenated oils as their first ingredient, as these are higher in saturated fats. Our recipes use primarily olive and canola oils. When choosing a cooking oil spray, look for one that is olive or canola oil-based. Better yet, purchase a refillable oil spritzer from a gourmet shop and fill with your own olive or canola oil. Because our menus are so low in fat, they do allow a small amount of either margarine or butter. If you prefer to use diet margarine, you can generally double the quantity.

Week 1 —1,200 Calories

(Note: an asterisk * indicates that the recipe is included in this book)

Sunday

Breakfast
(230 calories, 2 grams fat)
1 slice Baked Apple French Toast*
1 tbsp reduced-calorie syrup

Lunch
(315 calories, 7 grams fat)
1 cup Orange Chicken Salad*
1 Corn Muffin*

Dinner
(370 calories, 10 grams fat)
3" x 4" piece Vegetable Lasagne*
1 whole wheat dinner roll
Green salad with 2 tbsp
Parmesan Salad Dressing*

Snack
(320 calories, 6 grams fat)
1 serving Favorite Chocolate Chip Cake*
1 cup skim milk

Monday

Breakfast
(270 calories, 3 grams fat)
1 Raisin Bran Muffin*
1 cup lite 90-calorie yogurt
$1/2$ cup orange or grapefruit juice

Lunch
(340 calories, 14 grams fat)
1 cup Black Bean and Corn Salad*
2 part-skim cheese sticks
4 reduced-fat wheat crackers

Dinner
(410 calories, 13 grams fat)
3 oz Herbed Pork Tenderloin*
$1/2$ cup Roasted New Potatoes*
$1/2$ cup steamed spinach
1 cup Cauliflower with Nutmeg*
Green salad with 2 tbsp
reduced-fat dressing

Snack
(190 calories, 1 gram fat)
1 cup skim milk
1 banana

Tuesday

Breakfast
(220 calories, 2 grams fat)
1 slice wheat toast with
1 tsp fruit spread
1 cup skim milk
1 cup cantaloupe or
honeydew melon cubes

Lunch
(360 calories, 10 grams fat)
2 oz lean roast beef on
2 slices wheat bread
with lettuce, tomato, and
1 tbsp low-fat mayonnaise
1 cup vegetable soup

Dinner
(415 calories, 7 grams fat)
1¼ cups Colorful Pasta with
Pesto and White Beans*
Green salad with 2 tbsp
reduced-fat dressing
6 raw baby carrots

Snack
(215 calories, 1 gram fat)
½" slice No-Oil Zucchini Bread*
½ cup grapes
⅔ cup fat-free cottage cheese

Wednesday

Breakfast
(215 calories, 1 gram fat)
½" slice No-Oil Zucchini Bread*
½ grapefruit
1 cup skim milk

Lunch
(345 calories, 8 grams fat)
1 Tangy Tuna Melt*
1 apple

Dinner
(405 calories, 8 grams fat)
3 oz Turkey Cutlet*
½ cup Bow Ties Aglio Olio*
½ cup cooked brussels sprouts
½ cup steamed yellow squash
1 tsp margarine or butter

Snack
(225 calories, 5 grams fat)
3 cups lite popcorn
1 cup skim milk with 1½ tbsp
chocolate syrup

Thursday

Breakfast
(220 calories, 1 gram fat)
½ cup Raisin Bran cereal
1 cup skim milk
½ cup orange or grapefruit juice

Lunch
(350 calories, 7 grams fat)
1½ cups Chicken Vegetable Soup*
2 tbsp hummous
1 small pita bread
½ cup Summer Cucumber and
Tomato Salad*

Dinner
(420 calories, 9 grams fat)
4 oz Veal Parmigiana*
1 serving Polenta Presto*
1 cup steamed green beans
with lemon juice
½ cup Summer Cucumber
and Tomato Salad*

Snack
(225 calories, 4 grams fat)
½ banana
1 cup skim milk
5 vanilla wafers

Friday

Breakfast
(225 calories, 1 gram fat)
½ cinnamon raisin bagel
(or flavor of choice)
1 tsp apple butter
½ cup nonfat cottage cheese
½ cup orange or grapefruit juice

Lunch
(355 calories, 7 grams fat)
1 cup New Style
Macaroni and Cheese*
½ cup Zucchini Rosso*

Dinner
(420 calories, 9 grams fat)
3 oz Flounder Pomodoro*
½ cup cooked noodles
½ cup cooked peas
1 tsp butter or margarine
1 serving Sunshine Salad*

Snack
(220 calories, 1 gram fat)
1 cup skim milk
1 slice angel food cake
½ cup peach slices
(juice or light-syrup pack)

Saturday

Breakfast
(250 calories, 6 grams fat)
1 Mary's Morning Muffin*
1 cup skim milk

Lunch
(330 calories, 6 grams fat)
1 Pita Pizza*
1 orange

Dinner
(460 calories, 11 grams fat)
1 cup Candlelight Crab
  and Shrimp Soup*
1⅔ cup Sweet and Sour Pork
  and Veggies*
½ cup cooked rice

Snack
(170 calories, 0 fat)
1 apple
1 cup lite 90-calorie yogurt

Week 2—1,200 Calorie Meal Plan

Sunday

Breakfast
(235 calories, 6 grams fat)
$^1/_4$ cup cholesterol-free egg
substitute and 1 oz low-fat cheese
cooked in nonstick skillet; served on
  1 slice whole-wheat toast
$^1/_2$ cup orange or grapefruit juice

Lunch
(340 calories, 8 grams fat)
1 Bean Burrito*
$^1/_2$ cup frozen corn kernels, cooked
Green salad with 2 tbsp lite dressing

Dinner
(450 calories, 12 grams fat)
1 serving Balsamic Chicken*
$^1/_2$ cup Rush Hour Risotto*
$^1/_2$ cup Savory Spinach*
1 whole-wheat dinner roll with
  1 tsp butter or margarine

Snack
(200 calories, 3 grams fat)
2" x 2" piece Zucchini Cocoa Cake*
1 cup skim milk

Monday

Breakfast
(270 calories, 3 grams fat)
1 cup Yummie Yogurt*
1 cup cantaloupe or
  honeydew cubes

Lunch
(350 calories, 4 grams fat)
1 serving Nifty Nuggets*
2 tbsp catsup
$^1/_2$ cup roasted New Potatoes*
$^1/_2$ cup steamed zucchini

Dinner
(410 calories, 7 grams fat)
1$^1/_2$ cups cooked macaroni with
$^1/_2$ cup Tomato Cream Sauce*
1 tbsp grated Parmesan cheese
Green salad with 2 tbsp lite dressing

Snack
(190 calories, 1 gram fat)
15 minipretzels
1 cup skim milk
$^1/_2$ cup grapes

Tuesday

Breakfast
(220 calories, 1 gram fat)
1 1/4 cups Puffed Wheat
5 strawberries
1 cup skim milk
1/2 cup orange or grapefruit juice

Lunch
(365 calories, 3 grams fat)
1 cup Vegetarian Split Pea Soup*
2 tbsp Spinach Dip*
4 whole-wheat breadsticks or
8 reduced-fat wheat crackers
1 apple

Dinner
(405 calories, 8 grams fat)
2 cups Stir-Fried Beef*
1/2 cup cooked rice
1 cup sugar-free gelatin

Snack
(220 calories, no fat)
1/2 cup Berries in Zinfandel*
3/4 cup fat-free frozen yogurt

Wednesday

Breakfast
(270 calories, 3 grams fat)
1/2 cup Stick-to-Your-Ribs Oatmeal*
1 cup skim milk
1/2 cup orange or grapefruit juice

Lunch
(330 calories, 7 grams fat)
1 cup cooked macaroni with 1 tbsp
Low-Fat Pesto Sauce*
topped with 1/2 cup rinsed
and drained canned shrimp
and 1 tbsp Parmesan cheese
1/2 cup fruit salad

Dinner
(420 calories, 10 grams fat)
1 cup Commuter Chili*
1/2 cup cooked rice
Green salad with 2 tbsp lite dressing

Snack
(190 calories, no fat)
1 Cranberry Baked Apple*
1 cup lite 90-calorie yogurt

Thursday

Breakfast
(255 calories, 4 grams fat)
$^1/_2$ bagel, toasted
1 tbsp lite cream cheese
$^1/_2$ grapefruit
1 cup skim milk

Lunch
(320 calories, 10 grams fat)
2 oz lean turkey on 2 slices
whole-wheat bread
with 1 tbsp lite mayonnaise,
lettuce, and tomato
2 tbsp Hot Artichoke Dip*
12 raw baby carrots

Dinner
(400 calories, 10 grams fat)
1 serving Spaghetti
with Broccoli Sauce*
1 slice French bread with
1 tsp butter or margarine
Green salad with 2 tbsp lite dressing

Snack
(245 calories, 7 grams fat)
1 pear
1 part-skim mozzarella stick
5 breadsticks or
10 reduced-fat wheat crackers

Friday

Breakfast
(250 calories, 2 grams fat)
1 Deliteful Danish*
1 cup skim milk
$^1/_2$ cup orange or grapefruit juice

Lunch
(295 calories, 3 grams fat)
$1^1/_2$ cups Seafood Pasta*
$^1/_2$ cup Sesame Snow Peas*
1 cup grapes

Dinner
(430 calories, 16 grams fat)
2 slices thin-crust cheese pizza
Green salad with
2 tbsp fat-free dressing or vinegar

Snack
(230 calories, 2 grams fat)
20 baked tortilla chips
2 tbsp Fresh Salsa*
1 Fruit Kabob

Saturday

Breakfast
(260 calories, 4 grams fat)
1 Cranberry Orange Muffin*
1 cup skim milk
$\frac{1}{2}$ cup melon cubes

Lunch
(350 calories, 10 grams fat)
$\frac{1}{4}$ Mushroom Frittata*
$\frac{1}{2}$ cup Savory Spinach
1 toasted English muffin
with 1 tsp butter or margarine

Dinner
(405 calories, 11 grams fat)
4 Oriental Steamed Dumplings*
1 serving Oriental Monkfish*
$\frac{1}{2}$ cup mashed butternut squash
8 steamed asparagus spears
1 tsp butter or margarine

Snack
(210 calories, 1 gram fat)
3" x 3" piece Ice Box Cake*
1 cup skim milk

Week 3—1,200 Calories

Sunday

Breakfast
(255 calories, 3 grams fat)
2 Zucchini Pancakes*
with 1 tbsp lite syrup
1 cup skim milk
$1/2$ cup fruit salad

Lunch
(335 calories, 6 grams fat)
$1^1/2$ cups Tuna Macaroni Toss*
2 celery stalks
2 tbsp Yogurt Mustard Dip*

Dinner
(400 calories, 8 grams fat)
2 Veal Meatballs*
1 cup cooked spaghetti with
$1/2$ cup Basic Marinara Sauce*
1 tbsp Parmesan cheese
Green salad with 2 tbsp
fat-free dressing

Snack
(230 calories, 4 grams fat)
1 Cranberry Orange Muffin*
1 cup skim milk

Monday

Breakfast
(225 calories, 2 grams fat)
1 cup lite 90-calorie yogurt with
$1/4$ cup low-fat granola
$1/2$ cup melon cubes

Lunch
(340 calories, 9 grams fat)
2 Veal Meatballs* on kaiser roll
with $1/4$ cup Basic Marinara Sauce*
$2/3$ cup Broccoli with
Lemon and Pepper*

Dinner
(415 calories, 11 grams fat)
4 stuffed Mushrooms*
3 oz Baked Scallops*
$1/2$ cup Brussels sprouts
1 medium baked potato
1 tsp butter or margarine

Snack
(220 calories, 2 grams fat)
1 cup skim milk
$3/4$ cup Cheerios
$1/2$ banana

Tuesday

Breakfast
(220 calories, 1 gram fat)
$^1/_2$ English muffin, toasted
1 tsp apple butter
1 cup skim milk
$^1/_2$ cup orange or grapefruit juice

Lunch
(375 calories, 7 grams fat)
1 veggie burger on kaiser roll
with 1 tbsp catsup, pickle slices,
and lettuce
$^1/_2$ cup Curried Cauliflower
and Potato Salad*

Dinner
(440 calories, 14 grams fat)
1 Turkey Stuffed Pepper*
$^1/_2$ cup corn niblets
Green salad with 2 tbsp
low-calorie dressing
1 slice whole-wheat bread
1 tsp butter or margarine

Snack
(200 calories, 0 fat)
1 cup fat-free vanilla frozen yogurt
2 tbsp Raspberry Topping*

Wednesday

Breakfast
(225 calories, 1 gram fat)
1 low-fat frozen waffle with
1 tbsp lite syrup
and 1 cup strawberries, sliced
1 cup skim milk

Lunch
(350 calories, 17 grams fat)
2 hard-boiled eggs
$^3/_4$ cup Rice Salad*
$^1/_2$ cup roasted red peppers
with $^1/_2$ tsp olive oil

Dinner
(440 calories, 14 grams fat)
3 oz Honey Dijon Chicken*
$^2/_3$ cup baked beans
$^1/_2$ cup French cut green beans
Green salad with 2 tbsp
Parmesan Salad Dressing*
1 tsp butter or margarine

Snack
(210 calories, 7 grams fat)
12 reduced-fat wheat crackers
1 oz low-fat mozzarella
$^1/_2$ cup apple juice

Thursday

Breakfast
(230 calories, 1 gram fat)
²/₃ cup Cream of Wheat
¹/₂ cup orange or grapefruit juice
1 cup skim milk

Lunch
(330 calories, 7 grams fat)
2 oz lean ham on 2 slices rye bread
with lettuce and mustard
1 cup coleslaw

Dinner
(455 calories, 4 grams fat)
1¹/₂ cups Vegetarian Chili Casserole*
1 Corn Muffin*
Green salad with 2 tbsp
fat-free dressing

Snack
(200 calories, 1 gram fat)
¹/₂" slice Better Banana Bread*
1 cup lite 90-calorie yogurt

Friday

Breakfast
(255 calories, 1 gram fat)
¹/₂" slice Better Banana Bread*
1 cup skim milk
¹/₂ cup fruit salad

Lunch
(300 calories, 12 grams fat)
2 cups Chicken Corn Soup
with Asparagus*
6 multigrain saltines
1 tbsp natural peanut butter

Dinner
(440 calories, 10 grams fat)
1 serving Clams with Linguine*
1 tbsp Parmesan cheese
1 slice garlic bread
Green salad with balsamic vinegar

Snack
(225 calories, 4 grams fat)
5 vanilla wafers
1 cup skim milk
¹/₂ cup unsweetened applesauce

Saturday

Breakfast
(230 calories, 1 gram fat)
12 oz Café Latte*
$^1/_2$ cinnamon raisin English Muffin
1 tsp marmalade or jam
$^1/_2$ cup orange or grapefruit juice

Lunch
(335 calories, 13 grams fat)
1 cup Basic Pasta Salad* with
2 oz part-skim mozzarella cheese
on bed of greens
$^1/_2$ cup diet gelatin

Dinner
(425 calories, 13 grams fat)
3 oz Succulent Broiled Steak*
$^1/_2$ cup Sautéed Mushrooms
$^1/_2$ cup Roasted Garlic
Mashed Potatoes*
$^1/_2$ cup peas
1 tsp butter or margarine
1 serving Sunshine Salad*

Snack
(245 calories, 2 grams fat)
$^1/_2$ cup Bread Pudding*
1 cup skim milk

Week 1—1,500 Calories

Sunday

Breakfast
(290 calories, 2 grams fat)
1 slice Baked Apple French Toast*
1 tbsp reduced-calorie syrup
½ cup orange or grapefruit juice

Lunch
(410 calories, 10 grams fat)
1½ cups Orange Chicken Salad*
1 corn muffin

Dinner
(475 calories, 14 grams fat)
3" x 4" piece Vegetable Lasagne*
1 whole-wheat dinner roll with
   1 tsp butter or margarine
   green salad with 2 tbsp
Parmesan Salad Dressing*
   1 cup fruit salad

Snack
(320 calories, 6 grams fat)
1 serving Favorite
Chocolate Chip Cake*
1 cup skim milk

Monday

Breakfast
(340 calories, 5 grams fat)
1 Raisin Bran Muffin*
¾ cup low-fat vanilla yogurt
½ cup orange or grapefruit juice

Lunch
(420 calories, 15 grams fat)
1½ cups Black Bean and Corn Salad*
2 part-skim cheese sticks
5 reduced-fat wheat crackers

Dinner
(470 calories, 13 grams fat)
3 oz Herbed Pork Tenderloin*
½ cup Roasted New Potatoes*
½ cup steamed spinach
1 cup Cauliflower with Nutmeg*
   green salad with 2 tbsp
   reduced-fat dressing
   1 popsicle

Snack
(310 calories, 4 grams fat)
1 cup skim milk
1 banana
4 square graham crackers

Tuesday

Breakfast
(300 calories, 3 grams fat)
2 slices wheat toast with
1 tbsp fruit spread
1 cup skim milk
1 cup cantaloupe or
honeydew melon cubes

Lunch
(390 calories, 11 grams fat)
3 oz lean roast beef on
2 slices wheat bread
with lettuce, tomato, and
1 tbsp low-fat mayonnaise
1 cup vegetable soup

Dinner
(500 calories, 8 grams fat)
1 $\frac{1}{2}$ cups Colorful Pasta
with Pesto and White Beans*
green salad with 2 tbsp
reduced-fat dressing
10 raw baby carrots
2 plums

Snack
(305 calories, 1 gram fat)
1" slice No-Oil Zucchini Bread*
$\frac{1}{2}$ cup grapes
$\frac{2}{3}$ cup fat-free cottage cheese

Wednesday

Breakfast
(310 calories, 1 gram fat)
1" slice No-Oil Zucchini Bread*
$\frac{1}{2}$ grapefruit
1 cup skim milk

Lunch
(430 calories, 9 grams fat)
1 Tangy Tuna Melt* with
extra slice rye toast on top
1 apple

Dinner
(485 calories, 8 grams fat)
3 oz Turkey Cutlet*
$\frac{1}{2}$ cup Bow Ties Aglio Olio*
$\frac{1}{2}$ cup cooked Brussels sprouts
$\frac{1}{2}$ cup steamed yellow squash
1 tsp margarine or butter
$\frac{1}{2}$ cup apricots in light syrup

Snack
(300 calories, 5 grams fat)
5 cups lite popcorn
1 cup skim milk with
2 tbsp chocolate syrup

Thursday

Breakfast
(300 calories, 1 gram fat)
1 cup Raisin Bran cereal
1 cup skim milk
½ cup orange or grapefruit juice

Lunch
(415 calories, 10 grams fat)
1½ cups Chicken Vegetable Soup*
4 tbsp Hummus*
1 small pita bread
½ cup Summer Cucumber
and Tomato Salad*

Dinner
(470 calories, 9 grams fat)
4 oz Veal Parmigiana*
1 serving Polenta Presto*
1 cup steamed green beans
with lemon juice
½ cup Summer Cucumber and
Tomato Salad*
½ cup applesauce

Snack
(330 calories, 6 grams fat)
1 banana
1 cup skim milk
8 vanilla wafers

Friday

Breakfast
(345 calories, 1 gram fat)
1 cinnamon raisin bagel
(or flavor of choice)
2 tsp apple butter
½ cup nonfat cottage cheese
½ cup orange or grapefruit juice

Lunch
(395 calories, 11 grams fat)
1 cup New Style Macaroni
and Cheese*
½ cup Zucchini Rosso*
6 olives

Dinner
(475 calories, 10 grams fat)
3 oz Flounder Pomodoro*
¾ cup cooked noodles
½ cup cooked peas
1 tsp butter or margarine
1 serving Sunshine Salad*

Snack
(310 calories, 1 gram fat)
1 cup skim milk
1 slice angel food cake
1 cup peach slices
(juice or light syrup pack)
2 tbsp Raspberry Topping*

Saturday

Breakfast
(310 calories, 6 grams fat)
1 Mary's Morning Muffin*
1 cup skim milk
$^{1}/_{2}$ cup unsweetened juice

Lunch
(395 calories, 9 grams fat)
1 Pita Pizza*
1 orange
green salad with 2 tbsp
reduced-fat dressing

Dinner
(485 calories, 11 grams fat)
1 cup Candlelight Crab and
  Shrimp Soup*
$1^{2}/_{3}$ cups Sweet and Sour Pork
  and Veggies*
$^{1}/_{2}$ cup cooked rice
1 fortune cookie

Snack
(330 calories, 4 fat)
1 apple
1 cup lite 90-calorie yogurt
5 square graham crackers

Week 2—1,500 Calorie Meal Plan

Sunday

Breakfast
(305 calories, 8 grams fat)
^{1}/4 cup cholesterol-free egg
   substitute and 1 oz. low-
      fat cheese
cooked in nonstick skillet;
served on 2 slices whole-wheat toast
^{1}/2 cup orange or grapefruit juice

Lunch
(405 calories, 8 grams fat)
1 Bean Burrito*

1 cup frozen corn kernels, cooked
Green salad with 2 tbsp lite dressing

Dinner
(500 calories, 12 grams fat)
1 serving Balsamic Chicken*
^{1}/2 cup Rush Hour Risotto*
^{1}/2 cup Savory Spinach*
1 whole-wheat dinner roll with
   1 tsp butter or margarine
1 cup unsweetened raspberries

Snack
(280 calories, 3 grams fat)
2" x 2" piece Zucchini Cocoa Cake*
   ^{3}/4 cup fat-free frozen yogurt

Monday

Breakfast
(345 calories, 4 grams fat)
1 cup Yummie Yogurt*
1 slice raisin toast, plain or with
   1 tsp fruit spread
1 cup cantaloupe or
   honeydew cubes

Lunch
(400 calories, 8 grams fat)
1 serving Nifty Nuggets*
2 tbsp catsup
^{1}/2 cup Roasted New Potatoes*
1 cup steamed zucchini with
   1 tsp margarine or butter

Dinner
(490 calories, 8 grams fat)
1^1/2 cups cooked macaroni
   with ^{1}/3 cup Tomato Cream Sauce*
1 tbsp grated Parmesan cheese
Green salad with 2 tbsp lite dressing
   1 cup blueberries

Snack
(275 calories, 5 grams fat)
30 minipretzels
1 cup skim milk
^{2}/3 cup grapes

Tuesday

Breakfast
(300 calories, 2 gram fat)
1¼ cups puffed wheat
5 strawberries
1 cup skim milk
½ cup orange or grapefruit juice
1 slice whole-wheat toast with
2 tsp fruit spread

Lunch
(410 calories, 4 grams fat)
1 cup Vegetarian Split Pea Soup*
4 tbsp Spinach Dip*
6 whole-wheat breadsticks or
12 reduced-fat wheat crackers
1 apple

Dinner
(495 calories, 8 grams fat)
2 cups Stir-Fried Beef*
¾ cup cooked rice
1 cup sugar-free gelatin
with fruit added

Snack
(305 calories, no fat)
½ cup Berries in Zinfandel*
1 cup fat-free frozen yogurt

Wednesday

Breakfast
(330 calories, 5 grams fat)
¾ cup Stick-to-Your-Ribs Oatmeal*
1 cup skim milk
½ cup orange or grapefruit juice

Lunch
(395 calories, 10 grams fat)
1¼ cups cooked macaroni with
2 tbsp Low-Fat Pesto Sauce*
topped with ½ cup rinsed
and drained canned shrimp
and 1 tbsp Parmesan cheese
6 baby carrots

Dinner
(495 calories, 10 grams fat)
1 cup Commuter Chili*
½ cup cooked rice
green salad with 2 tbsp lite dressing
1 cup fruit salad

Snack
(305 calories, 3 grams fat)
1 Cranberry Baked Apple*
1 cup lite 90-calorie yogurt
4 square graham crackers

Thursday

Breakfast
(350 calories, 4 grams fat)
1 bagel, toasted
1 tbsp lite cream cheese
$\frac{1}{2}$ grapefruit
1 cup skim milk

Lunch
(370 calories, 11 grams fat)
3 oz lean turkey on 2 slices
whole-wheat bread
with 1 tbsp lite mayonnaise,
lettuce, and tomato
4 tbsp Hot Artichoke Dip*
12 raw baby carrots

Dinner
(485 calories, 10 grams fat)
1 serving Spaghetti with
Broccoli Sauce*
1 slice French bread with
1 tsp butter or margarine
green salad with 2 tbsp lite dressing
1 apple

Snack
(280 calories, 8 grams fat)
1 pear

1 part-skim mozzarella stick
8 breadsticks or 15
reduced-fat wheat crackers

Friday

Breakfast
(355 calories, 3 grams fat)
2 Deliteful Danish*
$\frac{3}{4}$ cup skim milk
$\frac{1}{2}$ cup orange or grapefruit juice

Lunch
(380 calories, 4 grams fat)
2 cups Seafood Pasta*
$\frac{1}{2}$ cup Sesame Snow Peas*
1 cup grapes

Dinner
(635 calories, 24 grams fat)
3 slices thin crust cheese pizza
green salad with 2 tbsp fat-free
dressing or vinegar

Snack
(190 calories, 1 grams fat)
15 baked tortilla chips
2 tbsp Fresh Salsa*
1 Fruit Kabob*

Saturday

Breakfast
(290 calories, 4 grams fat)
1 Cranberry Orange Muffin*
1 cup skim milk
1 cup melon cubes

Lunch
(395 calories, 11 grams fat)
$\frac{1}{3}$ Mushroom Frittata*
$\frac{1}{2}$ cup Savory Spinach*
1 toasted English muffin with
1 tsp butter or margarine

Dinner
(475 calories, 11 grams fat)
4 Oriental Steamed Dumplings*
1 serving Oriental Monkfish*
$\frac{3}{4}$ cup mashed butternut squash
8 steamed asparagus spears
1 tsp butter or margarine
1 Fruit Kabob*

Snack
(295 calories, 2 grams fat)
4" x 4" piece Ice Box Cake*
1 cup skim milk
1 cup strawberries

Week 3—1,500 Calories

Sunday

Breakfast
(305 calories, 4 grams fat)
3 Zucchini Pancakes* with 1 tbsp
lite syrup
1 cup skim milk
½ cup fruit salad

Lunch
(400 calories, 7 grams fat)
1¾ cups Tuna Macaroni Toss*

3 celery stalks
3 tbsp Yogurt Mustard Dip*

Dinner
(470 calories, 10 grams fat)
3 Veal Meatballs*
1 cup cooked spaghetti with
½ cup Basic Marinara Sauce*
1 tbsp Parmesan cheese
½ cup steamed yellow squash
Green salad with 2 tbsp
fat-free dressing

Snack
(310 calories, 4 grams fat)
1 Cranberry Orange Muffin*
1 cup skim milk
¾ cup unsweetened applesauce

Monday

Breakfast
(330 calories, 3 grams fat)
1 cup lite 90-calorie yogurt with
½ cup low-fat granola
½ cup melon cubes

Lunch
(395 calories, 11 grams fat)
3 Veal Meatballs* on kaiser roll
with ¼ cup Basic Marinara Sauce*
⅔ cup Broccoli with Lemon
and Pepper*

Dinner
(490 calories, 11 grams fat)
4 Stuffed Mushrooms*
3 oz Baked Scallops*
½ cup brussels sprouts
1 medium baked potato with
1 tsp butter or margarine
½ cup pineapple canned in juice

Snack
(300 calories, 3 grams fat)
1 cup skim milk
1 cup Cheerios
1 banana

Tuesday

Breakfast
(300 calories, 2 grams fat)
1 English muffin, toasted
2 tsp apple butter
1 cup skim milk
1/2 cup orange or grapefruit juice

Lunch
(390 calories, 7 grams fat)
1 veggie burger on kaiser roll
with 2 tbsp catsup, pickle
slices, and lettuce
1/2 cup Curried Cauliflower
and Potato Salad*

Dinner
(500 calories, 14 grams fat)
1 Turkey Stuffed Pepper*
1/2 cup corn niblets
Green salad with 2 tbsp
low-calorie dressing
1 slice whole-wheat bread
with 1 tsp butter or margarine
1 orange

Snack
(305 calories, 4 grams fat)
1 cup fat-free vanilla frozen yogurt
2 tbsp Raspberry Topping*
6 vanilla wafers

Wednesday

Breakfast
(320 calories, 1 gram fat)
2 low-fat frozen waffles
with 2 tbsp lite syrup
and 1 cup strawberries, sliced
1 cup skim milk

Lunch
(405 calories, 19 grams fat)
2 hard-boiled eggs
1 cup Rice Salad*
1/2 cup roasted red peppers
with 1/2 tsp olive oil

Dinner
(480 calories, 14 grams fat)
3 oz Honey Dijon Chicken*
2/3 cup baked beans
1/2 cup French-cut green beans
Green salad with 2 tbsp Parmesan
Salad Dressing*
1 tsp butter or margarine
1 fresh peach

Snack
(300 calories, 12 grams fat)
15 reduced-fat wheat crackers
2 oz low-fat mozzarella
1/2 cup apple juice

Thursday

Breakfast
(275 calories, 1 gram fat)
1 cup cream of wheat
½ cup orange or grapefruit juice
1 cup skim milk

Lunch
(420 calories, 13 grams fat)
2 oz lean ham and 1 oz low-fat
cheese on 2 slices rye bread
with lettuce and mustard
1 cup coleslaw

Dinner
(500 calories, 4 grams fat)
1½ cups Vegetarian Chili Casserole*
1 Corn Muffin*
Green salad with 2 tbsp
fat-free dressing
½ cup unsweetened applesauce

Snack
(305 calories, 2 grams fat)
1" slice Better Banana Bread*
1 cup lite 90-calorie yogurt

Friday

Breakfast
(340 calories, 2 grams fat)
1" slice Better Banana Bread*
1 cup skim milk
½ cup fruit salad

Lunch
(405 calories, 20 grams fat)
2 cups Chicken Corn Soup
with Asparagus*
8 multigrain saltines
2 tbsp natural peanut butter

Dinner
(470 calories, 10 grams fat)
1 serving Clams with Linguine*
1 tbsp Parmesan cheese
1 slice garlic bread
Green salad with balsamic vinegar
½ cup grapes

Snack
(315 calories, 7 grams fat)
10 vanilla wafers
1 cup skim milk
½ cup unsweetened applesauce

Saturday

Breakfast
(315 calories, 2 grams fat)
12 oz Café Latte*
1 cinnamon raisin English muffin
2 tsp marmalade or jam
$\frac{1}{2}$ cup orange or grapefruit juice

Lunch
(405 calories, 13 grams fat)
1 cup Basic Pasta Salad* with
2 oz part-skim mozzarella cheese
on a bed of greens
1 popsicle

Dinner
(470 calories, 13 grams fat)
3 oz Succulent Broiled Steak*
$\frac{1}{2}$ cup Sautéed Mushrooms*
$\frac{1}{2}$ cup Roasted Garlic Mashed
Potatoes*
$\frac{1}{2}$ cup peas
1 tsp butter or margarine
1 serving Sunshine Salad*
$\frac{1}{2}$ cup blueberries

Snack
(340 calories, 3 grams fat)
$\frac{1}{2}$ cup Bread Pudding*
1 cup skim milk

14

Main Dishes

POULTRY

Balsamic Chicken

1 tbsp flour	1 tsp olive oil
⅛ tsp salt	2 green onions
⅛ tsp pepper	4 oz presliced mushrooms
1 tsp dried rosemary leaves	1 tbsp water
1 tsp dried thyme leaves	⅓ cup balsamic vinegar
1 lb boneless skinless chicken breast	½ tsp sugar

Preheat oven to 375 degrees.

Combine flour, salt, pepper, and herbs on a flat plate. Rinse chicken and pat dry; cut into 4 pieces and trim off any excess fat. Lightly dredge chicken in the flour mixture.

Heat the olive oil in an 8- to 10-in nonstick skillet. Add chicken and brown on both sides.

Transfer the chicken to a baking dish suitable for serving and place chicken in preheated oven, covered, for about 20 minutes, or until chicken is no longer pink inside. Set skillet aside for the next step, reserving any remaining juices.

While the chicken is baking, chop the tops and bulbs of the green onions into ¼-in pieces. Wash mushrooms. Place mushrooms and onion into the skillet with 1 tablespoon of water and cook until mushrooms are wilted. Add vinegar and sugar; simmer until liquid is reduced by ½ the volume.

Spoon sauce into serving dish over chicken pieces and serve.

Makes 4 servings.

Nutrition Facts

Serving Size 1 Serving
Servings Per Recipe 4

Amount Per Serving

Calories 160	Calories from Fat 40

	% Daily Value*
Total Fat 4g	6 %
Saturated Fat 1g	5 %
Cholesterol 70mg	23 %
Sodium 135mg	6 %
Total Carbohydrate 4g	1 %
Dietary Fiber 1g	4 %
Sugars 1g	
Protein 26g	

Vitamin A 0%	•	Vitamin C 2%
Calcium 2%	•	Iron 10%

*Percent Daily Values are based on a 2,000 calorie diet.

Honey Dijon Chicken

¼ cup strong brewed tea
1 tbsp honey
1 tbsp lime juice
1 tbsp cider vinegar
1 tsp canola oil

1 tbsp Dijon mustard
1 tsp dried tarragon
½ tsp dried thyme
1 lb boneless skinless chicken breast

Combine all ingredients except chicken. Warm the mixture in a small microwaveable bowl or saucepan to dissolve the honey and blend well.

Cut any excess fat from chicken. If chicken pieces are large, cut in half.

Marinate chicken in honey Dijon mixture for several hours or overnight in a nonmetallic container.

Nutrition Facts

Serving Size 1 Serving
Servings Per Recipe 4

Amount Per Serving

Calories 150	Calories from Fat 60

	% Daily Value*
Total Fat 6g	9 %
Saturated Fat 1.5g	8 %
Cholesterol 50mg	17 %
Sodium 65mg	3 %
Total Carbohydrate 5g	2 %
Dietary Fiber 0g	0 %
Sugars 4g	
Protein 19g	

Vitamin A 2%	•	Vitamin C 0%
Calcium 0%	•	Iron 6%

*Percent Daily Values are based on a 2,000 calorie diet.

Broil until chicken is no longer pink inside and juices run clear, turning pieces during broiling and basting with extra marinade.

Makes 4 servings.

You can also prepare this marinade without the chicken and serve chilled as a salad dressing.

Nifty Nuggets

olive oil cooking spray
1 tbsp water
¾ cup plain breadcrumbs
⅛ tsp salt

¼ tsp paprika
3 tbsp nonfat plain yogurt
1 lb boneless skinless chicken
tenders

These chicken nuggets are healthier than any frozen product you can find and are sure to please both kids and adults! Make a double recipe ahead of time and store in the freezer for a quick meal.

Preheat oven to 425 degrees. Spray a large baking sheet with olive oil; set aside.

Combine breadcrumbs, salt, and paprika in a shallow bowl. Set aside.

Mix yogurt and water together. Cut chicken into bite-size pieces (1 lb will give you 40 to 48 pieces) and drop into yogurt mixture. After all of the chicken pieces are coated with the yogurt mixture, drop a few pieces at a time into the breadcrumbs and roll until the pieces are lightly coated.

Nutrition Facts		
Serving Size 10 - 12 pieces Servings Per Recipe 4		
Amount Per Serving		
Calories 200	Calories from Fat 35	
		% Daily Value*
Total Fat 4g		6 %
Saturated Fat 1g		5 %
Cholesterol 70mg		23 %
Sodium 290mg		12 %
Total Carbohydrate 14g		5 %
Dietary Fiber 1g		4 %
Sugars 1g		
Protein 28g		
Vitamin A 0%	•	Vitamin C 0%
Calcium 8%	•	Iron 10%
*Percent Daily Values are based on a 2,000 calorie diet.		

Place breaded chicken on baking sheet and then spray the tops lightly with olive oil spray.

Bake at 425 degrees for about 5 minutes; turn pieces and spray again lightly with olive oil. Bake another 5 minutes, until chicken is no longer pink inside.

Makes 4 servings (10–12 pieces per serving). Serve with a dab of catsup.

If desired, freeze nuggets on their baking sheet and then store in a plastic container for future use. The frozen nuggets can be microwaved until warmed through.

Turkey Cutlets

olive oil cooking spray
⅔ cup Italian seasoned breadcrumbs
1 tsp dried rosemary leaves
¼ tsp dried crushed sage

¼ cup nonfat milk
1 lb turkey breast cutlets
4 lemon wedges

This is an easy way to prepare turkey or veal cutlets without frying them.

Spray a roasting pan with olive oil cooking spray. Preheat oven to 375 degrees.

Combine the breadcrumbs with the rosemary and sage. Pour milk and breadcrumbs into two separate shallow bowls for dipping meat. Dip each cutlet into milk, then lightly coat on both sides with breadcrumbs. Arrange in roasting pan; cover with foil and bake for 10 minutes. Increase oven temperature to 425 degrees, remove cover, and bake for an additional 10–15 minutes, until lightly browned on top but still moist.

Nutrition Facts

Serving Size 1 Serving
Servings Per Recipe 4

Amount Per Serving	
Calories 190	Calories from Fat 10

	% Daily Value*
Total Fat 1g	2 %
Saturated Fat 0g	0 %
Cholesterol 70mg	23 %
Sodium 580mg	24 %
Total Carbohydrate 15g	5 %
Dietary Fiber 0g	0 %
Sugars 1g	
Protein 29g	

Vitamin A 0%	•	Vitamin C 0%
Calcium 6%	•	Iron 10%

*Percent Daily Values are based on a 2,000 calorie diet.

Serve with lemon wedges and a fresh parsley garnish.

Makes 4 servings.

Commuter Chili

1 lb lean ground turkey
2 15-oz cans kidney beans
16 oz bag frozen chopped
   peppers and onions (4 cups)
28 oz can diced tomatoes in juice
6 oz tomato paste
2 cloves garlic, crushed

1 tbsp ground cumin
3 tbsp chili powder
¼ tsp cayenne pepper, optional
¼ tsp ground coriander
1 tsp oregano
½ tsp salt

This chili is so simple that you can put it together after work and take a few minutes to relax while it's cooking! If time permits, brown the meat the night before.

Brown the ground turkey in a nonstick skillet over medium-high heat. Pat with paper towels to remove any excess fat. Drain kidney beans and rinse. In a 6-quart saucepan, combine all ingredients and heat on high until simmering.

Nutrition Facts
Serving Size 1 Cup
Servings Per Recipe 8

Amount Per Serving	
Calories 260	Calories from Fat 70

	% Daily Value*
Total Fat 7g	11%
Saturated Fat 2g	10%
Cholesterol 45mg	15%
Sodium 820mg	34%
Total Carbohydrate 29g	10%
Dietary Fiber 10g	40%
Sugars 6g	
Protein 18g	

Vitamin A 25%	•	Vitamin C 45%	
Calcium 10%	•	Iron 30%	

*Percent Daily Values are based on a 2,000 calorie diet.

Reduce heat and simmer on medium-low for 30–45 minutes, stirring occasionally, until flavors are well blended.

Makes 8 cups.

Serve over rice with a sprinkling of low-fat cheddar and a side salad.

Turkey Stuffed Peppers

2 tbsp chopped onion
2 carrots, finely chopped
2 stalks celery, finely chopped
4 bell peppers
¾ lb lean ground turkey
1 garlic clove, crushed
1 tsp dried basil

8 oz tomato sauce
¼ cup white wine
⅓ cup water
½ cup uncooked rice
¼ tsp salt
freshly ground pepper
4 tsp grated Parmesan cheese

Preheat oven to 375 degrees.

Chop vegetables in a food processor or prepare them ahead of time.

Wash peppers and cut off tops. Remove seeds. Steam peppers for approximately 5 minutes in a steamer or microwave, until tender.

Place peppers in a baking dish and set aside.

In a skillet, brown turkey and drain off any excess fat. Add remaining ingredients except cheese and simmer, covered, for approximately 20 minutes or until rice is cooked. Add extra water if necessary to keep mixture moist.

Fill each pepper with turkey and rice mixture. Top each with 1 teaspoon of cheese. Bake until lightly brown on top.

Nutrition Facts

Serving Size 1 Pepper
Servings Per Recipe 4

Amount Per Serving	
Calories 210	Calories from Fat 60

	% Daily Value*
Total Fat 7g	11 %
Saturated Fat 2g	10 %
Cholesterol 55mg	18 %
Sodium 340mg	14 %
Total Carbohydrate 22g	7 %
Dietary Fiber 4g	16 %
Sugars 7g	
Protein 14g	

Vitamin A 110%	•	Vitamin C 230%
Calcium 8%	•	Iron 15%

*Percent Daily Values are based on a 2,000 calorie diet.

Orange Chicken Salad

1 lb boneless skinless chicken breast
1 head broccoli
8 oz can sliced water chestnuts
11 oz can mandarin oranges in water
½ cup chopped purple onion
1 red bell pepper, chopped
¼ cup chopped fresh parsley

¼ cup chopped fresh parsley
¼ cup broth saved from cooking chicken
2 tsp sesame oil
2 tbsp soy sauce
1 tbsp cider vinegar
½ tsp freshly grated ginger root

Cover chicken with cold water in a sauce pan and simmer until no longer pink inside. Reserve broth. Cool chicken and chop into ¾-in chunks.

Chop broccoli into small florets. Steam just until barely tender and bright green. Plunge into ice water to chill and stop cooking.

Drain water chestnuts and mandarin oranges; set aside.

Chop the purple onion, red pepper, and parsley. Combine cooled chicken chunks with broccoli, onion, pepper, parsley, and water chestnuts. Gently mix in mandarin oranges.

To prepare dressing, combine ¼ cup reserved chicken broth, sesame oil, soy sauce, vinegar, and grated ginger. Chill. Toss dressing with salad just before serving.

Makes 5 1-cup servings.

Nutrition Facts

Serving Size 1 Cup
Servings Per Recipe 5

Amount Per Serving	
Calories 200	Calories from Fat 45

	% Daily Value*
Total Fat 5g	8 %
Saturated Fat 1g	5 %
Cholesterol 55mg	18 %
Sodium 490mg	20 %
Total Carbohydrate 14g	5 %
Dietary Fiber 4g	16 %
Sugars 3g	
Protein 24g	

Vitamin A 15%	•	Vitamin C 180%
Calcium 6%	•	Iron 10%

*Percent Daily Values are based on a 2,000 calorie diet.

FISH AND SEAFOOD

Flounder Pomodoro

1 lb flounder fillets
14½ oz can stewed tomatoes

1 tsp dried oregano
1 tsp dried basil

This is an extremely quick way to prepare fresh fish! You can substitute any type of white fish fillet that you have available.

Place flounder in a microwavable dish. Cover with the stewed tomatoes; sprinkle with oregano and basil.

Cover dish with wax paper and microwave on high for 6–8 minutes, or until fish flakes easily.

Makes 4 servings.

Nutrition Facts	
Serving Size 1 Serving	
Servings Per Recipe 4	

Amount Per Serving	
Calories 140	Calories from Fat 15

	% Daily Value*
Total Fat 1.5g	2 %
Saturated Fat 0g	0 %
Cholesterol 60mg	20 %
Sodium 340mg	14 %
Total Carbohydrate 9g	3 %
Dietary Fiber 1g	4 %
Sugars 5g	
Protein 22g	

Vitamin A 10%	•	Vitamin C 15%
Calcium 6%	•	Iron 8%

*Percent Daily Values are based on a 2,000 calorie diet.

Oriental Monkfish

1 tsp freshly grated ginger root
1 garlic clove, crushed
1 tsp sesame oil
2 tsp sugar

1 tbsp soy sauce or tamari
12 oz monkfish
1 green onion, sliced for garnish

This dish is delicious with monkfish, but removing the skin and membrane from the monkfish pieces can be quite time-consuming. If you want a quicker meal, substitute salmon or even chicken tenders, adjusting cooking time as needed.

For this recipe, authentic "thin soy" sauce from a Chinese grocery store or a good-quality tamari sauce will produce better results than ordinary grocery store soy sauce, if you have these items available.

In a small bowl, combine the grated ginger, crushed garlic, and sesame oil. Stir in sugar and soy sauce.

Remove skin and membrane from monkfish. Rinse and place in a shallow baking dish. Brush lightly with ginger and soy sauce mixture, reserving any extra sauce for basting.

Broil on high for 12–15 minutes until monkfish flesh is white, basting with extra sauce halfway through.

Serve garnished with sliced green onions (green and white parts).

Makes 2 servings.

Nutrition Facts
Serving Size 1 Serving
Servings Per Recipe 2

Amount Per Serving

Calories 170	Calories from Fat 45

	% Daily Value*
Total Fat 5g	8 %
Saturated Fat 1g	5 %
Cholesterol 45mg	16 %
Sodium 550mg	23 %
Total Carbohydrate 6g	2 %
Dietary Fiber 0g	0 %
Sugars 4g	
Protein 25g	

Vitamin A 2%	•	Vitamin C 4%
Calcium 2%	•	Iron 4%

*Percent Daily Values are based on a 2,000 calorie diet.

Baked Scallops

1¼ lb sea scallops
2 tsp lemon juice
2 tbsp reduced-calorie mayonnaise
¼ cup plain breadcrumbs

⅛ tsp paprika
1 tbsp fresh chopped or 1 tsp dried parsley

Preheat oven to 450 degrees.

Rinse the scallops and pat dry. Mix scallops, lemon juice, and mayonnaise together. Spread scallops in a single layer in a glass pie plate or 2-quart casserole. Spread breadcrumbs evenly over scallops. Sprinkle with paprika and parsley.

Bake, uncovered, for 10–12 minutes or until the scallops turn opaque. Serve with lemon wedges.

Makes 4 servings.

Nutrition Facts
Serving Size 1 Serving
Servings Per Recipe 4

Amount Per Serving

Calories 160	Calories from Fat 20

	% Daily Value*
Total Fat 2g	3 %
Saturated Fat 0g	0 %
Cholesterol 45mg	16 %
Sodium 310mg	13 %
Total Carbohydrate 9g	3 %
Dietary Fiber 0g	0 %
Sugars 0g	
Protein 25g	

Vitamin A 4%	•	Vitamin C 8%
Calcium 6%	•	Iron 6%

*Percent Daily Values are based on a 2,000 calorie diet.

Clams with Linguine

2 6.5-oz cans chopped clams
1 tbsp olive oil
2 medium cloves garlic, crushed
½ cup bottled clam juice
¼ cup white wine
1 tbsp lemon juice

1 tsp dried oregano
¼ tsp black pepper
2 tbsp chopped fresh parsley
8 oz dry linguine
grated Parmesan cheese (optional)

Drain the canned clams and add the liquid from the cans to the bottled clam juice. Set the drained clams aside.

In a medium saucepan, heat the oil and add crushed garlic. Stir until garlic begins to turn light brown. Remove from heat.

Add the clam juices, white wine, lemon juice, oregano and pepper to the pan with the garlic. Bring to a boil; reduce heat, and simmer, uncovered, for 5–7 minutes.

Nutrition Facts
Serving Size 1 Serving
Servings Per Recipe 4

Amount Per Serving	
Calories 270	Calories from Fat 40

	% Daily Value*
Total Fat 4.5g	7 %
Saturated Fat 0.5g	3 %
Cholesterol 0mg	0 %
Sodium 680mg	28 %
Total Carbohydrate 43g	14 %
Dietary Fiber 3g	12 %
Sugars 2g	
Protein 14g	

Vitamin A 0%	•	Vitamin C 6%
Calcium 2%	•	Iron 20%

*Percent Daily Values are based on a 2,000 calorie diet.

Meanwhile, bring pasta water to a boil and cook linguine according to package directions.

While linguine is cooking, add clams and fresh parsley to the clam juice mixture. Cook on low heat for an additional 5 minutes, but do not allow to boil, as this will make the clams tough.

Drain the linguine and transfer to a serving platter. Spoon clams and sauce evenly over the top.

Serve with a touch of grated Parmesan if desired.

Makes 4 servings, about 1 cup of linguine and ½ cup of sauce each.

Alaskan Seafood Salad

½ lb imitation crab meat
½ cup chopped celery
¼ cup chopped red bell pepper
1 tbsp chopped fresh parsley
2 tsp olive oil

2 tbsp red wine vinegar
1 tsp lemon juice
1 tsp Dijon mustard
⅛ tsp white pepper
lemon wedges for garnish

Chop seafood into 1-in chunks. Mix together the seafood, chopped celery, red pepper, and chopped parsley.

In a small bowl, combine olive oil, red wine vinegar, lemon juice, mustard, and pepper. Stir with a fork or a whisk. Pour over the seafood mixture and mix until salad is evenly coated. Serve chilled with fresh lemon wedges.

This recipe uses imitation crabmeat for convenience, but can be prepared with fresh steamed seafood of your choice to significantly reduce the sodium.

Makes 2 1-cup servings.

Nutrition Facts

Serving Size 1 Cup
Servings Per Recipe 2

Amount Per Serving	
Calories 190	Calories from Fat 60

	% Daily Value*
Total Fat 7g	11 %
Saturated Fat 1g	5 %
Cholesterol 40mg	13 %
Sodium 850mg	35 %
Total Carbohydrate 16g	5 %
Dietary Fiber 1g	4 %
Sugars 1g	
Protein 15g	

Vitamin A 10%	•	Vitamin C 100%
Calcium 6%	•	Iron 8%

*Percent Daily Values are based on a 2,000 calorie diet.

Tuna Macaroni Toss

3 cups uncooked elbow macaroni
6 oz jar roasted pepper, drained and cut into ½-in pieces
4 oz feta cheese
6 oz can water-packed white tuna
¼ cup hot water

½ cup frozen peas, thawed
2 tbsp lemon juice
1 tbsp fresh chopped or 1 tsp dried parsley
1 tbsp fresh chopped or 1 tsp dried basil

Cook macaroni according to package directions.

While pasta is cooking, chop roasted pepper into ½-in pieces. Crumble feta cheese. Lightly drain and flake tuna.

Drain macaroni, reserving ¼ cup of cooking liquid to use for the ¼ cup hot water. Return macaroni to pan and combine with all ingredients except cheese. Combine and stir over a low flame to heat through. Toss in crumbled feta cheese and serve.

Makes about 10 cups, or 6 1½-cup servings. Can be served warm or chilled.

Nutrition Facts	
Serving Size 1 1/2 cups	
Servings Per Recipe 6	
Amount Per Serving	
Calories 300	**Calories from Fat** 50
	% Daily Value*
Total Fat 6g	9 %
Saturated Fat 3g	15 %
Cholesterol 30mg	10 %
Sodium 340mg	14 %
Total Carbohydrate 44g	15 %
Dietary Fiber 3g	12 %
Sugars 3g	
Protein 18g	
Vitamin A 6% • Vitamin C 40%	
Calcium 10% • Iron 20%	
*Percent Daily Values are based on a 2,000 calorie diet.	

Tangy Tuna Melts

6 oz can white tuna in water
2 tbsp salsa
2 tsp reduced-fat mayonnaise

2 slices rye bread
¼ cup shredded reduced-fat cheddar cheese

Drain tuna and flake. Mix tuna, salsa, and mayonnaise together.

Toast bread. Top each slice of bread with half of the tuna mixture and 2 tbsp of shredded reduced-fat cheddar.

Broil for approximately 2 minutes or until cheese is slightly browned. If desired, top with additional salsa.

Serves 2.

Nutrition Facts

Serving Size 1 Serving
Servings Per Recipe 2

Amount Per Serving

Calories 260	Calories from Fat 70

	% Daily Value*
Total Fat 8g	12 %
Saturated Fat 3g	15 %
Cholesterol 45mg	15 %
Sodium 730mg	30 %
Total Carbohydrate 17g	6 %
Dietary Fiber 0g	0 %
Sugars 1g	
Protein 29g	

Vitamin A 8%	•	Vitamin C 4%
Calcium 15%	•	Iron 10%

*Percent Daily Values are based on a 2,000 calorie diet.

VEGETARIAN

New Style Macaroni and Cheese

5 oz ⅓-less-fat sharp cheddar cheese
2 oz reduced fat cream cheese
2 cups uncooked elbow macaroni
2 tsp cornstarch
¼ tsp parprika

½ tsp salt
¼ tsp dry mustard
2 cups skim milk
2 tbsp cornflake crumbs

Nutrition Facts

Serving Size 1 Cup
Servings Per Recipe 5

Amount Per Serving

Calories 310	Calories from Fat 80

	% Daily Value*
Total Fat 9g	14 %
Saturated Fat 4.5g	23 %
Cholesterol 30mg	10 %
Sodium 510mg	21 %
Total Carbohydrate 39g	13 %
Dietary Fiber 1g	4 %
Sugars 0g	
Protein 18g	

Vitamin A 10%	•	Vitamin C 0%
Calcium 35%	•	Iron 15%

*Percent Daily Values are based on a 2,000 calorie diet.

Preheat oven to 350 degrees. Shred cheddar cheese and cut cream cheese into small chunks; set aside.

Boil water for macaroni in a 6-quart saucepan. Cook macaroni according to package directions. Drain; rinse briefly with cool water. Pour drained macaroni into a 1½- or 2-quart casserole and set aside.

In a small bowl, mix together cornstarch, paprika, salt, and mustard; add ¼ cup of the milk a little at a time and stir until smooth. Set aside.

Heat the remaining 1¾ cups of the milk until just before it boils. Stir in cornstarch mixture and continue to heat and stir until slightly thickened. Stir in shredded cheese and cream cheese.

Pour the cheese sauce over the cooked macaroni in the casserole dish and stir till combined. Top with cornflake crumbs.

Bake, covered, for 25 minutes. Sauce will thicken during baking.

Makes about 5 cups. Compared to a traditional macaroni and cheese recipe, this dish will save you 270 calories and 25 grams of fat per cup!

Mushroom Frittata

olive or canola cooking oil spray
3 cups presliced mushrooms
3 green onions, sliced
¾ tsp dried basil
16 oz cholesterol-free egg substitute

2 eggs
¼ cup skim milk
⅛ tsp salt
⅛ tsp pepper
½ cup shredded low-fat cheese

Spray a 12-in nonstick skillet with cooking oil spray. Add sliced mushrooms, green onions, and basil; sauté until mushrooms are tender. Beat together egg substitute, eggs, milk, salt, and pepper. Pour into pan with mushrooms, distributing mushrooms evenly through egg mixture.

Cook over medium-high heat, using a spatula to lift the edges of the cooked egg, allowing the

Nutrition Facts

Serving Size 1/4 Frittata
Servings Per Recipe 4

Amount Per Serving	
Calories 140	Calories from Fat 30

	% Daily Value*
Total Fat 3.5g	5 %
Saturated Fat 1.5g	8 %
Cholesterol 110mg	37 %
Sodium 330mg	14 %
Total Carbohydrate 6g	2 %
Dietary Fiber 1g	4 %
Sugars 3g	
Protein 20g	

Vitamin A 15%	•	Vitamin C	4%
Calcium 20%	•	Iron	15%

*Percent Daily Values are based on a 2,000 calorie diet.

uncooked egg to run underneath and cook. Continue to cook until egg is mostly set.

Remove skillet from the heat and loosen the edges of the egg. Lay a large plate over the egg mixture. Hold your hand on the bottom of the plate and carefully invert the frittata onto the plate. Slide the frittata back into the pan, cooked side up. Sprinkle with shredded cheese and cover the pan with a lid. Cook over low heat until the bottom of the frittata is cooked and the cheese is melted.

Serves 4.

Vegetarian Chili Casserole

1 red or green bell pepper
2⅔ cups veggie burger crumbles
15 oz can black beans, drained and rinsed
8 oz can no-salt-added tomato sauce
8 oz water
¾ cup mild salsa
½ cup frozen corn

½ cup elbow macaroni, uncooked
1 tbsp chili powder
1 tsp cumin
1 tbsp lime juice
2 tbsp fresh chopped cilantro (optional)

This is a tasty recipe that requires very little effort to prepare. If you don't have a fresh bell pepper in your refrigerator, you can substitute 1 cup of fresh or frozen zucchini, green beans, or mushrooms. If you cannot find vegetable burger crumbles in your grocer's freezer, you can crumble your favorite brand of veggie burgers.

Chop pepper into ¾-in cubes. Combine all ingredients except lime juice in a large skillet. Bring to a boil, then simmer, covered, for 15–20 minutes until macaroni is tender. Stir several times during cooking.

Nutrition Facts

Serving Size 1 1/2 cups
Servings Per Recipe 4

Amount Per Serving

Calories 280	Calories from Fat 5

	% Daily Value*
Total Fat 1g	2 %
Saturated Fat 0g	0 %
Cholesterol 0mg	0 %
Sodium 680mg	28 %
Total Carbohydrate 46g	15 %
Dietary Fiber 13g	52 %
Sugars 8g	
Protein 23g	

Vitamin A 15%	•	Vitamin C 80%
Calcium 15%	•	Iron 30%

*Percent Daily Values are based on a 2,000 calorie diet.

When chili is cooked, stir in lime juice. Top with fresh chopped cilantro if desired.

Makes 6 cups, or 4 1½-cup servings.

Bean Burritos

½ cup shredded low-fat cheese
1 cup shredded lettuce
16 oz can fat-free refried beans
½ tsp ground cumin
½ tsp lime juice (optional)

½ cup salsa
8 low-fat flour tortillas,
  6-in diameter
½ cup fat-free sour cream

Choose mild, medium, or hot salsa, according to how much heat you like! You can also add chopped green jalapeño peppers or cayenne pepper to individual servings for those with different taste preferences.

Wrap tortilla shells in aluminum foil and place in a 350-degree oven for 5 minutes to warm and soften. Shred cheese (low-fat cheddar or mozzarella) and lettuce; set aside.

Nutrition Facts

Serving Size 1 Burrito
Servings Per Recipe 8

Amount Per Serving	
Calories 180	Calories from Fat 20

	% Daily Value*
Total Fat 2g	3 %
Saturated Fat 0.5g	3 %
Cholesterol 0mg	0 %
Sodium 570mg	24 %
Total Carbohydrate 31g	10 %
Dietary Fiber 2g	8 %
Sugars 2g	
Protein 9g	

Vitamin A 4%	•	Vitamin C 6%
Calcium 15%	•	Iron 15%

*Percent Daily Values are based on a 2,000 calorie diet.

In a small saucepan, combine the refried beans, cumin, lime juice, and salsa. Stir over medium-high heat to warm and soften. If necessary, add a teaspoon or two of water.

To assemble burritos, spread ¼ cup of the bean mixture, 1 tbsp of the shredded cheese, and 2 tbsp of the shredded lettuce in a line down the center of each tortilla shell. Fold both sides of the shell to the center, overlapping edges in the middle.

Place burritos close together in a baking dish and return to the oven to warm through for five to ten minutes. Top each burrito with 1 tbsp fat-free sour cream to serve.

Pita Pizza

1 whole-wheat pita (approx 6-in)
¼ cup Chunky Vegetable Sauce*
¼ cup shredded lite mozzarella

oregano
vegetables for pizza topping

Preheat oven to 400 degrees. Spread sauce over pita bread. Top with shredded cheese and sprinkle with oregano.

Bake for 7 minutes, until cheese bubbles. Serves 1.

If desired, add presliced mushrooms, peppers, or onions prior to baking. These toppings will add minimal calories—use them instead of pepperoni, sausage, or extra cheese.

*See recipe or use low-fat marinara or vegetable sauce from a jar.

Nutrition Facts
Serving Size 1 Pizza
Servings Per Recipe 1

Amount Per Serving	
Calories 250	Calories from Fat 45

	% Daily Value*
Total Fat 5g	8 %
Saturated Fat 0g	0 %
Cholesterol 10mg	3 %
Sodium 480mg	20 %
Total Carbohydrate 37g	12 %
Dietary Fiber 5g	20 %
Sugars 0g	
Protein 15g	

Vitamin A 10%	•	Vitamin C 0%
Calcium 25%	•	Iron 15%

*Percent Daily Values are based on a 2,000 calorie diet.

Vegetable Lasagne

2 qt Chunky Vegetable Sauce (see recipe)
15 oz fat-free ricotta
1 egg white
2 tbsp chopped fresh parsley
⅓ cup grated Parmesan cheese

⅛ tsp freshly ground black pepper
9 no-bake lasagne noodles
6 oz part-skim Swiss cheese, shredded

Prepare Chunky Vegetable Sauce ahead of time according to directions. Preheat oven to 350 degrees. Spray a 9 x 13-inch pan with olive oil cooking oil spray.

Combine ricotta, egg white, parsley, and ¼ cup of parmesan cheese. Season with freshly ground black pepper.

Spread ¼ of the sauce/vegetable mixture over the bottom of your 9 x 13-in pan. Cover with 3 no-bake lasagne noodles (they will expand during baking, so don't worry if they don't touch). Spread ⅓ of the ricotta mixture and ¼ of the Swiss cheese over the noodles. Repeat layers twice (sauce, noodles, ricotta, Swiss). Top with the last ¼ of sauce, ¼ of Swiss cheese, and remaining Parmesan cheese.

Nutrition Facts	
Serving Size 3" x 4" piece	
Servings Per Recipe 9	
Amount Per Serving	
Calories 150	Calories from Fat 20
	% Daily Value*
Total Fat 2.5g	**4 %**
Saturated Fat 1.5g	**8 %**
Cholesterol 15mg	**5 %**
Sodium 400mg	**17 %**
Total Carbohydrate 16g	**5 %**
Dietary Fiber 1g	**4 %**
Sugars 3g	
Protein 16g	
Vitamin A 6% • Vitamin C 0%	
Calcium 45% • Iron 6%	
*Percent Daily Values are based on a 2,000 calorie diet.	

Cover with foil and bake at 350 degrees for 35–40 minutes, or until noodles are tender. Uncover during the last 10 minutes of baking to brown.

Makes 9 servings.

Colorful Pasta with Pesto and White Beans

6 tbsp Low-Fat Pesto Sauce (see recipe)
12 oz uncooked vegetable spirals
6 tbsp water

15 oz can cannellini beans
1 tsp grated Parmesan cheese
black pepper, freshly ground

Prepare pesto sauce ahead of time.

Cook and drain veggie spirals according to package directions. While they are cooking, combine pesto and water; heat in microwave and stir until blended. Rinse and drain beans.

Toss pasta and pesto sauce, then fold in beans and stir to coat pasta and beans well.

Nutrition Facts	
Serving Size 1 Cup	
Servings Per Recipe 7	
Amount Per Serving	
Calories 260	Calories from Fat 25
	% Daily Value*
Total Fat 3g	**5 %**
Saturated Fat 0g	**0 %**
Cholesterol 0mg	**0 %**
Sodium 80mg	**3 %**
Total Carbohydrate 47g	**16 %**
Dietary Fiber 5g	**20 %**
Sugars 1g	
Protein 11g	
Vitamin A 2% • Vitamin C 4%	
Calcium 6% • Iron 20%	
*Percent Daily Values are based on a 2,000 calorie diet.	

Serve hot with a teaspoon of grated Parmesan and freshly ground black pepper. Makes 7 cups.

Spaghetti with Broccoli Sauce

1 clove garlic, crushed
1 tsp olive oil
¼ tsp red pepper flakes
13¾ oz can reduced-salt
  chicken broth
1 tbsp lemon juice
½ tsp sugar
¼ cup white wine
lemon slices

1 tsp dried basil
1 head broccoli, cut into
  florets
2 tbsp chopped fresh parsley
4 cups cooked spaghetti
  (about 12 oz dry)
black pepper, freshly ground

In a 4-quart saucepan, heat garlic in oil; add red pepper flakes and stir until garlic is medium brown. Remove any fat from the can of broth and pour into saucepan with garlic and oil mixture. Add lemon, sugar, wine, and basil.

Simmer sauce, uncovered, for 10 minutes. Add broccoli and parsley and cook for 3–5 more minutes.

While you are preparing the sauce, boil water for spaghetti. Cook spaghetti according to package directions and drain.

Nutrition Facts		
Serving Size 1 Serving		
Servings Per Recipe 4		
Amount Per Serving		
Calories 240	Calories from Fat 20	
		% Daily Value*
Total Fat 2.5g		4%
Saturated Fat 0g		0%
Cholesterol 0mg		0%
Sodium 45mg		2%
Total Carbohydrate 45g		15%
Dietary Fiber 5g		20%
Sugars 4g		
Protein 10g		
Vitamin A 10%	•	Vitamin C 110%
Calcium 6%	•	Iron 15%
*Percent Daily Values are based on a 2,000 calorie diet.		

Serve 1 cup of spaghetti with ½ cup of sauce. Top with freshly ground black pepper and garnish with a lemon slice, if desired.

For a higher-protein dish, add a can of drained water-packed white tuna to the sauce.

BEEF, PORK, AND VEAL

Succulent Broiled Steak

3 tbsp cider vinegar	1½ tsp sugar
2 tbsp orange juice	½ tsp seasoned salt
1½ tsp Worcestershire sauce	1 garlic clove, crushed
1 tsp olive oil	1 lb top round steak for
	London broil

Mix all ingredients except beef in a heavy zipper plastic bag or a nonmetal bowl. Trim any excess fat from the meat and pierce several holes in it to allow marinade to soak in. Add meat to marinade and allow to soak for 2–3 hours or overnight.

Broil or grill the meat to desired doneness. While meat is cooking, pour leftover marinade into a small saucepan and add 2 tbsp of water. Simmer, covered, for 5 minutes.

Slice the meat thinly on the diagonal and spoon cooked marinade and pan juices over the meat before serving.

If desired, top with Sautéed Mushrooms (see recipe).

Makes 4 3-oz servings.

Nutrition Facts

Serving Size 1 Serving
Servings Per Recipe 4

Amount Per Serving

Calories 140	Calories from Fat 45

	% Daily Value*
Total Fat 5g	8 %
Saturated Fat 1.5g	8 %
Cholesterol 55mg	18 %
Sodium 250mg	10 %
Total Carbohydrate 3g	1 %
Dietary Fiber 0g	0 %
Sugars 2g	
Protein 21g	

Vitamin A 0%	•	Vitamin C 10%
Calcium 0%	•	Iron 10%

*Percent Daily Values are based on a 2,000 calorie diet.

Stir-Fried Beef

8 oz top round, partially frozen
2 tbsp dry sherry, divided
2 tbsp low-sodium soy sauce, divided
1 tsp brown sugar
2 tsp sesame oil, divided
1 tsp fresh grated ginger root
1 clove garlic, crushed
1 cup broccoli florets
1 red bell pepper, sliced

1 cup sliced zucchini
1 carrot, sliced thinly on diagonal
1 stalk celery, chopped
1 cup sliced mushrooms
2 tbsp hoisin sauce
3 tbsp water
1 tsp cornstarch
2 green onions, chopped

Slice beef into ⅛-in thick strips on the diagonal. Combine in nonmetal bowl with 1 tbsp sherry, 1 tbsp soy sauce, and brown sugar; marinate for 2 hours or overnight.

Heat 1 tsp sesame oil in a nonstick frying pan. Sauté the ginger and garlic until fragrant. Add the beef strips and stir-fry until cooked through. Remove meat from pan but reserve juices in pan.

Nutrition Facts	
Serving Size 2 Cups	
Servings Per Recipe 2	
Amount Per Serving	
Calories 290	Calories from Fat 70
	% Daily Value*
Total Fat 8g	12 %
Saturated Fat 1.5g	8 %
Cholesterol 50mg	17 %
Sodium 720mg	30 %
Total Carbohydrate 25g	8 %
Dietary Fiber 6g	24 %
Sugars 15g	
Protein 32g	
Vitamin A 110% • Vitamin C 200%	
Calcium 8% • Iron 25%	
*Percent Daily Values are based on a 2,000 calorie diet.	

Have vegetables chopped ahead of time (you can use your own mixture or chopped salad bar veggies, as long as you start with about 4–5 cups of raw sliced veggies).

Add 1 tsp sesame oil and 1 tbsp sherry to pan and heat. Add vegetables and steam/sauté until tender. Add meat back to pan.

Mix the hoisin sauce, water, 1 tbsp soy sauce, and cornstarch together. Stir until cornstarch is well dissolved. Add to meat and vegetables and heat until well coated with thickened sauce.

Garnish with sliced green onions. Serve over rice.

Makes 2 2-cup servings.

Sweet and Sour Pork and Veggies

½ lb pork loin strips for stir fry
2 tbsp soy sauce, divided
3 tbsp red wine vinegar, divided
clove garlic, crushed
1 tsp freshly grated ginger root
4 oz pineapple juice
2 tbsp brown sugar
1½ tsp cornstarch

1 tsp sesame oil
1 red bell pepper, sliced into ½-in chunks
1 green bell pepper, sliced into ½-in chunks
1 cup presliced mushrooms
8 oz can sliced water chestnuts

If you can, try to buy lean pork strips that are already sliced for stir fry. Otherwise, take a piece of pork loin or tenderloin and freeze partially; then slice in small strips ⅛-in thick. This recipe works equally well with chicken breast.

Combine 1 tbsp soy sauce, 1 tbsp vinegar, garlic, and ginger in a small nonmetal bowl. Add pork strips. Marinate in the refrigerator at least 30 minutes or overnight.

Nutrition Facts

Serving Size 1 2/3 cups
Servings Per Recipe 3

Amount Per Serving	
Calories 260	Calories from Fat 80

	% Daily Value*
Total Fat 9g	14 %
Saturated Fat 2.5g	13 %
Cholesterol 35mg	12 %
Sodium 740mg	31 %
Total Carbohydrate 27g	9 %
Dietary Fiber 4g	16 %
Sugars 15g	
Protein 18g	

Vitamin A 4%	•	Vitamin C 80%
Calcium 4%	•	Iron 10%

*Percent Daily Values are based on a 2,000 calorie diet.

Mix pineapple juice, remaining tablespoon of soy sauce and 2 tablespoons of vinegar, brown sugar, and cornstarch. Stir until cornstarch is fully dissolved. Set aside.

Heat sesame oil in a nonstick skillet. Add meat and stir-fry until lightly browned. Add the sliced peppers and mushrooms; stir-fry until vegetables start to get tender.

Stir the pineapple juice and cornstarch mixture. Add drained water chestnuts and cornstarch mixture to skillet. Continue cooking over medium heat until sauce thickens and vegetables are desired tenderness.

Serve over ⅓ cup rice. Makes about 5 cups, or 3 1⅔-cup servings.

This recipe freezes well and also makes good leftovers!

Herbed Pork Tenderloin

16 oz pork tenderloin	**1 tsp dried thyme**
1 tbsp lemon juice	**1 tsp dried sage**
1 tsp dried rosemary leaves	**lemon slices**

Pork tenderloin is quite low in fat and easy to prepare. It usually comes packaged as two pieces that weigh less than 16 oz each, so you may have to use a slightly smaller piece of meat. Once the meat is thinly sliced, however, it will look like plenty on the plate.

Rinse tenderloin and pat dry. "Butterfly" the tenderloin by slicing down the center without separating the halves; spread halves open like a butterfly. Rub with lemon juice and sprinkle with herbs on both sides.

Broil on high for 10 minutes each side or until an internal temperature of 160 degrees. Garnish with 3–4 lemon slices and broil an additional 2 minutes until lemons begin to wilt.

Makes 4 3-oz servings.

Nutrition Facts

Serving Size 1 Serving
Servings Per Recipe 4

Amount Per Serving

Calories 180	Calories from Fat 80

	% Daily Value*
Total Fat 8g	**12 %**
Saturated Fat 3g	**15 %**
Cholesterol 60mg	**20 %**
Sodium 60mg	**3 %**
Total Carbohydrate 2g	**1 %**
Dietary Fiber 0g	**0 %**
Sugars 0g	
Protein 24g	

Vitamin A 0%	•	Vitamin C 20%
Calcium 2%	•	Iron 8%

*Percent Daily Values are based on a 2,000 calorie diet.

Veal Meatballs

1 lb ground veal	¼ tsp salt
1 slice bread, finely crumbled	¼ tsp dried minced garlic
2 egg whites	¼ tsp pepper
½ tsp oregano	2 tbsp chopped fresh or 2 tsp
½ tsp dried sage	dried parsley
¼ tsp nutmeg	2 tbsp fat-free grated Parmesan cheese

These meatballs are tasty for pasta meals or sandwiches. You can make them slightly smaller for parties and serve with a toothpick. Meatballs can be frozen individually after baking for convenience.

Combine all ingredients and mix thoroughly. Use a tablespoon to form meatballs about 1½ in. in diameter; pat meatballs tightly with your hands. One pound of veal will make 12–13 meatballs.

Nutrition Facts

Serving Size 2 Meatballs
Servings Per Recipe 6

Amount Per Serving

Calories 110	Calories from Fat 40
	% Daily Value*
Total Fat 4.5g	**7 %**
Saturated Fat 2g	**10 %**
Cholesterol 60mg	**20 %**
Sodium 190mg	**8 %**
Total Carbohydrate 3g	**1 %**
Dietary Fiber 0g	**0 %**
Sugars 0g	
Protein 16g	

Vitamin A 0%	•	Vitamin C 0%
Calcium 2%	•	Iron 4%

*Percent Daily Values are based on a 2,000 calorie diet.

Spray a broiler pan with cooking spray. Arrange meatballs on broiler pan and broil for 3–4 minutes until lightly browned. Flip meatballs and broil another 3–4 minutes. Cover meatballs with foil and bake at 350 degrees for an additional 5–10 minutes, until no longer pink inside.

Remove meatballs from broiler pan and pat with paper towels to remove any excess grease. Meatballs can be eaten as is provided that they are cooked thoroughly, or simmered in a low-fat tomato sauce.

Makes 6 servings (2 meatballs per person).

Veal Parmigiana

olive oil cooking spray
¼ cup nonfat milk
½ cup Italian seasoned bread
   crumbs
1 lb veal cutlets
1 cup basic marinara sauce

½ cup shredded part-skim
   mozzarella
1 tbsp grated Parmesan
   cheese
dried oregano

This is a baked version of a dish that is normally loaded with fat. You can use homemade marinara sauce or a low-fat marinara from a jar.

Preheat oven to 375 degrees. Spray a large roasting pan with olive oil cooking spray.

Pour milk and breadcrumbs into separate shallow bowls and set aside.

Place veal cutlets between pieces of plastic wrap and pound to ⅛-in thickness with a meat mallet. Dip each cutlet into milk, then coat both sides lightly with breadcrumbs. Place in roasting pan. When all of the cutlets are in the roasting pan, spray the tops lightly with olive oil spray.

Cover roasting pan with foil and bake cutlets for 10 minutes. Increase the oven temperature to 425 degrees, remove cover, and bake for an additional 10–12 minutes until lightly browned.

Remove cutlets to an oven-proof serving platter. Spread sauce over meat and sprinkle with mozzarella, Parmesan, and oregano. Return to the oven for another 3–5 minutes at 425 degrees until warmed through and cheese bubbles.

Makes 4 servings, about 4 oz each.

Nutrition Facts	
Serving Size 1 Serving	
Servings Per Recipe 4	
Amount Per Serving	
Calories 250	Calories from Fat 60
	% Daily Value*
Total Fat 7g	11%
Saturated Fat 3g	15%
Cholesterol 95mg	32%
Sodium 760mg	32%
Total Carbohydrate 16g	5%
Dietary Fiber 1g	4%
Sugars 1g	
Protein 32g	
Vitamin A 10% • Vitamin C 25%	
Calcium 20% • Iron 10%	
*Percent Daily Values are based on a 2,000 calorie diet.	

15

Side Dishes

STARCHES

Polenta Presto

13¾ oz can lower-salt chicken broth
⅔ cup fine yellow corn meal

1 tbsp grated Parmesan
cheese

Traditional polenta is prepared over a low flame and requires almost constant attention and stirring. This simple version nearly cooks itself and is ready in a flash!

In a 1½- or 2-quart microwavable dish, combine broth and cornmeal. Microwave on high, covered, for 2 mintues. Remove from oven and stir.

Microwave uncovered for 4–6 more minutes, until firm. Sprinkle with grated Parmesan and serve.

These instructions are for a 700-watt microwave oven. If your power is different, cooking times will vary.

Serves 4.

Nutrition Facts	
Serving Size 1 Serving	
Servings Per Recipe 4	
Amount Per Serving	
Calories 90	Calories from Fat 5
	% Daily Value*
Total Fat 1g	2 %
Saturated Fat 0g	0 %
Cholesterol 0mg	0 %
Sodium 50mg	2 %
Total Carbohydrate 18g	6 %
Dietary Fiber 2g	8 %
Sugars 0g	
Protein 3g	
Vitamin A 0% • Vitamin C 0%	
Calcium 2% • Iron 0%	

Percent Daily Values are based on a 2,000 calorie diet.

Rush Hour Risotto

1½ cups chicken broth
½ cup water
½ cup dry white wine

1 cup Arborio or long-grain rice
2 tbsp grated Parmesan cheese

Traditional risotto requires a lot of attention during cooking and can be time-consuming to make. Here is a simple and quick version of this popular dish. It is tastier with Arborio rice, but you can use regular rice if that's all you have available. Homemade chicken stock or broth that comes packaged in a carton rather than a can has a better flavor and will give you a nicer product.

Nutrition Facts

Serving Size 1/2 cup
Servings Per Recipe 6

Amount Per Serving

Calories 120	Calories from Fat 5

	% Daily Value*
Total Fat 0.5g	1%
Saturated Fat 0g	0%
Cholesterol 0mg	0%
Sodium 60mg	3%
Total Carbohydrate 25g	8%
Dietary Fiber 1g	4%
Sugars 0g	
Protein 4g	

Vitamin A 0%	•	Vitamin C 0%
Calcium 4%	•	Iron 8%

*Percent Daily Values are based on a 2,000 calorie diet.

Bring broth, water, and wine to a boil in a medium saucepan. Add rice; cover and simmer 20 minutes or until liquid is absorbed.

Stir in Parmesan cheese and serve.

Makes 3 cups, or 6 half-cup servings.

Bow Ties Aglio Olio

½ lb bow tie pasta
1 tsp olive oil
1 clove garlic, crushed

¼ cup chopped fresh parsley
1 tbsp grated Parmesan cheese

Prepare bow ties according to package directions. Reserve ¼ cup of cooking water when pasta is drained.

In a small fry pan, heat oil over medium-high heat. Toast crushed garlic in the oil until light brown and fragrant. Add parsley and stir briefly; then combine with cooked pasta. Stir in ¼ cup reserved hot water and then toss with cheese.

Makes 4 cups, or 8 half-cup servings.

Nutrition Facts

Serving Size 1/2 cup
Servings Per Recipe 8

Amount Per Serving

Calories 120	Calories from Fat 20

	% Daily Value*
Total Fat 2.5g	4 %
Saturated Fat 0g	0 %
Cholesterol 35mg	12 %
Sodium 20mg	1 %
Total Carbohydrate 20g	7 %
Dietary Fiber 1g	4 %
Sugars 1g	
Protein 4g	

Vitamin A 0%	•	Vitamin C 4%
Calcium 0%	•	Iron 6%

*Percent Daily Values are based on a 2,000 calorie diet.

Garlic Mashed Potatoes

1½ lbs golden potatoes	**1 cup skim milk**
1 tsp butter or margarine	**¼ tsp salt**
2 large or 3 small cloves garlic	**⅛ tsp white pepper**

Wash and peel potatoes. Chop into quarters and cook in boiling water until tender, about 10 minutes. Drain and set aside.

While potatoes are cooking, melt butter over medium heat in a small saucepan. Peel and crush the garlic, then add to the butter and cook until lightly browned. Add the milk, salt, and pepper and heat through.

Nutrition Facts

Serving Size 1/2 cup
Servings Per Recipe 10

Amount Per Serving

Calories 70	Calories from Fat 5

	% Daily Value*
Total Fat 0.5g	1 %
Saturated Fat 0g	0 %
Cholesterol 0mg	0 %
Sodium 80mg	3 %
Total Carbohydrate 13g	4 %
Dietary Fiber 1g	4 %
Sugars 1g	
Protein 2g	

Vitamin A 0%	•	Vitamin C 20%
Calcium 4%	•	Iron 6%

*Percent Daily Values are based on a 2,000 calorie diet.

Combine mashed potatoes, garlic, buttermilk, salt, and pepper. Beat with an electric mixer until fluffy.

Makes 5 cups, or 10 half-cup servings.

Roasted New Potatoes

1½ lbs tiny new potatoes
¼ tsp seasoned salt
1 tsp dried dill

1 tbsp chopped fresh or 1 tsp
 dried parsley
olive oil cooking spray

Preheat oven to 450 degrees.

Wash new potatoes and cut into quarters (or if using larger potatoes, cut into ½-in chunks). Sprinkle with seasoned salt and herbs; toss to coat.

Spray a baking sheet with olive oil cooking spray. Spread potatoes onto sheet and add more olive oil spray.

Bake for 30 minutes, stirring once or twice so that potatoes brown evenly.

Nutrition Facts	
Serving Size 1/2 cup	
Servings Per Recipe 6	
Amount Per Serving	
Calories 120	Calories from Fat 0
	% Daily Value*
Total Fat 0g	0 %
Saturated Fat 0g	0 %
Cholesterol 0mg	0 %
Sodium 70mg	3 %
Total Carbohydrate 26g	9 %
Dietary Fiber 0g	0 %
Sugars 2g	
Protein 3g	
Vitamin A 0% • Vitamin C 30%	
Calcium 0% • Iron 8%	
*Percent Daily Values are based on a 2,000 calorie diet.	

Makes 6 half-cup servings. Use your favorite seasonings to change the flavor of this recipe!

Black Bean and Corn Salad

15 oz can black beans
1½ cups frozen corn niblets
1 green pepper, cut into
  ½-in chunks
1 large tomato or 1 cup
  canned chunks
½ cup mild salsa

1 tbsp lime juice or cider
  vinegar
¼ tsp salt
1 tsp ground cumin
2 tbsp chopped fresh
  cilantro
green onions (optional)

Drain and rinse black beans; set aside. Thaw corn in a strainer under running water. Seed and chop the pepper and tomato (you can use drained, chopped, canned tomatoes if fresh are out of season). Combine all ingredients in a bowl. Mix well; chill before serving. Garnish with additional chopped cilantro and 2 tbsp green onions, if desired.

Nutrition Facts	
Serving Size 1/2 cup	
Servings Per Recipe 8	
Amount Per Serving	
Calories 80	Calories from Fat 5
	% Daily Value*
Total Fat 0.5g	1%
Saturated Fat 0g	0%
Cholesterol 0mg	0%
Sodium 180mg	8%
Total Carbohydrate 15g	5%
Dietary Fiber 4g	16%
Sugars 3g	
Protein 4g	
Vitamin A 4% • Vitamin C 50%	
Calcium 0% • Iron 6%	
*Percent Daily Values are based on a 2,000 calorie diet.	

Rice Salad

1 cup converted rice
2 oz sharp provolone cheese
2 oz prosciutto ham

½ cup frozen petite peas
1 tbsp olive oil
¼ cup chopped fresh parsley

This salad is good with a few capers sprinkled on top, if you have them handy. It is nice for a party or lunchtime leftovers.

Prepare rice according to package directions. Cool. Chop cheese and ham into ¼-in pieces. Mix together cooked rice, cheese, ham, peas, and oil. Chill before serving. Garnish with chopped parsely.

Makes about 5 cups, or 10 half-cup servings.

Nutrition Facts

Serving Size 1/2 cup
Servings Per Recipe 10

Amount Per Serving

Calories 110	Calories from Fat 30

	% Daily Value*
Total Fat 3g	**5 %**
Saturated Fat 1.5g	**8 %**
Cholesterol 5mg	**2 %**
Sodium 105mg	**4 %**
Total Carbohydrate 16g	**5 %**
Dietary Fiber 0g	**0 %**
Sugars 0g	
Protein 4g	

Vitamin A 4%	•	Vitamin C 15%
Calcium 6%	•	Iron 6%

*Percent Daily Values are based on a 2,000 calorie diet.

Basic Pasta Salad

1 cup sliced zucchini
1 cup sliced yellow squash
½ cup broccoli florets
½ cup sliced carrots
1 red pepper, sliced into ¾" pieces
6 oz uncooked pasta
1½ tbsp olive oil
1½ tbsp cold water
1 tbsp fresh chopped basil, or
   1 tsp dried

1 tbsp chopped fresh parsley,
   or 1 tsp dried
¼ tsp black pepper
2 oz feta cheese, crumbled
1 cup chopped ripe tomato
1 tbsp lemon juice
1 tbsp balsamic vinegar

You can vary this recipe by using whatever variety of vegetables or pasta you have on hand.

Chop vegetables and set aside, keeping tomato separate. Cook pasta according to package directions. During the last minute of cooking, add the vegetables, except the tomato, to the boiling water to blanch vegeta-

Nutrition Facts

Serving Size 1/2 cup
Servings Per Recipe 14

Amount Per Serving

Calories 80	Calories from Fat 25

	% Daily Value*
Total Fat 2.5g	**4 %**
Saturated Fat 1g	**5 %**
Cholesterol 5mg	**2 %**
Sodium 55mg	**2 %**
Total Carbohydrate 12g	**4 %**
Dietary Fiber 1g	**4 %**
Sugars 2g	
Protein 3g	

Vitamin A 25%	•	Vitamin C 30%
Calcium 4%	•	Iron 4%

*Percent Daily Values are based on a 2,000 calorie diet.

bles lightly. Drain pasta and vegetables and rinse with cold water to begin cooling.

Toss the pasta mixture, oil, water, basil, parsley, and pepper together. Stir in feta cheese and tomatoes. Chill well. Just before serving, add lemon juice and balsamic vinegar and mix well.

Makes about 7 cups, or 14 half-cup servings.

Curried Cauliflower and Potato Salad

1 lb potatoes, cut into 1-in chunks
2 cups raw cauliflower florets
¼ cup nonfat plain yogurt
1 tbsp low-fat mayonnaise
1 tsp curry powder

¼ tsp salt
1 tsp mustard seeds
½ cup frozen peas, thawed
2 green onions, chopped

Bring 2 quarts of water to a boil in a sauce pan. Add potatoes and cook for 3 minutes, then add cauliflower to pan and return to boil. Cook until potatoes are tender, about 3–4 more minutes after the water returns to a boil. Pour potatoes and cauliflower into a colander; drain. Cover with ice cubes to chill quickly. Set aside.

Mix together yogurt, mayonnaise, curry powder, salt, and mustard seeds. Toss potatoes, cauliflower, frozen peas, and green onions together. Stir in yogurt/mayonnaise dressing. Serve chilled.

Nutrition Facts	
Serving Size 1/2 cup	
Servings Per Recipe 8	
Amount Per Serving	
Calories 80	Calories from Fat 10
	% Daily Value*
Total Fat 1g	2 %
Saturated Fat 0g	0 %
Cholesterol 0mg	0 %
Sodium 125mg	5 %
Total Carbohydrate 15g	5 %
Dietary Fiber 2g	8 %
Sugars 2g	
Protein 3g	
Vitamin A 0% • Vitamin C 40%	
Calcium 4% • Iron 6%	
*Percent Daily Values are based on a 2,000 calorie diet.	

Makes about 5 cups, or 10 half-cup servings.

VEGETABLES

Cauliflower with Nutmeg

4 cups raw cauliflower
½ cup chicken broth

nutmeg, preferably freshly
ground

Freshly ground nutmeg really makes this recipe if you have it. If not, substitute ground nutmeg from the grocery store.

Wash and cut cauliflower into florets. Steam until tender but still crisp, about 5–7 minutes. Warm the broth in a microwavable cup or small saucepan. Toss the steamed cauliflower with the warm chicken broth and sprinkle with ground nutmeg to taste.

Makes 4 servings, about 1 cup each.

Nutrition Facts
Serving Size 1 Cup
Servings Per Recipe 4

Amount Per Serving	
Calories 40	Calories from Fat 5

	% Daily Value*
Total Fat 0.5g	1%
Saturated Fat 0g	0%
Cholesterol 0mg	0%
Sodium 40mg	2%
Total Carbohydrate 5g	2%
Dietary Fiber 3g	12%
Sugars 0g	
Protein 3g	

Vitamin A 2%	•	Vitamin C 90%
Calcium 2%	•	Iron 2%

*Percent Daily Values are based on a 2,000 calorie diet.

Broccoli with Lemon and Pepper

3 cups raw broccoli florets
1 tsp olive oil
1 clove garlic, peeled

¼ tsp hot red pepper flakes
1 tbsp lemon juice
2 tbsp water

Wash and cut broccoli into florets. Steam to desired crispness.

In a small frying pan, heat olive oil with whole garlic clove until garlic is lightly browned. Add hot pepper flakes and stir for 30 seconds to 1 minute over low heat. Remove from heat as soon as pepper flakes begin to turn brown.

Stir in lemon juice and water. Remove garlic clove and toss oil mixture with broccoli.

Serve hot or chilled. Makes 4 servings, about ⅔ cup each.

Nutrition Facts	
Serving Size 2/3 cup	
Servings Per Recipe 4	
Amount Per Serving	
Calories 35	Calories from Fat 10
	% Daily Value*
Total Fat 1.5g	**2%**
Saturated Fat 0g	**0%**
Cholesterol 0mg	**0%**
Sodium 20mg	**1%**
Total Carbohydrate 4g	**1%**
Dietary Fiber 2g	**8%**
Sugars 1g	
Protein 2g	
Vitamin A 10% • Vitamin C 100%	
Calcium 4% • Iron 4%	
*Percent Daily Values are based on a 2,000 calorie diet.	

Savory Spinach

10 oz prewashed fresh spinach leaves
¼ cup golden raisins

½ cup water
1 tbsp slivered almonds, toasted

Rinse spinach and remove any tough ends. Set aside. In a 4-quart saucepan, bring raisins and water to a boil. Cover and reduce heat; simmer for approximately 5 minutes or until raisins are tender.

Add spinach leaves to pan. Cover and continue to cook, allowing spinach to steam for about 1 minute. Stir and continue to cook, uncovered, for 1–2 more minutes or until spinach is wilted.

Serve sprinkled with toasted slivered almonds. Makes 4 half-cup servings.

Nutrition Facts	
Serving Size 1/2 cup	
Servings Per Recipe 4	
Amount Per Serving	
Calories 50	Calories from Fat 10
	% Daily Value*
Total Fat 1g	**2%**
Saturated Fat 0g	**0%**
Cholesterol 0mg	**0%**
Sodium 5mg	**0%**
Total Carbohydrate 9g	**3%**
Dietary Fiber 1g	**4%**
Sugars 7g	
Protein 1g	
Vitamin A 4% • Vitamin C 0%	
Calcium 0% • Iron 2%	
*Percent Daily Values are based on a 2,000 calorie diet.	

Sautéed Mushrooms

8 oz presliced mushrooms
olive oil cooking spray
1 clove garlic, crushed
1 tsp Worcestershire sauce

1 tbsp fresh or 1 tsp dried parsley
1 tsp fresh or ½ tsp dried
 rosemary
1 tbsp water

Wash mushrooms. Heat cooking spray and garlic in a nonstick skillet until garlic begins to brown.

Add mushrooms and remaining ingredients to skillet. Sauté over medium-high heat for approximately 5 minutes, until mushrooms are tender but not dry. (If mushrooms do become dry, add another tablespoon of water.)

Makes 1 cup, or 2 half-cup servings.

Can be used as a side dish or as a topping for meat, poultry, pizza, etc.

Nutrition Facts

Serving Size 1/2 cup
Servings Per Recipe 2

Amount Per Serving

Calories 40	Calories from Fat 5

	% Daily Value*
Total Fat 0.5g	1 %
Saturated Fat 0g	0 %
Cholesterol 0mg	0 %
Sodium 30mg	1 %
Total Carbohydrate 7g	2 %
Dietary Fiber 1g	4 %
Sugars 2g	
Protein 3g	

Vitamin A 0%	•	Vitamin C 20%
Calcium 0%	•	Iron 10%

*Percent Daily Values are based on a 2,000 calorie diet.

Sesame Snow Peas

2 tsp sesame seeds
½ lb snow peas
1 tsp reduced-sodium soy sauce

1 tsp cider vinegar
½ tsp sugar
¼ tsp sesame oil

Toast sesame seeds in a 400-degree oven for 3–5 minutes, stirring halfway through, until golden brown.

Steam snow peas for approximately 4–5 minutes until desired degree of tenderness.

Mix together soy sauce, vinegar, sugar, and sesame oil. Toss snow peas, soy sauce mixture, and toasted sesame seeds together until well coated.

Makes 3 cups, or 6 half-cup servings.

Nutrition Facts

Serving Size 1/2 cup
Servings Per Recipe 6

Amount Per Serving

Calories 35	Calories from Fat 5

	% Daily Value*
Total Fat 0.5g	**1%**
Saturated Fat 0g	**0%**
Cholesterol 0mg	**0%**
Sodium 40mg	**2%**
Total Carbohydrate 5g	**2%**
Dietary Fiber 2g	**8%**
Sugars 1g	
Protein 2g	

Vitamin A 0%	•	Vitamin C 45%
Calcium 2%	•	Iron 2%

*Percent Daily Values are based on a 2,000 calorie diet.

Zucchini Rosso

2 tbsp tomato paste
½ cup water
½ tsp instant minced onion
1 tsp frozen apple juice concentrate
⅛ tsp salt

2 whole cloves
1 lb zucchini (2 medium)
½ tsp dried basil
black pepper

Combine tomato paste, water, onion, apple juice concentrate, salt, black pepper, dried basil, and cloves in a medium saucepan. Stir together over medium-high heat. When mixture comes to a boil, reduce heat and simmer, covered, for 5 minutes.

Cut zucchini in half lengthwise and then cut into ¼-in slices. Add to tomato mixture and stir to coat zucchini. Return to a simmer and cover again.

Nutrition Facts

Serving Size 1/2 cup
Servings Per Recipe 4

Amount Per Serving

Calories 30	Calories from Fat 0

	% Daily Value*
Total Fat 0g	**0%**
Saturated Fat 0g	**0%**
Cholesterol 0mg	**0%**
Sodium 100mg	**4%**
Total Carbohydrate 6g	**2%**
Dietary Fiber 2g	**8%**
Sugars 3g	
Protein 2g	

Vitamin A 4%	•	Vitamin C 20%
Calcium 2%	•	Iron 4%

*Percent Daily Values are based on a 2,000 calorie diet.

Simmer for 10 minutes, or until zucchini are tender.

Remove cloves before serving.

Makes 4 half-cup servings.

Summer Cucumber and Tomato Salad

2½ cups seeded, chopped tomato
1 cucumber, peeled and chopped
2 tbsp chopped green onion
2 tbsp chopped fresh parsley
2 tbsp chopped fresh basil
2 tbsp balsamic vinegar

2 tsp red wine vinegar
1½ tsp olive oil
⅛ tsp salt
freshly ground black pepper
low-fat mozzarella, as desired

Chop tomato and cucumber into ¾-in chunks; set aside. In a serving bowl, mix together remaining ingredients. If you do not have all of the fresh herbs available, you can improvise—but do try to use fresh basil if you can get it. If you use dried herbs, cut the amount in half. Add chopped tomato and cucumber; toss to mix well. Serve chilled.

Makes about 4 cups, or 8 half-cup servings.

For a main dish salad, add chunks of low-fat mozzarella.

Nutrition Facts		
Serving Size 1/2 cup		
Servings Per Recipe 8		
Amount Per Serving		
Calories 30	Calories from Fat 10	
		% Daily Value*
Total Fat 1g		2 %
Saturated Fat 0g		0 %
Cholesterol 0mg		0 %
Sodium 45mg		2 %
Total Carbohydrate 4g		1 %
Dietary Fiber 1g		4 %
Sugars 2g		
Protein 1g		
Vitamin A 6%	• Vitamin C 25%	
Calcium 0%	• Iron 2%	
*Percent Daily Values are based on a 2,000 calorie diet.		

Sunshine Salad

3 cups mixed greens or chopped lettuce   **1 tbsp slivered almonds**
2 clementines or tangerines   **2 tbsp raspberry vinegar, or to taste**

This salad works well with spring mixed greens, alone or mixed with chopped lettuce. If your grocery store does not carry spring mix, you can use plain chopped romaine or leaf lettuce.

Wash lettuce, tear into small pieces, and divide evenly between two salad plates. Peel clementines and arrange wedges on top of the lettuce (if using tangerines you will have to remove their seeds). Sprinkle each salad with ½ tbsp slivered almonds and raspberry vinegar to taste.

Serve chilled. Makes 2 servings.

Nutrition Facts
Serving Size 1 Serving
Servings Per Recipe 2

Amount Per Serving

Calories 80	Calories from Fat 25

	% Daily Value*
Total Fat 2.5g	4 %
Saturated Fat 0g	0 %
Cholesterol 0mg	0 %
Sodium 10mg	0 %
Total Carbohydrate 12g	4 %
Dietary Fiber 4g	16 %
Sugars 7g	
Protein 2g	

Vitamin A 20%	•	Vitamin C 60%
Calcium 8%	•	Iron 8%

*Percent Daily Values are based on a 2,000 calorie diet.

16

Appetizers and Dips

Oriental Steamed Dumplings

Dumplings:

 1 tsp sesame oil
 1 tbsp freshly grated ginger
 2 green onions, chopped
 2½ cups shredded cabbage
 ½ cup shredded carrots
 1 tsp soy sauce
 2 tbsp dry sherry or 2 tbsp water
 2 dozen wonton wrappers
 cooking spray

Dipping Sauce:

 1 tbsp soy sauce
 2 tbsp water
 2 tsp brown sugar
 1 tsp rice or wine vinegar

This recipe takes a bit of effort, but is very tasty and worth the time if you have it. As a shortcut, use preshredded cole slaw mix without the dressing instead of shredding your own carrots and cabbage. Authentic "thin soy" sauce from a Chinese grocery store or good-quality tamari sauce will produce better results than ordinary soy sauce, if you can get it.

Nutrition Facts

Serving Size 4 Dumplings
Servings Per Recipe 6

Amount Per Serving

Calories 120	Calories from Fat 10

	% Daily Value*
Total Fat 1.5g	**2 %**
Saturated Fat 0g	**0 %**
Cholesterol 5mg	**2 %**
Sodium 430mg	**18 %**
Total Carbohydrate 23g	**8 %**
Dietary Fiber 1g	**4 %**
Sugars 3g	
Protein 4g	

Vitamin A 25%	•	Vitamin C 20%
Calcium 4%	•	Iron 8%

*Percent Daily Values are based on a 2,000 calorie diet.

In a nonstick skillet, heat sesame oil and sauté ginger and green onions until fragrant. Add shredded cabbage and carrots, 1 tsp soy sauce, and sherry or water. Sauté for about 5–7 minutes until cabbage is tender and excess moisture is gone.

Place about 1 tbsp of cabbage mixture in each wonton wrapper. Fold wrapper into a triangle and fold corners of triangle to the center of the wonton. Seal seams with wet fingertips (the wonton package should have directions).

Spray a steamer with cooking spray and place a few dumplings at a time into the steamer, seam side up, and steam for 5 minutes. Alternately, the dumplings can be dropped into simmering broth for 5 minutes.

Mix together 1 tbsp of soy sauce, water, brown sugar, and vinegar. Stir until sugar is well dissolved. Serve dumplings warm with soy sauce mixture as a dipping sauce.

Makes about 24 dumplings, or 6 4-dumpling portions.

Stuffed Mushrooms

14 oz large mushrooms for stuffing	olive oil cooking spray
1 slice whole wheat bread	2 tbsp white wine
1 garlic clove, crushed	2 oz crumbled blue cheese

Wash mushrooms and remove stems. Steam mushroom caps upside down in a steamer or microwave for 5 minutes, or until tender.

Trim ends from mushroom stems. Place trimmed stems and bread (tear the slice into pieces) in a food processor and process until finely chopped.

In a nonstick sauté pan, brown the garlic in cooking spray. Add mushroom/breadcrumb mixture and wine. Cook over medium heat until all of the wine has evaporated.

Place about a tablespoon of stuffing into each mushroom cap, dividing stuffing evenly between the mushrooms. Press stuffing into mushroom caps with the back of a spoon.

Sprinkle stuffed mushrooms with blue cheese and broil until cheese is melted.

Makes about 16 stuffed mushrooms, or 4 portions.

Nutrition Facts

Serving Size 4 Mushrooms
Servings Per Recipe 4

Amount Per Serving

Calories 90	Calories from Fat 35

	% Daily Value*
Total Fat 4g	6 %
Saturated Fat 1.5g	8 %
Cholesterol 5mg	2 %
Sodium 140mg	6 %
Total Carbohydrate 6g	2 %
Dietary Fiber 1g	4 %
Sugars 2g	
Protein 6g	

Vitamin A 0%	•	Vitamin C 0%
Calcium 4%	•	Iron 4%

*Percent Daily Values are based on a 2,000 calorie diet.

Hot Artichoke Dip

8½ oz can artichoke hearts
1 cup nonfat cottage cheese

½ cup fat-free grated Parmesan cheese
paprika

Drain artichoke hearts. Combine artichokes and cottage cheese in a food processor or blender; process until smooth. Stir in Parmesan, making sure there are no lumps from the cheese.

Pour into a heat-proof dish and microwave on high for 3 minutes. Stir the dip, then cook on 50% power for 5 minutes, until heated through. Sprinkle with paprika.

Nutrition Facts

Serving Size 2 Tbsp
Servings Per Recipe 20

Amount Per Serving

Calories 20	Calories from Fat 0

	% Daily Value*
Total Fat 0g	0 %
Saturated Fat 0g	0 %
Cholesterol 0mg	0 %
Sodium 90mg	4 %
Total Carbohydrate 2g	1 %
Dietary Fiber 0g	0 %
Sugars 1g	
Protein 3g	

Vitamin A 0%	•	Vitamin C 0%
Calcium 0%	•	Iron 0%

*Percent Daily Values are based on a 2,000 calorie diet.

This recipe can also be baked at 375 degrees until heated through.

Makes about 2½ cups, or 20 2-tbsp servings.

Spinach Dip

10 oz frozen chopped spinach, thawed
1 cup plain nonfat yogurt
4 tbsp dry vegetable soup mix

½ cup chopped fresh parsley
4 green onions, chopped
2 tbsp lemon juice

Thaw spinach. Drain well and pat with paper towels to squeeze out extra moisture.

Blend yogurt and soup mix together. Combine with remaining ingredients and drained spinach; mix well. Let chill several hours or overnight to allow flavors to blend.

Makes 2 cups, or 16 2-tbsp servings.

Nutrition Facts

Serving Size 2 Tbsp
Servings Per Recipe 16

Amount Per Serving	
Calories 15	Calories from Fat 0

	% Daily Value*
Total Fat 0g	0 %
Saturated Fat 0g	0 %
Cholesterol 0mg	0 %
Sodium 95mg	4 %
Total Carbohydrate 3g	1 %
Dietary Fiber 0g	0 %
Sugars 1g	
Protein 1g	

Vitamin A 10%	•	Vitamin C 8%
Calcium 4%	•	Iron 0%

*Percent Daily Values are based on a 2,000 calorie diet.

Hummus

15 oz can garbanzo beans
2 tbsp tahini (sesame butter)
4 tbsp water

1 clove garlic
2 tbsp lemon juice
¼ tsp ground cumin

This recipe makes a tasty dip for raw vegetables or pita triangles. It also serves as a nutritious sandwich spread!

Drain garbanzo beans. Place all ingredients into a food processor or blender. Blend until smooth and creamy. Add another tablespoon of water and continue to blend if mixture is not smooth enough.

Use extra lemon or a dash of hot sauce if desired.

Makes $1\frac{1}{4}$ cups, or 10 2-tbsp servings.

Nutrition Facts

Serving Size 2 Tbsp
Servings Per Recipe 10

Amount Per Serving

Calories 70	Calories from Fat 25

	% Daily Value*
Total Fat 3g	5 %
Saturated Fat 0g	0 %
Cholesterol 0mg	0 %
Sodium 170mg	7 %
Total Carbohydrate 8g	3 %
Dietary Fiber 2g	8 %
Sugars 2g	
Protein 3g	

Vitamin A 0%	•	Vitamin C 4%
Calcium 2%	•	Iron 6%

*Percent Daily Values are based on a 2,000 calorie diet.

Fresh Salsa

28 oz can of diced tomatoes
1 cup raw or frozen chopped green pepper
$\frac{1}{2}$ cup chopped onion
1 clove garlic, crushed
1 can (4 oz) diced jalapeño peppers

1 tsp ground cumin
$\frac{1}{2}$ tsp Louisiana hot sauce
1 tbsp lime juice
$\frac{1}{4}$ tsp ground red pepper
1 tbsp chopped fresh cilantro

Even though ready-made salsa is widely available in grocery stores, this recipe is easy to fix and a sure crowd pleaser. It is also lower in sodium than most commercial salsas. Fresh cilantro adds a lot to this dish—it's worth the effort to find it if you can.

Combine all ingredients in large microwavable bowl. Microwave on high 10 minutes, or until flavors blend. Chill at least 4 hours before serving. If desired, add extra ground red pepper and lime juice to taste when chilled.

Nutrition Facts

Serving Size 2 Tbsp
Servings Per Recipe 32

Amount Per Serving

Calories 10	Calories from Fat 0

	% Daily Value*
Total Fat 0g	0 %
Saturated Fat 0g	0 %
Cholesterol 0mg	0 %
Sodium 60mg	3 %
Total Carbohydrate 2g	1 %
Dietary Fiber 0g	0 %
Sugars 1g	
Protein 0g	

Vitamin A 4%	•	Vitamin C 15%
Calcium 0%	•	Iron 0%

*Percent Daily Values are based on a 2,000 calorie diet.

Makes about 4 cups or 32 2-tbsp servings.

Yogurt Mustard Dip

1 cup plain yogurt
2 tbsp Dijon mustard

Blend well and chill. Makes a delicious dip for raw vegetables or steamed asparagus. You can also use on sandwiches.

Makes 8 2-tbsp servings.

Nutrition Facts
Serving Size 2 Tbsp
Servings Per Recipe 8

Amount Per Serving

Calories 20	Calories from Fat 0

% Daily Value*

Total Fat 0g	0 %
Saturated Fat 0g	0 %
Cholesterol 0mg	0 %
Sodium 40mg	2 %
Total Carbohydrate 3g	1 %
Dietary Fiber 0g	0 %
Sugars 1g	
Protein 2g	

Vitamin A 0%	•	Vitamin C 0%
Calcium 6%	•	Iron 0%

*Percent Daily Values are based on a 2,000 calorie diet.

Herb Vinaigrette Dressing

2 tbsp red wine vinegar
2 tbsp lemon juice
1 tbsp olive oil
2 tbsp strong brewed tea
1 tbsp maple syrup
1/4 tsp salt
1/4 tsp pepper
1/2 tsp dried basil
1/2 tsp dried oregano
1/2 tsp dried thyme

Whisk all ingredients together and chill well. Stir or shake well before serving.

Makes about 1/2 cup, or 4 2-tbsp servings.

Nutrition Facts
Serving Size 2 Tbsp
Servings Per Recipe 4

Amount Per Serving

Calories 45	Calories from Fat 30

% Daily Value*

Total Fat 3.5g	5 %
Saturated Fat 0g	0 %
Cholesterol 0mg	0 %
Sodium 150mg	6 %
Total Carbohydrate 4g	1 %
Dietary Fiber 0g	0 %
Sugars 3g	
Protein 0g	

Vitamin A 0%	•	Vitamin C 4%
Calcium 0%	•	Iron 2%

*Percent Daily Values are based on a 2,000 calorie diet.

17

Soups and Sauces

Candlelight Crab and Shrimp Soup

6 cups reduced salt chicken broth
¾-in slice ginger root, peeled
2 green onions
6 oz can crabmeat

½ lb raw shrimp
¼ lb snow peas
1 cup sliced mushrooms
1–2 tbsp fresh chopped
   cilantro

This recipe was first prepared during a power outage, thus its name!

Remove fat from the top of chicken broth cans. Peel ginger root and cut into two pieces. Slice green onions, tops and bulbs, on the diagonal in ¼-in pieces. Pour broth into a 4-quart saucepan and add ginger and green onions. Simmer, covered, for 30 minutes. Remove ginger.

Rinse crabmeat and remove any shells. Add crab, snow peas, and mushrooms to hot broth. Simmer until mushrooms begin to wilt.

Nutrition Facts

Serving Size 1 Cup
Servings Per Recipe 6

Amount Per Serving	
Calories 100	Calories from Fat 20

	% Daily Value*
Total Fat 2g	3 %
Saturated Fat 1g	5 %
Cholesterol 100mg	33 %
Sodium 300mg	13 %
Total Carbohydrate 3g	1 %
Dietary Fiber 1g	4 %
Sugars 1g	
Protein 17g	

Vitamin A 4%	•	Vitamin O 13%
Calcium 6%	•	Iron 10%

*Percent Daily Values are based on a 2,000 calorie diet.

Clean and devein shrimp. Peel, leaving tails on. Add to soup and heat just until shrimp are bright pink (do not overcook as shrimp will become tough).

Serve immediately. To serve, distribute shrimp evenly in bowls, then pour soup over shrimp. Garnish with a sprinkling of fresh chopped cilantro.

Makes 6 1-cup servings.

Chicken Corn Soup with Asparagus

4 green onions, tops and bulbs
olive or canola cooking oil spray
1 cup chopped carrots (2–3 whole)
²⁄₃ cup chopped celery (2 stalks)
4 cups water
1 tsp salt
¼ tsp pepper

2 bay leaves
2½ tsp thyme leaves
½ tsp basil leaves
12 oz boneless skinless
    chicken breast
1½ cups frozen white corn,
    thawed
12 oz fresh asparagus

Chop green onions, celery, and carrots into small slices ahead of time.

Sauté onions in a 4-quart sauce pan in cooking oil spray until tender. Add carrot and celery and stir until mixed. Add water, salt, pepper, and spices; cover and bring to a boil.

When boiling, add whole chicken pieces. Turn heat to medium and simmer for 10–15 minutes, until chicken is no longer pink inside. Remove chicken to a plate to cool.

Nutrition Facts	
Serving Size 1 Cup	
Servings Per Recipe 8	
Amount Per Serving	
Calories 70	Calories from Fat 10
	% Daily Value*
Total Fat 1g	2 %
Saturated Fat 0g	0 %
Cholesterol 15mg	5 %
Sodium 340mg	14 %
Total Carbohydrate 6g	2 %
Dietary Fiber 2g	8 %
Sugars 3g	
Protein 8g	
Vitamin A 40% • Vitamin C 25%	
Calcium 2% • Iron 4%	

*Percent Daily Values are based on a 2,000 calorie diet.

Trim tough ends from asparagus and cut spears into ¾-in pieces. Add asparagus and corn niblets to the soup.

Chop cooled chicken into small pieces and add back to soup. Simmer for another 5–10 minutes, until asparagus is tender. Remove bay leaves and discard.

Serve hot. Makes 8 1-cup servings.

Chicken Vegetable Soup

2 13-oz cans reduced-salt chicken broth
½ lb boneless skinless chicken breast
½ cup chopped onion
1 bay leaf
½ tsp thyme
½ tsp rosemary leaves

3 cups water
1 14-oz can diced tomatoes in juice
1 lb frozen soup mix vegetables
1 cup fine egg noodles, dry
½ cup chopped fresh flat leaf parsley

This is an easy way to make homemade chicken soup without spending hours in the kitchen. You can add your own chopped vegetables if you have the time.

Remove fat from top of cans of chicken broth. In a large pot, simmer chicken breast pieces, onion, bay leaf, thyme, and rosemary in chicken broth and water for 15–20 minutes. Remove chicken and reserve.

Nutrition Facts		
Serving Size 1 Cup		
Servings Per Recipe 10		
Amount Per Serving		
Calories 90	Calories from Fat 10	
		% Daily Value*
Total Fat 1g		2 %
Saturated Fat 0g		0 %
Cholesterol 20mg		7 %
Sodium 350mg		15 %
Total Carbohydrate 11g		4 %
Dietary Fiber 1g		4 %
Sugars 0g		
Protein 9g		
Vitamin A 20%	•	Vitamin C 25%
Calcium 2%	•	Iron 6%
*Percent Daily Values are based on a 2,000 calorie diet.		

Add canned tomatoes and frozen vegetables to pot. While bringing back to a simmer, cut chicken into tiny pieces. Add back to pot. Simmer, partially covered, for another 15–20 minutes.

Add noodles and chopped parsley. Cook until noodles are done. Remove bay leaves before serving.

Makes 10 cups.

Vegetarian Split Pea Soup

11–13 cups water (for soaking and
    simmering)
2 carrots
2 celery stalks
1 lb dried split peas

2 tsp dried minced onion
1¼ tsp salt
2 bay leaves
½ tsp ground coriander

Soak peas in 6–8 cups of water overnight (or bring to a boil first and then soak for 2 hours). Rinse and drain.

Chop carrots and celery into small pieces. Combine all ingredients and 5 cups water in a 6-quart saucepan and simmer, loosely covered, for 1½–2 hours, until fairly smooth and thick.

Makes 8 cups, or 16 half-cup servings.

Nutrition Facts

Serving Size 1/2 cup
Servings Per Recipe 8

Amount Per Serving

Calories 210	Calories from Fat 5

	% Daily Value*
Total Fat 0.5g	1 %
Saturated Fat 0g	0 %
Cholesterol 0mg	0 %
Sodium 390mg	16 %
Total Carbohydrate 37g	12 %
Dietary Fiber 15g	60 %
Sugars 6g	
Protein 14g	

Vitamin A 50%	•	Vitamin C 6%
Calcium 4%	•	Iron 15%

*Percent Daily Values are based on a 2,000 calorie diet.

Basic Marinara Sauce

1 tsp olive oil
1 clove peeled garlic, crushed
2 tbsp finely chopped onion
28 oz can tomato puree
28 oz can crushed tomato

2 tbsp chopped fresh basil
freshly ground black pepper
pinch of nutmeg (optional)
½ tsp sugar
⅛ tsp salt

In a 4-quart saucepan, sauté garlic and onion in olive oil until very lightly browned. Add tomatoes and stir. Add basil, pepper, and a pinch of nutmeg (freshly ground if possible). Simmer, loosely covered, for 1–2 hours. Stir frequently to prevent burning. If the sauce tastes very acidic, add ½ tsp sugar. You may also want to add about ⅛ tsp salt.

Makes about 5 cups (10 servings). Will keep in the refrigerator for 1 week; freezes well.

Nutrition Facts

Serving Size 1/2 cup
Servings Per Recipe 10

Amount Per Serving

Calories 45	Calories from Fat 5

	% Daily Value*
Total Fat 0.5g	1%
Saturated Fat 0g	0%
Cholesterol 0mg	0%
Sodium 340mg	14%
Total Carbohydrate 9g	3%
Dietary Fiber 2g	8%
Sugars 0g	
Protein 2g	

Vitamin A 10%	•	Vitamin C 50%
Calcium 0%	•	Iron 4%

*Percent Daily Values are based on a 2,000 calorie diet.

Variations (add while cooking):
  Add 1 can drained chick peas.
  Add ½ lb cooked and drained Italian turkey sausage.
  Add 2 cups finely chopped cauliflower or frozen mixed
     vegetables.
  Add ½ lb sliced mushrooms and ¼ cup dry red wine be-
     fore adding tomatoes; simmer until tender.

Chunky Vegetable Sauce

1 cup presliced mushrooms	28 oz can diced tomatoes
1 carrot, finely chopped	8 oz can tomato sauce
2 celery stalks, finely chopped	6 oz can tomato paste
4 medium zucchini, finely chopped	2 tsp dried basil
½ cup chopped onion	¼ tsp salt
1 clove garlic, crushed	¼ tsp freshly ground pepper
1 tbsp olive oil	½ tsp sugar
¼ cup dry white wine	

Chop vegetables finely by hand or with a food processor. In a 6-quart saucepan, lightly sauté onion and garlic in olive oil. Add remaining vegetables and wine; steam/sauté until vegetables are slightly tender.

Add tomatoes, sauce, paste, basil, salt, pepper, and sugar. Simmer 30 minutes, covered, and an additional 30–45 minutes uncovered, until sauce is thick.

Makes 2 quarts, or 16 half-cup servings.

Nutrition Facts	
Serving Size 1/2 cup	
Servings Per Recipe 16	
Amount Per Serving	
Calories 45	Calories from Fat 10
	% Daily Value*
Total Fat 1g	2%
Saturated Fat 0g	0%
Cholesterol 0mg	0%
Sodium 260mg	11%
Total Carbohydrate 8g	3%
Dietary Fiber 2g	8%
Sugars 4g	
Protein 2g	
Vitamin A 20% • Vitamin C 25%	
Calcium 4% • Iron 10%	
*Percent Daily Values are based on a 2,000 calorie diet.	

See recipes for Vegetable Lasagne and Pita Pizza for ideas on using this sauce, or serve on top of pasta.

Low-Fat Pesto Sauce

1½ cups fresh basil leaves, packed
½ cup flat parsley leaves, packed
¼ cup pine nuts or walnut pieces
3 cloves garlic, peeled
2 tbsp olive oil

2 tbsp water
⅛ tsp nutmeg
¼ tsp salt
½ cup grated nonfat Parmesan cheese

Chop basil, parsley, nuts, and garlic in a food processor. Add oil and water and blend until smooth.

Transfer to a bowl; stir in nutmeg, salt, and cheese. Store in the refrigerator.

When serving, mix in a teaspoon or two of boiling water per tablespoon of pesto to make it easier to spread.

Use on pasta, pizza, or sandwiches. See recipe for Colorful Pasta with Pesto and White Beans in the Vegetarian section of Chapter 14.

Makes 1 cup, or 16 1-tbsp portions.

Nutrition Facts

Serving Size 1 Tbsp
Servings Per Recipe 16

Amount Per Serving

Calories 40	Calories from Fat 25

	% Daily Value*
Total Fat 3g	5 %
Saturated Fat 0g	0 %
Cholesterol 0mg	0 %
Sodium 65mg	3 %
Total Carbohydrate 2g	1 %
Dietary Fiber 0g	0 %
Sugars 1g	
Protein 2g	

Vitamin A 2%	•	Vitamin C 6%
Calcium 0%	•	Iron 0%

*Percent Daily Values are based on a 2,000 calorie diet.

Roasted Pepper Sauce

12 oz jar roasted peppers and liquid
1 clove garlic, peeled and crushed
2 tsp dried oregano
½ tsp dried rosemary leaves
½ tsp black pepper

1½ tsp sugar
1 tbsp plus 1 tsp olive oil
2 tbsp hot water
⅛ tsp salt

Combine all ingredients in a food processor and process until smooth. Use on hot cooked pasta, fish, or meat, or use cold as a spread on sandwiches.

Makes 1½ cups, or 12 2-tbsp servings.

Nutrition Facts

Serving Size 2 Tbsp
Servings Per Recipe 12

Amount Per Serving

Calories 35	Calories from Fat 15

	% Daily Value*
Total Fat 1.5g	2 %
Saturated Fat 0g	0 %
Cholesterol 0mg	0 %
Sodium 85mg	4 %
Total Carbohydrate 6g	2 %
Dietary Fiber 0g	0 %
Sugars 1g	
Protein 0g	

Vitamin A 10%	•	Vitamin C 30%
Calcium 0%	•	Iron 0%

*Percent Daily Values are based on a 2,000 calorie diet.

18

Breakfasts, Breads, and Muffins

Zucchini Pancakes

1 cup whole-wheat pancake mix
1 cup skim milk
2 tsp canola oil
1 egg

1 cup shredded zucchini
1 tbsp golden raisins, chopped
½ tsp cinnamon
canola oil cooking spray

This recipe offers some extra nutrition and variety over plain pancakes. Shred and freeze zucchini in 1- or 2-cup portions during the summer and you'll have it available in the winter. Make the portions generous, as they will shrink when frozen and thawed.

Combine pancake mix, milk, oil, and egg; stir till combined. Fold in zucchini, chopped raisins, and cinnamon. Blend.

Spray a nonstick griddle with canola oil cooking spray and heat over medium-high heat. Pour 2 measuring tablespoons of pancake batter for each pancake onto the prepared griddle; cook pancakes according to package directions.

Makes about 16 3-in pancakes.

Nutrition Facts	
Serving Size 2 Pancakes	
Servings Per Recipe 8	

Amount Per Serving	
Calories 110	Calories from Fat 20

	% Daily Value*
Total Fat 2g	**3 %**
Saturated Fat 0g	**0 %**
Cholesterol 25mg	**8 %**
Sodium 310mg	**13 %**
Total Carbohydrate 18g	**6 %**
Dietary Fiber 2g	**8 %**
Sugars 5g	
Protein 5g	

Vitamin A 4%	•	Vitamin C 4%
Calcium 10%	•	Iron 8%

*Percent Daily Values are based on a 2,000 calorie diet.

Baked Apple French Toast

cooking spray
10 oz Italian bread
20 oz can lite apple pie filling
8 oz egg substitute
1 tsp vanilla extract
1¾ cup skim milk

1 tsp cinnamon
2 tbsp sugar
⅛ tsp salt

Nutrition Facts

Serving Size 1 Slice
Servings Per Recipe 8

Amount Per Serving	
Calories 210	Calories from Fat 20

	% Daily Value*
Total Fat 2.5g	4 %
Saturated Fat 0.5g	3 %
Cholesterol 0mg	0 %
Sodium 340mg	14 %
Total Carbohydrate 38g	13 %
Dietary Fiber 2g	8 %
Sugars 5g	
Protein 8g	

Vitamin A 10%	•	Vitamin C 0%	
Calcium 10%	•	Iron 10%	

*Percent Daily Values are based on a 2,000 calorie diet.

Spray the bottom of a 9 x 13-in pan with cooking spray. Preheat oven to 350 degrees. Spread apples in a thin layer over the bottom of the pan, cutting apples in half lengthwise if slices are thick. Apple pieces should be thin enough that they cover the bottom of the pan without a lot of gaps.

Slice bread into eight 1-in thick slices and arrange on top of the apples. Mix together remaining ingredients. Pour egg mixture over the bread slices, wetting each slice of bread.

Let stand for 10 minutes to allow the bread to soak up some of the egg mixture. If you wish, you can cover and refrigerate for up to 12 hours before baking. Bake, covered, for 45 minutes and uncovered an additional 10 minutes. The egg should be set and the tops of the bread very lightly browned.

Serve with low-calorie pancake syrup. To serve, remove each slice of bread and surrounding egg mixture with a spatula. Top the slice with any remaining apple from underneath.

Makes 8 servings, 1 slice each.

Stick-to-Your-Ribs Oatmeal

1 cup quick-cooking oats
1 cup skim milk
⅔ cup water
⅛ tsp salt

2 tsp natural peanut butter
1 tbsp raisins
2 tsp brown sugar
¼ tsp cinnamon

Combine all ingredients in a large microwavable bowl. Cook on high for 4–5 minutes, until oats are tender and fluid is absorbed. Stir well to blend peanut butter in.

This recipe can also be prepared on the stove top in a saucepan. Combine ingredients; simmer and stir as above.

Makes 2 cups, or 4 half-cup servings.

Nutrition Facts
Serving Size 1/2 cup
Servings Per Recipe 4

Amount Per Serving

Calories 130	Calories from Fat 25
	% Daily Value*
Total Fat 3g	5 %
Saturated Fat 0.5g	3 %
Cholesterol 0mg	0 %
Sodium 105mg	4 %
Total Carbohydrate 21g	7 %
Dietary Fiber 2g	8 %
Sugars 7g	
Protein 5g	

Vitamin A 4%	•	Vitamin C 0%
Calcium 8%	•	Iron 6%

*Percent Daily Values are based on a 2,000 calorie diet.

Deliteful Danish

¼ cup nonfat ricotta
1 tsp confectioners' sugar
2 slices raisin bread
2 tsp apricot or strawberry fruit
  spread
cinnamon

Mix ricotta and confectioners' sugar together until smooth. Toast raisin bread.

Spread each slice of toast with 2 tbsp of ricotta mixture. Top each piece with 1 tsp of fruit spread and sprinkle with cinnamon.

Makes 2.

Nutrition Facts
Serving Size 1 Piece
Servings Per Recipe 2

Amount Per Serving

Calories 110	Calories from Fat 10
	% Daily Value*
Total Fat 1.5g	2 %
Saturated Fat 0g	0 %
Cholesterol 5mg	2 %
Sodium 170mg	7 %
Total Carbohydrate 18g	6 %
Dietary Fiber 1g	4 %
Sugars 3g	
Protein 6g	

Vitamin A 4%	•	Vitamin C 0%
Calcium 15%	•	Iron 6%

*Percent Daily Values are based on a 2,000 calorie diet.

Better Banana Bread

3 tbsp ground walnuts
3 ripe bananas, mashed
½ cup granulated sugar
3 tbsp fruit-based fat replacement*
½ cup cholesterol-free egg substitute
1 tsp vanilla extract

1 cup all-purpose flour
¾ cup whole-wheat flour
1 tsp baking soda
1 tsp baking powder
½ tsp salt

Preheat oven to 350 degrees. Spray a 9-in loaf pan with cooking spray, then lightly flour the pan.

Place ground walnuts in a shallow pan and toast in the oven until lightly browned.

Combine mashed bananas, sugar, fruit-based fat replacement, egg, and vanilla in a small bowl. Mix together flours, baking soda, baking powder, and salt. Combine wet and dry ingredients, stirring only until combined. Fold in walnuts.

Nutrition Facts

Serving Size 1/2" slice
Servings Per Recipe 16

Amount Per Serving	
Calories 110	Calories from Fat 5

	% Daily Value*
Total Fat 1g	2 %
Saturated Fat 0g	0 %
Cholesterol 0mg	0 %
Sodium 190mg	8 %
Total Carbohydrate 23g	8 %
Dietary Fiber 1g	4 %
Sugars 10g	
Protein 3g	

Vitamin A 0%	•	Vitamin C 4%
Calcium 0%	•	Iron 4%

*Percent Daily Values are based on a 2,000 calorie diet.

Pour batter into prepared pan. Bake for 40–45 minutes, or until a toothpick inserted into the center comes out clean. Cover loosely with foil during the last 10 minutes of baking to prevent excessive browning on the top.

Allow bread to cool before slicing. Makes about 16 half-inch slices.

* This recipe was tested using Lighter Baker® by Sunsweet, a fruit puree fat replacement. Other brands of fruit-based fat replacement are available—they can be found in the baking section of grocery stores.

No-Oil Zucchini Bread

$1\frac{1}{2}$ cups sugar
$1\frac{1}{2}$ cups all-purpose flour
$1\frac{1}{2}$ cups whole-wheat flour
1 tsp salt
1 tsp baking powder
1 tsp baking soda
2 tsp cinnamon
$\frac{1}{2}$ tsp nutmeg

$\frac{1}{2}$ cup raisins
3 cups shredded zucchini
1 egg
2 egg whites
1 cup unsweetened applesauce
$\frac{1}{2}$ cup skim milk
2 tsp grated lemon rind
2 tsp vanilla extract

Preheat oven to 325 degrees. Grease and flour two 9 x 5-in loaf pans.

Combine dry ingredients and raisins in a bowl. Set aside.

Shred zucchini. Mix shredded zucchini, egg, applesauce, milk, lemon rind, and vanilla until well blended. Mix with dry ingredients.

Pour into loaf pans and bake for 1 hour or until knife inserted in center comes out clean. Allow to cool.

Nutrition Facts

Serving Size 1/2" slice
Servings Per Recipe 32

Amount Per Serving	
Calories 100	Calories from Fat 0

	% Daily Value*
Total Fat 0g	0 %
Saturated Fat 0g	0 %
Cholesterol 5mg	2 %
Sodium 135mg	6 %
Total Carbohydrate 21g	7 %
Dietary Fiber 1g	4 %
Sugars 11g	
Protein 2g	

Vitamin A 0%	•	Vitamin C 0%	
Calcium 2%	•	Iron 4%	

*Percent Daily Values are based on a 2,000 calorie diet.

To serve, slice each loaf into 16 $\frac{1}{2}$-in pieces. Wrap the unused portion tightly. For maximum freshness, may be stored in the freezer or refrigerator.

Cranberry Orange Muffins

1 cup cranberries, chopped
1 cup flour
1 cup rolled oats
¾ cup sugar
1½ tsp baking powder
1 tsp salt

½ tsp baking soda
1 tbsp grated orange rind
2 tbsp canola oil
¾ cup orange juice
1 egg

Preheat oven to 350 degrees. Line 12 muffin cups with paper or foil liners.

Wash cranberries and chop in food processor; set aside. Mix dry ingredients together in a bowl. Add orange rind, oil, juice, and beaten egg; stir until combined (do not beat). Fold in cranberries.

Fill muffin cups about ¾ full with batter. Bake for 20–30 minutes, until golden brown on top.

Makes 12 muffins.

Nutrition Facts

Serving Size 1 Muffin
Servings Per Recipe 12

Amount Per Serving	
Calories 150	Calories from Fat 30

	% Daily Value*
Total Fat 3.5g	5 %
Saturated Fat 0g	0 %
Cholesterol 20mg	7 %
Sodium 320mg	13 %
Total Carbohydrate 28g	9 %
Dietary Fiber 1g	4 %
Sugars 14g	
Protein 3g	

Vitamin A 4%	•	Vitamin C 15%
Calcium 4%	•	Iron 6%

*Percent Daily Values are based on a 2,000 calorie diet.

Raisin Bran Muffins

cooking spray
1 cup whole-wheat flour
1 cup all-purpose flour
½ cup rolled oats
¾ cup sugar
2½ tsp baking soda

½ tsp salt
4 cups raisin bran
2 cups low-fat buttermilk
¼ cup canola oil
4 egg whites

Preheat oven to 400 degrees. Spray a nonstick muffin pan with cooking spray; set aside. Stir together dry ingredients except raisin bran. In a separate bowl, whisk buttermilk, oil, and egg whites until smooth.

Stir in cereal and allow to soften for about 1 minute. Mix wet ingredients into dry, ⅓ at a time, stirring until just mixed each time. Fill muffin cups ⅔ of the way (use a scant ¼ cup batter per muffin).

Bake until golden, 15–20 minutes. Store extra batter in the refrigerator for up to 1 week.

Makes 24 muffins.

Nutrition Facts

Serving Size 1 Muffin
Servings Per Recipe 24

Amount Per Serving

Calories 130	Calories from Fat 25
	% Daily Value*
Total Fat 3g	5 %
Saturated Fat 0g	0 %
Cholesterol 0mg	0 %
Sodium 250mg	10 %
Total Carbohydrate 22g	7 %
Dietary Fiber 2g	8 %
Sugars 9g	
Protein 3g	

Vitamin A 0%	•	Vitamin C 0%
Calcium 4%	•	Iron 8%

*Percent Daily Values are based on a 2,000 calorie diet.

Mary's Morning Muffins

1¼ cups flour
1 tbsp baking powder
6 tbsp sugar
2 cups All-Bran cereal

1¼ cups skim milk
2 egg whites
3 tbsp canola oil
⅓ cup miniature chocolate chips

Preheat oven to 400 degrees. Line a 2½-inch muffin pan with 12 foil baking cups.

Stir together flour, baking powder, and sugar. Set aside.

Measure All-Bran cereal and milk into a mixing bowl. Stir to combine; let stand 1–2 minutes or until softened. Add egg whites and oil. Beat well.

Add dry ingredients to wet, stirring only until combined. Fold in minichips. Portion batter

Nutrition Facts

Serving Size 1 Muffin
Servings Per Recipe 12

Amount Per Serving

Calories 180	Calories from Fat 50
	% Daily Value*
Total Fat 5g	8 %
Saturated Fat 1g	5 %
Cholesterol 0mg	0 %
Sodium 210mg	9 %
Total Carbohydrate 29g	10 %
Dietary Fiber 4g	16 %
Sugars 12g	
Protein 5g	

Vitamin A 6%	•	Vitamin C 8%
Calcium 15%	•	Iron 15%

*Percent Daily Values are based on a 2,000 calorie diet.

evenly into baking cups. Bake for about 25 minutes or until muffins are golden brown.

These muffins freeze well. To defrost, microwave on high for 15 seconds after removing from foil cups.

Makes 12.

Corn Muffins

cooking spray
1 cup cornmeal
1 cup flour
2 tbsp sugar
3 tsp baking powder

½ tsp salt
2 tbsp canola oil
1 cup nonfat milk
2 egg whites
8 oz can creamed corn

Preheat oven to 425 degrees. Spray nonstick muffin tins with cooking spray. Combine dry ingredients. In a separate bowl, combine oil, milk, and egg whites. Beat until well blended. Stir in corn.

Stir together dry ingredients alternately with wet with a few swift strokes. Fill muffin tins ¾ full.

Bake for 20–25 minutes, or until golden on top.

Makes 12.

Nutrition Facts

Serving Size 1 Muffin
Servings Per Recipe 12

Amount Per Serving	
Calories 130	Calories from Fat 25

	% Daily Value*
Total Fat 2.5g	4 %
Saturated Fat 0g	0 %
Cholesterol 0mg	0 %
Sodium 240mg	10 %
Total Carbohydrate 22g	7 %
Dietary Fiber 1g	4 %
Sugars 3g	
Protein 4g	

Vitamin A 0%	•	Vitamin C 6%	
Calcium 10%	•	Iron 6%	

*Percent Daily Values are based on a 2,000 calorie diet.

Yummie Yogurt

8 oz nonfat plain yogur
1 tsp natural peanut butter
2 tsp honey
¼ cup bran cereal

Stir yogurt, peanut butter, and honey together until well blended. Mix in bran cereal or cereal of your choice. Enjoy!

Makes 1 serving.

Nutrition Facts
Serving Size 1 Cup
Servings Per Recipe 1

Amount Per Serving	
Calories 230	Calories from Fat 25

	% Daily Value*
Total Fat 2.5g	4 %
Saturated Fat 0g	0 %
Cholesterol 0mg	0 %
Sodium 230mg	10 %
Total Carbohydrate 39g	13 %
Dietary Fiber 2g	8 %
Sugars 27g	
Protein 13g	

Vitamin A 10%	•	Vitamin C 8%
Calcium 35%	•	Iron 15%

*Percent Daily Values are based on a 2,000 calorie diet.

Café Latte

8 oz skim milk
4 oz brewed espresso
ground cinnamon

If you're not a milk drinker, try this European coffee concoction instead!

Pour milk into a large coffee mug and heat in a microwave until very hot but not boiling, about 1½ minutes. If the milk boils, it will develop a skin on top, which should be removed. Whip warmed milk by hand with a small wire whisk until lightly frothed. Add espresso and stir. Top with ground cinnamon.

Serves 1.

Nutrition Facts
Serving Size 12 ounces
Servings Per Recipe 1

Amount Per Serving	
Calories 90	Calories from Fat 0

	% Daily Value*
Total Fat 0g	0 %
Saturated Fat 0g	0 %
Cholesterol 5mg	2 %
Sodium 130mg	6 %
Total Carbohydrate 13g	4 %
Dietary Fiber 0g	0 %
Sugars 11g	
Protein 9g	

Vitamin A 15%	•	Vitamin C 4%
Calcium 30%	•	Iron 2%

*Percent Daily Values are based on a 2,000 calorie diet.

Desserts

19

Desserts

Favorite Chocolate Chip Cake

2 tbsp finely ground walnuts
2 tbsp canola oil
¼ cup fruit-based fat replacement*
½ cup sugar
½ cup brown sugar
1 egg
2 egg whites

1 tsp vanilla extract
1 cup nonfat milk
2 cups all-purpose flour
1 tsp baking powder
1 tsp baking soda
½ tsp salt
1 cup miniature semisweet
   chocolate chips

Preheat oven to 350 degrees. Grease and flour a bundt pan or 9-in tube pan.

Place walnuts in a shallow baking pan and toast in the oven until lightly browned.

Combine next 8 ingredients in a bowl. Beat until smooth. Combine flour, baking powder, baking soda, and salt in a separate small bowl; mix until combined. Add flour mixture to first bowl, ⅓ at a time, mixing only until combined.

Nutrition Facts

Serving Size 1/12 of cake
Servings Per Recipe 12

Amount Per Serving	
Calories 250	Calories from Fat 50

	% Daily Value*
Total Fat 6g	9 %
Saturated Fat 1.5g	8 %
Cholesterol 20mg	7 %
Sodium 260mg	11 %
Total Carbohydrate 44g	15 %
Dietary Fiber 1g	4 %
Sugars 23g	
Protein 5g	

Vitamin A 0%	•	Vitamin C 0%	
Calcium 6%	•	Iron 8%	

*Percent Daily Values are based on a 2,000 calorie diet.

Fold in chocolate chips and walnuts. Pour batter into prepared baking pan.

Bake at 350 degrees for 45–50 minutes, or until a knife inserted in the center comes out clean. Do not overbake. Cool in pan for about 10 minutes. Loosen the edges of the cake with a knife and then transfer the cake to a baking rack to cool.

Serves 12.

*This recipe was tested using Lighter Bake® by Sunsweet.

Berries in Zinfandel

2 cups fresh strawberries or raspberries
2 tbsp sugar

6 oz white zinfandel wine
fresh mint

Toss berries and sugar together. Pour wine over berries. Let stand 1 hour then toss again, using care not to bruise the berries. Serve in chilled wineglasses with a sprig of fresh mint. Makes 4 servings, ½ cup each.

This recipe works nicely with either wine, champagne, or non-alcoholic champagne.

Nutrition Facts

Serving Size 1/2 cuo
Servings Per Recipe 4

Amount Per Serving

Calories 60	Calories from Fat 0

	% Daily Value*
Total Fat 0g	0 %
Saturated Fat 0g	0 %
Cholesterol 0mg	0 %
Sodium 0mg	0 %
Total Carbohydrate 14g	5 %
Dietary Fiber 4g	16 %
Sugars 12g	
Protein 1g	

Vitamin A 0%	•	Vitamin C 25%
Calcium 0%	•	Iron 2%

*Percent Daily Values are based on a 2,000 calorie diet.

Fruit Kabobs

1 cup cubed honeydew melon
1 cup cubed cantaloupe
1 cup halved strawberries
8 oz can pineapple chunks in juice
½ cup seedless green grapes

pineapple juice from
  canned chunks
2 tbsp frozen orange juice
  concentrate

Thread fruit onto 12-in wooden skewers, alternating types of fruits as you go along.

Mix pineapple juice with orange juice concentrate.

Drizzle juice over kabobs. Makes 8.

You can substitute other fruits depending on availability; the key to this recipe is having a variety of colors.

Nutrition Facts	
Serving Size 1 Kabob	
Servings Per Recipe 8	
Amount Per Serving	
Calories 60	Calories from Fat 0
	% Daily Value*
Total Fat 0g	0 %
Saturated Fat 0g	0 %
Cholesterol 0mg	0 %
Sodium 0mg	0 %
Total Carbohydrate 13g	4 %
Dietary Fiber 1g	4 %
Sugars 11g	
Protein 1g	
Vitamin A 6% • Vitamin C 60%	
Calcium 0% • Iron 0%	
*Percent Daily Values are based on a 2,000 calorie diet.	

Cranberry Baked Apples

3 baking apples
¾ cup chopped cranberries
1 tsp grated orange peel

1 tsp cinnamon
6 tbsp maple syrup
vanilla yogurt

Preheat oven to 350 degrees. Choose a baking apple such as Rome or Granny Smith.

Cut apples in half across the middle (top and bottom halves). Remove seeds and cores. Place in baking dish. Pour ½ cup water into the bottom of the baking dish around the apples.

Chop cranberries finely in a food processor. Mix together cranberries, orange peel, and cinnamon. Top each apple half with about 2 tablespoons of cranberry mixture. Drizzle 1 tablespoon maple syrup over each apple half. Bake for 30–40 minutes, or until apples are tender (baking time will vary according to the variety of apple you use). Serve warm with a dollop of low-fat vanilla yogurt, if desired. Makes 6 servings, one-half apple each.

Nutrition Facts

Serving Size 1/2 apple
Servings Per Recipe 6

Amount Per Serving

Calories 100	Calories from Fat 0

	% Daily Value*
Total Fat 0g	0 %
Saturated Fat 0g	0 %
Cholesterol 0mg	0 %
Sodium 0mg	0 %
Total Carbohydrate 25g	8 %
Dietary Fiber 3g	12 %
Sugars 21g	
Protein 0g	

Vitamin A 0%	•	Vitamin C 10%
Calcium 4%	•	Iron 2%

*Percent Daily Values are based on a 2,000 calorie diet.

Chocolate Raspberry Cake

1½ cups flour
1 cup sugar
3 tbsp baking cocoa
1 tsp baking soda
½ tsp salt

3 tbsp canola oil
2 tbsp raspberry vinegar
1 tsp vanilla extract
1 cup water

Preheat oven to 350 degrees. In an 8 x 8-in pan, combine flour, sugar, cocoa, baking soda, and salt. Mix well; then make 3 wells (holes) in the mixture. Measure oil into one well, vinegar into the next, and vanilla into the third. Pour in water. Stir until thoroughly mixed (do not beat or overmix). Bake for 30–35 minutes, or until edges start to pull

Nutrition Facts

Serving Size 1/16 cake
Servings Per Recipe 16

Amount Per Serving

Calories 110	Calories from Fat 25

	% Daily Value*
Total Fat 2.5g	4 %
Saturated Fat 0g	0 %
Cholesterol 0mg	0 %
Sodium 150mg	6 %
Total Carbohydrate 21g	7 %
Dietary Fiber 0g	0 %
Sugars 12g	
Protein 1g	

Vitamin A 0%	•	Vitamin C 0%
Calcium 0%	•	Iron 2%

*Percent Daily Values are based on a 2,000 calorie diet.

away from the pan and a toothpick inserted into the center comes out clean.

Cool and cut into 2-in squares. Dust with powdered sugar if desired.

Makes 16 pieces.

Ice Box Cake

9½ low-fat graham crackers (5 in. long)   1 1.4-oz box vanilla fat/
1 1.4-oz box chocolate fat/sugar-free   sugar-free pudding mix
    pudding mix   3½ cups nonfat milk

You can select devil's food or chocolate fudge instead of plain chocolate and white chocolate instead of vanilla, or choose flavors that are altogether different. You can also substitute the plain fat-free mixes if you don't care to use artificial sweeteners, although the calories will be higher.

Lay 4½ crackers in a flat layer in the bottom of a 9-in square pan. Prepare the vanilla pudding mix using 1¾ cups milk. Pour over crackers and let stand for a minute or two to set.

Layer another 4½ crackers over the first layer of pudding and then prepare the chocolate pudding mix with the remaining 1¾ cups of milk. Pour over the first layer of pudding and crackers.

Crush the remaining ½ graham cracker into crumbs and sprinkle over the top layer of pudding.

Let chill for several hours until pudding has set and graham crackers have softened.

Makes 9 3 x 3-in pieces.

Nutrition Facts		
Serving Size 3" x 3" piece		
Servings Per Recipe 9		
Amount Per Serving		
Calories 120	Calories from Fat 10	
		% Daily Value*
Total Fat 1g		2 %
Saturated Fat 0g		0 %
Cholesterol 0mg		0 %
Sodium 150mg		6 %
Total Carbohydrate 25g		8 %
Dietary Fiber 0g		0 %
Sugars 9g		
Protein 4g		
Vitamin A 0%	•	Vitamin C 0%
Calcium 10%	•	Iron 4%
*Percent Daily Values are based on a 2,000 calorie diet.		

Bread Pudding

3 cinnamon raisin English muffins, stale
1½ cups nonfat milk
1 egg
2 egg whites
¼ cup honey

2 tsp vanilla extract
⅛ tsp nutmeg
½ tsp grated orange peel
vanilla yogurt (optional)

Preheat oven to 350 degrees. Cut stale or lightly toasted English muffins into ½-in cubes. Place in the bottom of a 1½-qt baking dish. If you don't have English muffins handy, substitute 3 cups of cubed raisin bread.

Mix together remaining ingredients, beating until honey is well dissolved. Pour over muffin or bread cubes, thoroughly saturating all of the cubes.

Bake for 40–45 minutes, or until a knife inserted in the center comes out clean.

Makes 6 servings, about half-cup each. Serve plain or topped with a spoonful of vanilla yogurt.

Nutrition Facts

Serving Size 1/2 cup
Servings Per Recipe 6

Amount Per Serving

Calories 160   Calories from Fat 15

	% Daily Value*
Total Fat 2g	3 %
Saturated Fat 0g	0 %
Cholesterol 35mg	12 %
Sodium 190mg	8 %
Total Carbohydrate 29g	10 %
Dietary Fiber 0g	0 %
Sugars 14g	
Protein 6g	

Vitamin A 6%	•	Vitamin C	0%
Calcium 10%	•	Iron	4%

*Percent Daily Values are based on a 2,000 calorie diet.

Raspberry Topping

1 cup apple juice
2 tsp sugar-free raspberry gelatin mix

1 cup frozen raspberries, unsweetened

Heat apple juice to boiling. Stir in gelatin mix until fully dissolved. Combine juice, gelatin, and raspberries in a blender and blend until smooth.

Strain mixture through a sieve to remove seeds. Chill well. Mixture will thicken, so stir well before using to loosen the sauce.

Serve over angel food cake, fresh fruit, or frozen yogurt.

Store in the refrigerator. Makes about 1¼ cups, or 10 2-tbsp servings.

Nutrition Facts

Serving Size 2 Tbsp
Servings Per Recipe 10

Amount Per Serving

Calories 20	Calories from Fat 0

	% Daily Value*
Total Fat 0g	0 %
Saturated Fat 0g	0 %
Cholesterol 0mg	0 %
Sodium 0mg	0 %
Total Carbohydrate 4g	1 %
Dietary Fiber 1g	4 %
Sugars 4g	
Protein 0g	

Vitamin A 0%	•	Vitamin C 20%
Calcium 0%	•	Iron 0%

*Percent Daily Values are based on a 2,000 calorie diet.

APPENDIX I

Information for Your Doctor

If you are interested in starting to take one of the prescription medications, you need to discuss your decision with your doctor. For some physicians, the use of diet drugs for weight control is part of their regular practice. However, some doctors may have less experience using diet drugs or may not be familiar with all of the information from the latest studies. This appendix was written with that in mind. I have written an open letter to your doctor to introduce myself and the concepts of this book. Copy this section and give it to your doctor. Be sure to include Table I.1. He or she may find this information helpful in treating your weight problem.

Dear Doctor:

Your patient is interested in taking medication for weight loss. I usually consider patients candidates for diet medication if they have not been successful at losing and maintaining weight loss with standard techniques—diet, exercise, and behavior modification, and have a BMI>30.

$$\text{Body Mass Index (BMI)} = \frac{\text{weight (kg)}}{\text{height (meters)}^2}$$

For your convenience in determining the BMI of your patient, see the accompanying table.

The indication for diet medication is even more imperative in women with a waist circumference >35 inches and in men with waist circumference >40 inches. People exceeding these measurements have been demonstrated to develop coronary artery disease, diabetes, hyperlipidemia, and many other obesity-related health risks including death at a higher incidence than people with a normal waist circumference.

If your patient already has one or more complications of obesity, many experts, including myself, would initiate diet medication if his or her BMI is >27. In general, the risks involved with taking diet drugs are less than those associated with remaining obese.

Of course, the decision to prescribe antiobesity drugs is yours alone. Some physicians have avoided using diet drugs since the problems associated with fenfluramine (Pondomin and Redux) were uncovered. There is no convincing evidence, however, that any of the drugs currently available for the treatment of obesity cause valvular heart disease or pulmonary hypertension. Other physicians have limited experience with diet medications and are, therefore, reluctant to use them. For those individuals, I have written an overview of the dietary program found in my book, *The Complete Book of Diet Drugs.* I explain indications and contraindications for using antiobesity drugs, outline specific dosing schedules, make recommendations for length of treatment, and offer guidelines for maintenance therapy. I suggest methods for monitoring your patients, provide information on the possible side effects associated with the drugs, and list selected references for further reading.

Now that relatively safe and effective drug regimens are

available for weight control, many physicians have found that using these drugs has substantially improved the lives of their patients. We still have useful tools (some old, some new) for treating what has been one of the most vexing problems we physicians see on a daily basis.

Sincerely yours,
STEVEN R. PEIKIN, MD

Professor of Medicine
Head, Division of Gastroenterology and Liver Diseases
Cooper Hospital/University Medical Center
Robert Wood Johnson Medical School at Camden
University of Medicine and Dentistry of New Jersey

Basic Principles of Prescribing Diet Medication

Pharmacologic management of obesity should always be used in conjunction with the conventional treatments of calorie reduction, behavior modification, and exercise. *The Complete Book of Diet Drugs* includes a detailed, comprehensive regimen for your patient in all three categories. You may prefer to give your patient your own diet and exercise guidelines or modify my recommendations. Although *The Complete Book of Diet Drugs* attempts to individualize treatment as best as possible, nothing can compare to the care given with a one-on-one doctor/patient relationship. Here is a summary of the conventional treatment used in *The Complete Book of Diet Drugs*.

Low-Calorie Diet

By individualizing calorie restriction, most participants on this program should have a calorie deficit of 500 to 1,000 calories per day (the calorie range of daily meal plans is 1,200 to 1,500 calories). This should result in a weight loss of 1 to 2 pounds per week (a deficit of 500 calories per day yields 3,500 calories a week, equaling approximately 1 pound of weight lost).

In order to calculate a daily calorie prescription, take the patient's weight in pounds and multiply the number by 13. Next subtract 500 if you want the patient to lose 1 pound per week or 1,000 if the goal is to lose 2 pounds per week (a safe rate of weight loss is 1 percent of body weight per week); if for example, a 160-pound woman wants to lose 1 pound per week, 160 x 13 = 2,080 - 500 = 1,580 calories per day.

The diet is balanced and based on the American Dietetic Association Exchange List for Meal Planning, with a macronutrient distribution of approximately 25–30 percent of calories from fat, 12–15 percent from protein and 55–63 percent from carbohydrates. The plan also includes 25–30 grams of fiber per day. The meal plans encourage people to eat cruciferous vegetables and fruit. The original recipes, designed by a registered dietitian, limit the use of saturated fats but include monounsaturated fats and fish oil. A vitamin and mineral supplement is recommended, especially for individuals receiving fewer than 1,500 calories per day and for those individuals using Xenical™ (orlistat).

Behavioral Modification

Standard techniques to modify eating behavior based on operant conditioning are suggested (e.g., eat only at a table set for dining; don't do anything else while you are eating, etc.). People are instructed to keep a record of their daily food intake. I also stress the importance of eating more of the right foods as well as eating less of the wrong ones. Tasty, nutritious snacks are recommended to replace standard calorie and fat-laden snacks.

Exercise

Several exercise options designed by a professor of exercise physiology are recommended in *The Complete Book of Diet Drugs*. Readers are advised to exercise at least three times a week for a minimum of 15–20 minutes at a time. Effort is graded and monitoring the pulse rate is recommended to avoid overexertion. Those over 45 years old and/or those who have risk factors for coronary artery disease are told to seek the guidance of a physician before commencing the exercise module.

Drug Therapy

As I mentioned in the cover letter, candidates for anti-obesity drug treatment should have a BMI>30 or BMI>27 if they have one or more health risks associated with obesity (see Table I.1).

Table I.1
How to Determine BMI

Height (Feet/Inches)

Weight (Pounds)	5'0"	5'1"	5'2"	5'3"	5'4"	5'5"	5'6"	5'7"	5'8"	5'9"	5'10"	5'11"	6'0"	6'1"	6'2"	6'3"	6'4"
100	20	19	18	18	17	17	16	16	15	15	14	14	14	13	13	12	12
105	21	20	19	19	18	17	17	16	16	16	15	15	14	14	13	13	13
110	21	21	20	19	19	18	18	17	17	16	16	15	15	15	14	14	13
115	22	22	21	20	20	19	19	18	17	17	17	16	16	15	15	14	14
120	23	23	22	21	21	20	19	19	18	18	17	17	16	16	15	15	15
125	24	24	23	22	21	21	20	20	19	18	18	17	17	16	16	16	15
130	25	25	24	23	22	22	21	20	20	19	19	18	18	17	17	16	16
135	26	26	25	24	23	22	22	21	21	20	19	19	18	18	17	17	16
140	27	26	26	25	24	23	23	22	21	21	20	20	19	18	18	17	17
145	28	27	27	26	25	24	23	23	22	21	21	20	20	19	19	18	18
150	29	28	27	27	26	25	24	23	23	22	22	21	20	20	19	19	18
155	30	29	28	27	27	26	25	24	24	23	22	22	21	20	20	19	19
160	31	30	29	28	27	27	26	25	24	24	23	22	22	21	21	20	19

Table I.1 (Cont.)
How to Determine BMI

Height (Feet/Inches)

Weight (Pounds)	5'0"	5'1"	5'2"	5'3"	5'4"	5'5"	5'6"	5'7"	5'8"	5'9"	5'10"	5'11"	6'0"	6'1"	6'2"	6'3"	6'4"
165	32	31	30	29	28	27	27	26	25	24	24	23	22	22	21	21	20
170	33	32	31	30	29	28	27	27	26	25	24	24	23	22	22	21	21
175	34	33	32	31	30	29	28	27	27	26	25	24	24	23	22	22	21
180	35	34	33	32	31	30	29	28	27	27	26	25	24	24	23	22	22
185	36	35	34	33	32	31	30	29	28	27	27	26	25	24	24	23	23
190	37	36	35	34	33	32	31	30	29	28	27	26	26	25	24	24	23
195	38	37	36	35	33	32	31	31	30	29	28	27	26	26	25	24	24
200	39	38	37	35	34	33	32	31	30	30	29	28	27	26	26	25	24
205	40	39	37	36	35	34	33	32	31	30	29	29	28	27	26	26	25
210	41	40	38	37	36	35	34	33	32	31	30	29	28	28	27	26	26
215	42	41	39	38	37	36	35	34	33	32	31	30	29	28	28	27	26
220	43	42	40	39	38	37	36	34	33	32	32	31	30	29	28	27	27
225	44	43	41	40	39	37	36	35	34	33	32	31	31	30	29	28	27
230	45	43	42	41	39	38	37	36	35	34	33	32	31	30	30	29	28
235	46	44	43	42	40	39	38	37	36	35	34	33	32	31	30	29	29
240	47	45	44	43	41	40	39	38	36	35	34	33	33	32	31	30	29
245	48	46	45	43	42	41	40	38	37	36	35	34	33	32	31	31	30
250	49	47	46	44	43	42	40	39	38	37	36	35	34	33	32	31	30
260	51	49	48	46	45	43	42	41	40	38	37	36	35	34	33	32	32
265	52	50	48	47	45	44	43	42	40	39	38	37	36	35	34	33	32
270	53	51	49	4	46	45	44	42	41	40	39	38	37	36	35	34	33
275	54	52	50	49	47	46	44	43	42	41	39	38	37	36	35	34	33
280	55	53	51	50	48	47	45	44	43	41	40	39	38	37	36	35	34
285	56	54	52	50	48	47	46	45	43	42	41	40	39	38	37	36	35
290	57	55	53	51	50	48	47	45	44	43	42	40	39	38	37	36	35
295	58	56	54	52	51	49	48	46	45	44	42	41	40	39	38	37	36
300	59	57	55	53	51	50	48	47	46	44	43	42	41	40	39	37	37
305	60	58	56	54	52	51	49	48	46	45	44	43	41	40	39	38	37
310	61	59	57	55	53	52	50	49	47	46	44	43	42	41	40	39	38
315	62	60	58	56	54	52	51	49	48	47	45	44	43	42	40	39	38
320	62	60	59	57	55	53	52	50	49	47	46	45	43	42	41	40	39
325	63	61	59	58	56	54	52	51	49	48	47	45	44	43	42	41	40

Table I.1 (Cont.)
How to Determine BMI

Height (Feet/Inches)

Weight (Pounds)	5'0"	5'1"	5'2"	5'3"	5'4"	5'5"	5'6"	5'7"	5'8"	5'9"	5'10"	5'11"	6'0"	6'1"	6'2"	6'3"	6'4"
330	64	62	60	58	57	55	53	52	50	49	47	46	45	44	42	41	40
335	65	63	61	59	58	56	54	52	51	49	48	47	45	44	43	42	41
340	66	64	62	60	58	57	55	56	52	50	49	47	46	45	44	42	41
345	676	5	63	61	59	57	56	54	52	51	50	48	47	46	44	43	42
350	68	66	64	62	60	58	56	55	53	52	50	49	47	46	45	44	43
355	69	67	65	63	61	59	57	56	54	52	51	50	48	47	46	44	43
360	70	68	66	64	62	60	58	56	55	53	52	50	49	47	46	45	44
365	71	69	67	65	63	61	59	57	55	54	52	51	50	48	47	46	44
370	72	70	68	66	64	62	60	58	56	55	53	52	50	49	48	46	45
375	73	71	69	66	64	62	61	59	57	55	54	52	51	49	48	47	46
380	74	72	70	67	65	63	61	60	58	56	55	53	52	50	49	47	46
385	75	73	70	68	66	64	62	60	58	57	55	56	52	51	49	48	47
390	76	74	71	69	67	65	62	61	59	58	56	54	53	51	50	49	47
395	77	75	72	70	68	66	64	62	60	58	57	55	54	52	51	49	48
400	78	76	73	71	69	67	65	63	61	59	57	56	54	53	51	50	49

For individuals not covered by this table, calculate BMI by converting pounds to kilograms (1 pound = 0.45 kilogram) and inches to meters (1 inch = .0254 meter). The equation for BMI is weight (in kilograms) divided by height (in meters) squared [kg/m2]. Source: *Shape Up America!*, 6707 Democracy Blvd., Suite 107, Bethesda, MD 20817.

Table 1.2 lists contraindications to diet medication.

Table I.2
Absolute Contraindications to Diet Drugs

Pregnancy	Concurrent use of MAO inhibitors or lithium*
Lactation	Development of primary pulmonary hypertension
Severe psychosis	Known allergy to specific diet drug
Anorexia nervosa	Severe uncontrolled hypertension*
Alcoholism	Heart, kidney or liver failure
Drug abuse	Concurrent use of migraine medication (sumatriptan, dehydroergotamine)*

Relative Contraindications to Diet Drugs

Poorly controlled hypertension*	Cardiac arrhythmia*
Glaucoma*	Symptomatic coronary artery disease*
Depression*	Concurrent use of serotonin selective reuptake
Anticipated surgery (should discontinue	inhibitors (Prozac™, Effexor™, Paxil™)*
drugs two weeks prior to surgery)*	

*Only contraindicated for use with Meridia™, phentermine, and related sympath-omimetic drugs (see Chapter 5). Xenical™ can still be used.

Drugs can effect weight loss by suppressing appetite, stimulating satiety, inducing thermogenesis or by impairing absorption of dietary nutrients. To date, the main mechanism of action for all over-the-counter and doctor-prescribed, prescription anti-obesity medication, is appetite suppression and stimulation of satiety. The only exception is Xenical™ (orlistat), a drug that works by interfering with the absorption of dietary fat.

Table I.3 outlines information for prescribing currently used diet drugs. With the exception of Prozac™ (fenfluramine), a specific serotonergic reuptake inhibitor (SSRI), and Xenical™ (orlistat), a carboxylipase inhibitor, most diet medications fall under the class called sympathomimetics. While this class of drug is derived from the amphetamines, they have fewer side effects and are not addictive to any significant degree. Meridia™ (Sibutramine) is a special class of drug that has both serotonergic and sympathomimetic properties (specific serotonin and norepinephrine reuptake inhibitor or SNRI). Effexor™ (Venlafaxine) also has both serotonergic and sympathomimetic properties but the drug only weakly prevents the reuptake of norepinephrine compared to sibutramine. The most commonly used drugs are phenylpropanolamine (OTC), phentermine, sibutramine and orlistat.

Table I.3
Currently Used Diet Drugs

Name	Brand Name	Dosing Range (mg/day)	Starting Dose	Usual Dose	DEA Generic Schedule
Over-The-Counter					
Phenylpropanolamine	Dexatrim™ Acutrim™	75	75 mg	75 mg/day	NA
Prescription					
Phentermine	Ionomin™	15–30	15 mg/day in A.M	30 mg/day. in A.M	IV
	Fastin™	15–30	or		
	Adipex-P™	½ tab –37.5	½ Adipex-P in A.M.	37.5 mg/day in A.M.	IV
Mazindol	Mazinor™ Sanorex™	1–3	1 mg/day before lunch	2 mg/day before lunch	IV
Diethylproprion	Tenuate™	75	25 mg* 1 hr before meals	25 mg 1 hr before meals	IV
Sibutramine	Meridia™	10–15	10 mg/day in A.M.	10–15 mg/day in A.M.	IV
Orlistat	Xenical™	360	120 mg with each meal	120 mg with each meal	NA
Fluoxetine**	Prozac™	20–60	20 mg with breakfast	20 mg at breakfast and dinner	NA
Venlafaxine**	Effexor™	75–225	25 mg with meals	25 mg with meals	NA

* or 75mg sustained release in the morning.

** Not approved by the FDA for weight loss.

There are two major reasons why a combination of drugs may be useful. If monotherapy is not effective, adding a second drug with a different mechanism of action may increase efficacy. If monotherapy is effective but associated with troubling side effects, then the addition of another agent may permit a lower dose of the initial drug used. While drug combination therapy became popular with the phen/fen regimen, there is no convincing evidence that combinations of the drugs listed in Table I.3 work better than single-agent therapy for obesity. Studies using combinations of drugs (e.g., Xenical™ plus Meridia™) are under way, and new treatment options may be available in the future. I do not recommend any prescription drug combinations at this point.

Depending on your patient's initial starting weight, motivation, ability to exercise, and so forth, the goal of treatment will be either partial weight loss in order to treat or prevent obesity-related risk factors or the achievement of ideal body weight. The former goal is more realistic for most of your patients. Unless a person has a coexisting condition, such as diabetes, in addition to being overweight, it is not necessary to order routine laboratory work while your patient is taking antiobesity drugs. Monthly office visits during the first three months of treatment are recommended for monitoring vital signs and assessing drug side effects. If the patient is tolerating the drug well, less frequent visits may suffice. If a patient does not lose at least 4 pounds in the first month of treatment, the drug will probably not be effective in the long term either. Another drug class should be prescribed (e.g., switch from Meridia™ to Xenical™ or vice versa). Table I.4 outlines the management of obese patients in a weight loss drug program.

Table I.4
Managing Obese Patients*

Initial visit	Three months
Diet history	Evaluate response to treatment
Risk Assessment	Evaluate for side effects
-Age at onset of obesity	Brief exam
-BMI	Adjust plan
-Waist circumference	*Six months*
-Weight-related comorbidity	Most weight is lost

Complete physical exam	Same evaluation as before
Laboratory work and EKG (if indicated)	*Nine months*
Decide on treatment modality	Weight maintenance check
One month	Same evaluation as before
Evaluate response to treatment (weigh in)	*Twelve months*
Evaluate for side effects including decrease in	Weight maintenance check
exercise tolerance and shortness of breath	Same evaluation as before
Vital signs	
Adjust plan	

* Your patients will have more success if they can speak weekly with health care providers (e.g., dietitian, nurse, physician), and come in for regular weight checks. Using a diet diary may also be helpful.

After your patient achieves his or her goal weight, the next step is maintenance. Weight maintenance is the biggest stumbling block to a successful diet program. Although lifestyle changes are reinforced throughout the period of active weight loss, few people are able to change their eating behavior on a permanent basis. Furthermore, if drug therapy is discontinued, the majority of people will begin to regain their weight. This situation is no different with hypertensive or diabetic patients after cessation of treatment. Therefore, weight maintenance will be more successful if drug treatment is continued. Although some drugs are approved for only 3 months of treatment (e.g., phentermine), Meridia™ is approved for 1 year and Xenical™ is approved for 2 years. The drugs seem to work for as long as they are given (doses may need to be increased in some patients). The exception to this rule is Prozac™ (fluoxetine). With this drug, weight gain may occur after 6 months despite continuation of therapy.

We physicians prescribe many drugs beyond the FDA-recommended time period (e.g., omeprazole). This time limit means there is limited safety data submitted to the FDA beyond a certain length of treatment. It does not necessarily mean the drug is not safe to take in the long term. You will need to determine your own comfort level regarding length of treatment.

It is reasonable to stop medication after achieving the goal weight. Some patients are able to maintain their weight loss despite cessation of therapy, especially if they exercise frequently. If your patient gains more than 10 pounds above their goal weight, however, it is reasonable to restart drug therapy. In my opinion, it makes no sense to allow your patient to regain all the weight before starting drug treatment again. Consult Table I.5 for drug treatment options for weight maintenance.

Table I.5
Drug Treatment Options for Weight Maintenance

1. Continue same drug at same dose given for active weight loss.
2. Continue same drug at a lower dose than that required for active weight loss (step-down approach).
3. Give drug at the same dose or lower dose every other day.
4. Intermittent use of medication (drug holiday approach).

There are advantages and disadvantages to each of these approaches. As you might expect, Approach 1 is likely to be the most efficacious but not the safest. Approaches 2 and 3 make a lot of sense as long as they work. In some patients, the dose of medication needed to maintain weight loss will be the same dose needed to induce weight loss. Approach 4 may be the safest but it may not be as well tolerated by the patient. In this case, weight will tend to fluctuate more. More importantly, the patient may need to constantly re-acclimate to any side effects of the drug.

Table I.6 lists the more common diet drug side effects. For a more detailed list, consult your *PDR*. Since the above information is not meant to be a comprehensive review of the pharmacologic management of obesity, I encourage you to take a CME course on this topic and do further reading. For your convenience, I have listed selected references pertaining to drug therapy for obesity.

Table I.6
Potential Diet Drug Side Effects*

Body System	Symphathomimetics (e.g., phentermine)	SSRI/SNRI (e.g., Prozac™, Effexor™, Meridia™)	Lipas Inhibitor (e.g., Xenical™)
Neurologic	Stimulation	Insomnia	
	Restlessness	Nervousness	
	Sleep disturbance	Fatigue	
	Headache	Headache	
	Fatigue, drowsiness	Anxiety	
	Blurred vision	Tremor	
	Tremor	Dizziness	
Heart/Lung	Palpitations (fluttering feeling in chest)	Fast heart rate	
	Fast heart rate	High blood pressure	
	High blood pressure		
Digestive	Dry mouth	Dry mouth	Oily spotting
	Nausea	Nausea	Flatus with discharge
	Constipation	Constipation	Fatty/oily stool
	Diarrhea		Increased defecation

*Partial list.

Suggested Reading for Your Doctor

Crandall, C. "Managing obesity with drug therapy," pp. 37–60. *Internal Medicine,* Vol. 18, Jul. 1997.

Hollander, P., Elbein, S.C., Hirsch, I.B., et al. "Role of orlistat in the treatment of obese patients with type 2 diabetes," pp. 1288–1294. *Diabetes Care,* Vol. 21, No. 8, Aug. 1998.

Mantzoros, C.S. "The role of leptin in human obesity and disease: A review of current evidence," pp. 671–680. *Annals of Internal Medicine,* Vol. 130, No. 8, Apr. 1999.

McNeely, W., Benfield, P. "Orlistat," pp. 242–250. *New Drugs Profile,* Aug. 1998.

National Task Force on the Prevention and Treatment of Obesity. "Long-term pharmacotherapy in the management of obesity," pp. 1907–1915. *Pharmacotherapy for Obesity,* Vol. 276, No. 23, Dec. 1996.

North American Association for the Study of Obesity, *Obesity Research,* Vol. 6, Supp. 2, Sept. 1998.

North American Association for the Study of Obesity, *Obesity Research*, Vol. 7, No. 2, Mar. 1999.

North American Association for the Study of Obesity, *Obesity Research,* Vol. 7, No. 4, Jul. 1999.

Railey, M.T. "Evaluation and Treatment of Obesity," *Primary Care Reports,* Vol. 3, No. 14, Jul. 1997.

Shiffman, M. L., Kaplan, G. D., Brinkman-Kaplan, V., et al. "Prophylaxis against gallstone formation with ursodeoxycholic acid in patients participating in a very-low-calorie diet program," pp. 899–905. *Annals Intern Medicine,* 122, 1995.

Silverstone, T. "Clinical use of appetite suppressants," pp. 151–167. *Drug and Alcohol Dependence,* Vol. 17, 1986.

Sjostrom, L., Rissanen, A., Andersen, T., et al. "Randomized placebo-controlled trial of orlistat for weight loss and prevention of weight regain in obese patients," pp. 167–172. *The Lancet,* Vol. 352, No. 9123, July 1998.

World Health Organization, "Preventing and Managing the Global Epidemic," *Obesity,* June 1997.

APPENDIX II

Maintenance Meal Plans Based on the American Dietetic Association Exchange Lists for Meal Planning

Our maintenance meal plans are based on the American Dietetic Association Exchange Lists for meal planning. Exchange Lists are foods listed together because they are alike. Each serving of a food has about the same amount of carbohydrate, protein, fat, and number of calories as the other foods on that list. Any food on a list can be "exchanged" or traded for any other foods on that list. For example, you can trade the slice of bread you might eat for breakfast for one-half cup of cooked cereal. Each of these foods equals one starch choice.

Our meal plans list how many exchanges you are allowed for each meal. You look up the portion sizes using the lists in this Appendix. For instance, if you are allowed to have one fruit exchange at snack time, you refer to the fruit list and choose one of any fruit in the portion listed, such as one-half cup of unsweetened applesauce. If you were allowed to have two fruit exchanges, you could choose two different fruits or a double portion of one. All of our meal plans include examples to help illustrate use of the exchanges. While this system may take a little planning in the beginning, using the food exchanges will become second nature to you in a short time.

Exchange Lists for Meal Planning

STARCH LIST

Cereals, grains, pasta, breads, crackers, snacks, starchy vegetables, and cooked dried beans, peas, and lentils are starches. In general, one starch is:

- ½ cup of cereal, grain, pasta, or starchy vegetable,
- 1 ounce of a bread product, such as 1 slice of bread,
- ¾ to 1 ounce of most snack foods. (Some snack foods may also have added fat.)

Nutrition Tips

1. Most starch choices are good sources of B vitamins.
2. Foods made from whole grains are good sources of fiber.
3. Dried beans and peas are a good source of protein and fiber.

Selection Tips

1. Choose starches made with little fat as often as you can.
2. Starchy vegetables prepared with fat count as one starch and one fat.
3. Bagels or muffins can be 2, 3, or 4 ounces in size, and can, therefore, count as 2, 3, or 4 starch choices. Check the size you eat.

4. Dried beans, peas, and lentils are also found on the Meat and Meat Substitutes list.

5. Regular potato chips and tortilla chips are found on the Other Carbohydrates list.

6. Most of the serving sizes are measured after cooking.

7. Always check Nutrition Facts on the food label.

The Exchange Lists are the basis of a meal planning system designed by a committee of the American Diabetics Association and The American Dietetic Association. While designed primarily for people with diabetes and others who must follow special diets, the Exchange Lists are based on principles of good nutrition that apply to everyone. © 1995 American Diabetes Association Inc., The American Dietetic Association.

One Starch Exchange Equals
15 grams carbohydrate, 3 grams protein, 0–1 gram fat, and 80 calories.

Bread

Bagel	½ (1 oz)	Pita, 6 in across	½
Bread, reduced-calorie	2 slices (1½ oz)	Roll, plain, small	1 (1 oz)
Bread, white, whole-wheat, pumpernickel, rye	1 slice (1 oz)	Raisin bread, unfrosted	1 slice (1 oz)
Bread sticks, crisp, 4 in long x ½ in	2 (⅔ oz)	Tortilla, corn, 6 in across	1
English muffin	½	Tortilla, flour, 7–8 in across	1
Hot dog or hamburger bun	½ (1 oz)	Waffle, 4½-in square, reduced-fat	1

Cereals and Grains

Bran cereals	½ cup	Millet	¼ cup
Bulgur	½ cup	Muesli	¼ cup
Cereals	½ cup	Oats	½ cup
Cereals, unsweetened, ready-to-eat	¾ cup	Pasta	½ cup
Cornmeal (dry)	3 tbsp	Puffed cereal	1½ cups
Couscous	⅓ cup	Rice milk	½ cup
Flour (dry)	3 tbsp	Rice, white or brown	⅓ cup
Granola, low-fat	¼ cup	Shredded Wheat	½ cup
Grape-Nuts	¼ cup	Sugar-frosted cereal	½ cup
Grits	½ cup	Wheat germ	3 tbsp
Kasha	½ cup		

One Starch Exchange Equals

15 grams carbohydrate, 3 grams protein, 0–1 gram fat, and 80 calories.

Starchy Vegetables

Baked beans	⅓ cup	Plantain	½ cup
Corn	½ cup	Potato, baked or boiled	1 small (3 oz)
Corn on cob, medium	1 (5 oz)	Potato, mashed	½ cup
Mixed vegetables with corn, peas, or pasta	1 cup	Squash, winter (acorn, butternut)	1 cup
Peas, green	½ cup	Yam, sweet potato, plain	½ cup

Crackers and Snacks

Animal crackers	8	Popcorn (popped, no fat added or low-fat microwave)	3 cups
Graham crackers, 2½-in square	3		
Matzoh	¾ oz	Pretzels	¾ oz
Melba toast	4 slices	Rice cakes, 4 in across	2
Oyster crackers	24	Whole-wheat crackers, no fat added	2–5 (¾ oz)
Saltine-type crackers	6		
Snack chips, fat-free (tortilla, potato)	15–20 (¾ oz)		

Dried Beans, Peas, and Lentils

(Count as 1 starch exchange, plus 1 very lean meat exchange.)

Beans and peas (garbanzo, pinto, kidney, white, split, black-eyed)	½ cup	Lentils	½ cup
Lima beans	⅔ cup	Miso♦	3 tbsp

♦ = 400 mg or more of sodium per serving.

One Starch Exchange Equals

15 grams carbohydrate, 3 grams protein, 0–1 gram fat, and 80 calories.

Starchy Foods Prepared with Fat
(Count as 1 starch exchange, plus 1 fat exchange.)

Biscuit, 2½ in across	1	Pancake, 4 in across	2
Chow mein noodles	½ cup	Popcorn, microwave	3 cups
Corn bread, 2-in cube	1 (2 oz)	Sandwich crackers, cheese or peanut butter filling	3
Crackers, round butter type	6	Stuffing, bread (prepared)	⅓ cup
Croutons	1 cup	Taco shell, 6 in across	2
French-fried potatoes	16–25 (3 oz)	Waffle, 4½-in square	1
Granola	¼ cup	Whole-wheat crackers, fat added	4–6 (1 oz)
Muffin, small	1 (1½ oz)		

Starches often swell in cooking, so a small amount of uncooked starch will become a much larger amount of cooked food. The following table shows some of the changes.

Food (Starch Group)	Uncooked	Cooked
Oatmeal	3 tbsp	½ cup
Cream of Wheat	2 tbsp	½ cup
Grits	3 tbsp	½ cup
Rice	2 tbsp	⅓ cup
Spaghetti	¼ cup	½ cup
Noodles	⅓ cup	½ cup
Macaroni	¼ cup	½ cup
Dried beans	¼ cup	½ cup
Dried peas	¼ cup	½ cup
Lentils	3 tbsp	½ cup

Common Measurements

3 tsp = 1 tbsp	4 ounces = ½ cup
4 tbsp = ¼ cup	8 ounces = 1 cup
5⅓ tbsp = ⅓ cup	1 cup = ½ pint

FRUIT LIST

Fresh, frozen, canned, and dried fruits and fruit juices are on this list. In general, one fruit exchange is:

- 1 small to medium fresh fruit
- ½ cup of canned or fresh fruit or fruit juice
- ¼ cup of dried fruit

Nutrition Tips

1. Fresh, frozen, and dried fruits have about 2 grams of fiber per choice. Fruit juices contain very little fiber.
2. Citrus fruits, berries, and melons are good sources of vitamin C.

Selection Tips

1. Count ½ cup cranberries or rhubarb sweetened with sugar substitutes as free foods.
2. Read the Nutrition Facts on the food label. If one serving has more than 15 grams of carbohydrate, you will need to adjust the size of the serving you eat or drink.
3. Portion sizes for canned fruits are for the fruit and a small amount of juice.
4. Whole fruit is more filling than fruit juice and may be a better choice.
5. Food labels for fruits may contain the words "no sugar added" or "unsweetened." This means that no sucrose (table sugar) has been added.
6. Generally, fruit canned in extra light syrup has the same amount of carbohydrate per serving as the "no sugar added" or the juice pack. All canned fruits on the fruit list are based on one of these three types of pack.

One Fruit Exchange Equals

15 grams carbohydrate and 60 calories. The weight includes skin, core, seeds, and rind.

Fruit

Apple, unpeeled, small	1 (4 oz)	Kiwi	1 (3½ oz)
Applesauce, unsweetened	½ cup	Mandarin oranges, canned	¾ cup
Apples, dried	4 rings	Mango, small	½ fruit (5½ oz or ½ cup)
Apricots, fresh	4 whole (5½ oz)	Nectarine, small	1 (5 oz)
Apricots, dried	8 halves	Orange, small	1 (6½ oz)
Apricots, canned	½ cup	Papaya	½ fruit (8 oz) or 1 cup cubes
Banana, small	1 (4 oz)	Peach, medium, fresh	1 (6 oz)
Blackberries	¾ cup	Peaches, canned	½ cup
Blueberries	¾ cup	Pear, large, fresh	½ (4 oz)
Cantaloupe, small	⅓ melon (11 oz) or 1 cup cubes		
Cherries, sweet, fresh	12 (3 oz)	Pears, canned	½ cup
Cherries, sweet, canned	½ cup	Pineapple, fresh	¾ cup
Dates	3	Pineapple, canned	½ cup
Figs, fresh	1½ large or 2 medium (3½ oz)	Plums, small	2 (5 oz)
Figs, dried	1½	Plums, canned	½ cup
Fruit cocktail	½ cup	Prunes, dried	3
Grapefruit, large	½ (11 oz)	Raisins	2 tbsp
Grapefruit sections, canned	¾ cup	Raspberries	1 cup
Grapes, small	17 (3 oz)	Tangerines, small	2 (8 oz)
Honeydew melon	1 slice (10 oz) or 1 cup cubes	Watermelon	1 slice (13½ oz) or 1¼ cup cubes

Fruit Juice

Apple juice/cider	½ cup	Grapefruit juice	½ cup
Cranberry juice cocktail	⅓ cup	Orange juice	½ cup
Cranberry juice cocktail, reduced-calorie	1 cup	Pineapple juice	½ cup
Fruit juice blends, 100% juice	⅓ cup	Prune juice	⅓ cup
Grape juice	⅓ cup		

MILK LIST

Different types of milk and milk products are on this list. Cheeses are on the Meat list and cream and other dairy fats are on the Fat list. Based on the amount of fat they contain, milks are divided into skim/very low-fat milk, low-fat milk, and whole milk. One choice of these includes:

	Carbohydrate (g)	Protein (g)	Fat (g)	Calories
Skim/very low-fat	12	8	0–3	90
Low-fat	12	8	5	120
Whole	12	8	8	150

Nutrition Tips

1. Milk and yogurt are good sources of calcium and protein. Check the food label.
2. The higher the fat content of milk and yogurt, the greater the amount of saturated fat and cholesterol. Choose lower-fat varieties.
3. For those who are lactose intolerant, look for lactose-reduced or lactose-free varieties of milk.

Selection Tips

1. One cup equals 8 fluid ounces or ½ pint.
2. Look for chocolate milk, frozen yogurt, and ice cream on the Other Carbohydrates list.
3. Nondairy creamers are on the Free Foods list.
4. Look for rice milk on the Starch list.
5. Look for soy milk on the Medium-Fat Meat list.

One Milk Exchange equals
12 grams carbohydrate and 8 grams protein.

Skim and Very Low-Fat Milk
(0–3 grams fat per serving)

Skim milk	1 cup
½% milk	1 cup
1% milk	1 cup
Nonfat or low-fat buttermilk	1 cup
Evaporated skim milk	½ cup
Nonfat dry milk	⅓ cup dry
Plain nonfat yogurt	¾ cup
Nonfat or low-fat fruit-flavored yogurt sweetened with aspartame or with a nonnutritive sweetener	1 cup

Low-Fat
(5 grams fat per serving)

2% milk	1 cup
Plain low-fat yogurt	¾ cup
Sweet acidophilus milk	1 cup

Whole Milk
(8 grams fat per serving)

Whole milk	1 cup
Evaporated whole milk	½ cup
Goat's milk	1 cup
Kefir	1 cup

OTHER CARBOHYDRATES LIST

You can substitute food choices from this list for a starch, fruit, or milk choice on your meal plan. Some choices will also count as one or more fat choices.

Nutrition Tips

1. These foods can be substituted in your meal plan, even though they contain added sugars or fat. However, they do not contain as many important vitamins and minerals as the choices on the Starch, Fruit, or Milk list.
2. When planning to include these foods in your meal, be sure to include foods from all the lists to eat a balanced meal.

Selection Tips

1. Because many of these foods are concentrated sources of carbohydrate and fat, the portion sizes are often very small.
2. Always check Nutrition Facts on the food label. It will be your most accurate source of information.
3. Many fat-free or reduced-fat products made with fat replacers contain carbohydrate. When eaten in large amounts, they may need to be counted. Talk with your dietitian to determine how to count these in your meal plan.
4. Look for fat-free salad dressings in smaller amounts on the Free Foods list.

One Exchange Equals

15 grams carbohydrate, or 1 starch, or 1 fruit, or 1 milk.

Food	Serving Size	Exchanges per Serving
Angel food cake, unfrosted	¹⁄₁₂ cake	2 carbohydrates
Brownie, small, unfrosted	2-in square	1 carbohydrate, 1 fat
Cake, unfrosted	2-in square	1 carbohydrate, 1 fat
Cake, frosted	2-in square	2 carbohydrates, 1 fat
Cookie, fat-free	2 small	1 carbohydrate
Cookie or sandwich cookie with cream filling	2 small	1 carbohydrate, 1 fat
Cupcake, frosted	1 small	2 carbohydrates, 1 fat

Food	Serving Size	Exchanges per Serving
Cranberry sauce, jellied	¼ cup	2 carbohydrates
Doughnut, plain cake	1 medium (1½ oz)	1½ carbohydrates, 2 fats
Doughnut, glazed	3¾ in across (2 oz)	2 carbohydrates, 2 fats
Fruit juice bars, frozen, 100% juice	1 bar (3 oz)	1 carbohydrate
Fruit snacks, chewy (pureed fruit concentrate)	1 roll (¾ oz)	1 carbohydrate
Fruit spreads, 100% fruit	1 tbsp	1 carbohydrate
Gelatin, regular	½ cup	1 carbohydrate
Gingersnaps	3	1 carbohydrate

One Exchange Equals

15 grams carbohydrate, or 1 starch, or 1 fruit, or 1 milk.

Food	Serving Size	Exchanges per Serving
Granola bar	1 bar	1 carbohydrate, 1 fat
Granola bar, fat-free	1 bar	2 carbohydrates
Hummus	⅓ cup	1 carbohydrate, 1 fat
Ice cream	½ cup	1 carbohydrate, 2 fats
Ice cream, light	½ cup	1 carbohydrate, 1 fat
Ice cream, fat-free, no sugar added	½ cup	1 carbohydrate
Jam or jelly, regular	1 tbsp	1 carbohydrate
Milk, chocolate, whole	1 cup	2 carbohydrates, 1 fat
Pie, fruit, 2 crusts	⅙ pie	3 carbohydrates, 2 fats
Pie, pumpkin or custard	⅛ pie	1 carbohydrate, 2 fats
Potato chips	12–18 (1 oz)	1 carbohydrate, 2 fats
Pudding, regular (made with low-fat milk)	½ cup	2 carbohydrates
Pudding, sugar-free (made with low-fat milk)	½ cup	1 carbohydrate
Salad dressing, fat-free	¼ cup	1 carbohydrate
Sherbet, sorbet	½ cup	2 carbohydrates
Spaghetti or pasta sauce, canned	½ cup	1 carbohydrate, 1 fat
Sweet roll or Danish	1 (2½ oz)	2½ carbohydrates, 2 fats
Syrup, light	2 tbsp	1 carbohydrate
Syrup, regular	1 tbsp	1 carbohydrate
Syrup, regular	¼ cup	4 carbohydrates
Tortilla chips	6–12 (1 oz)	1 carbohydrate, 2 fats
Yogurt, frozen, low-fat, fat-free	⅓ cup	1 carbohydrate, 0–1 fat
Yogurt, frozen, fat-free, no sugar added	½ cup	1 carbohydrate
Yogurt, low-fat with fruit	1 cup	3 carbohydrates, 0–1 fat
Vanilla wafers	5	1 carbohydrate, 1 fat

VEGETABLE LIST

Vegetables that contain small amounts of carbohydrates and calories are on this list. Vegetables contain important nutrients. Try to eat at least 2 or 3 vegetable choices each day. In general, one vegetable exchange is:

- ½ cup of cooked vegetables or vegetable juice
- 1 cup of raw vegetables

If you eat 1 to 2 vegetable choices at a meal or snack, you do not have to count the calories or carbohydrates because they contain small amounts of these nutrients.

Nutrition Tips

1. Fresh and frozen vegetables have less added salt than canned vegetables. Drain and rinse canned vegetables if you want to remove some salt.
2. Choose more dark green and dark yellow vegetables, such as spinach, broccoli, romaine, carrots, chilies, and peppers.
3. Broccoli, brussels sprouts, cauliflower, greens, peppers, spinach, and tomatoes are good sources of vitamin C.
4. Vegetables contain 1 to 4 grams of fiber per serving.

Selection Tips

1. A 1-cup portion of broccoli is a portion about the size of a lightbulb.
2. Tomato sauce is different from spaghetti sauce, which is on the Other Carbohydrates list.
3. Canned vegetables and juices are available without added salt.
4. If you eat more than 4 cups of raw vegetables or 2 cups of cooked vegetables at one meal, count them as 1 carbohydrate choice.
5. Starchy vegetables such as corn, peas, winter squash, and potatoes that contain larger numbers of calories and amounts of carbohydrates are on the Starch list.

One Vegetable Exchange Equals

5 grams carbohydrate, 2 grams protein, 0 grams fat, and 25 calories.

Artichoke
Artichoke hearts
Asparagus
Beans (green, wax, Italian)
Bean sprouts
Beets
Broccoli
Brussels sprouts
Cabbage
Carrots
Cauliflower
Celery
Cucumber
Eggplant
Green onions or scallions
Greens (collard, kale, mustard, turnip)
Kohlrabi
Leeks
Mixed vegetables (without corn, peas, or pasta)

Mushrooms
Okra
Onions
Pea pods
Peppers (all varieties)
Radishes
Salad greens (endive, escarole, lettuce, romaine, spinach)
Sauerkraut◆
Spinach
Summer squash
Tomato
Tomatoes, canned
Tomato sauce◆
Tomato/vegetable juice◆
Turnips
Water chestnuts
Watercress
Zucchini

◆ = 400 mg or more sodium per exchange.

MEAT AND MEAT SUBSTITUTES LIST

Meat and meat substitutes that contain both protein and fat are on this list. In general, one meat exchange is:

- 1 oz meat, fish, poultry, or cheese,
- ½ cup dried beans.

Based on the amount of fat they contain, meats are divided into very lean, lean, medium-fat, and high-fat lists. This is done so you can see which ones contain the least amount of fat. One ounce (one exchange) of each of these includes:

	Carbohydrate (g)	Protein (g)	Fat (g)	Calories
Very lean	0	7	0–1	35
Lean	0	7	3	55
Medium-fat	0	7	5	75
High-fat	0	7	8	100

Nutrition Tips

1. Choose very lean and lean meat choices whenever possible. Items from the high-fat group are high in saturated fat, cholesterol, and calories and can raise blood cholesterol levels.
2. Meats do not have any fiber.
3. Dried beans, peas, and lentils are good sources of fiber.
4. Some processed meats, seafood, and soy products may contain carbohydrate when consumed in large amounts. Check the Nutrition Facts on the label to see if the amount is close to 15 grams. If so, count it as a carbohydrate choice as well as a meat choice.

Selection Tips

1. Weigh meat after cooking and removing bones and fat. Four ounces of raw meat is equal to 3 ounces of cooked meat. Some examples of meat portions are:
   - 1 ounce cheese = 1 meat choice and is about the size of a 1-inch cube.
   - 2 ounces meat = 2 meat choices, such as
        1 small chicken leg or thigh
        ½ cup cottage cheese or tuna
   - 3 ounces meat = 3 meat choices and is about the size of a deck of cards, such as

1 medium pork chop
1 small hambuger
½ of a whole chicken breast
1 unbreaded fish fillet

2. Limit your choices from the high-fat group to three times per week or less.
3. Most grocery stores stock Select and Choice grades of meat. Select grades of meat are the leanest meats. Choice grades contain a moderate amount of fat, and Prime cuts of meat have the highest amount of fat. Restaurants usually serve Prime cuts of meat.
5. "Hamburger" may contain added seasoning and fat, but ground beef does not.
6. Read labels to find products that are low in fat and cholesterol (5 grams or less of fat per serving).
7. Dried beans, peas, and lentils are also found on the Starch list.
8. Peanut butter, in smaller amounts, is also found on the Fats list.
9. Bacon, in smaller amounts, is also found on the Fats list.

Meal Planning Tips

1. Bake, roast, broil, grill, poach, steam, or boil these foods rather than frying.
2. Place meat on a rack so the fat will drain off during cooking.
3. Use a nonstick spray and a nonstick pan to brown or fry foods.
4. Trim off visible fat before or after cooking.
5. If you add flour, bread crumbs, coating mixes, fat, or marinados when cooking, ask your dietitian how to count them in your meal plan.

Very Lean Meat and Substitutes List

One exchange equals 0 grams carbohydrate, 7 grams protein, 0–1 gram fat, and 35 calories.

One, very lean meat exchange is equal to any of the following items:

Poultry: Chicken or turkey (white meat, no skin), Cornish hen (no skin)   1 oz

Fish: Fresh or frozen cod, flounder, haddock, halibut, trout; tuna fresh or canned in water   1 oz

Shellfish: Clams, crab, lobster, scallops, shrimp, imitation shellfish   1 oz

Game: Duck or pheasant (no skin) venison, buffalo, ostrich   1 oz

Cheese with 1 gram or less fat per ounce:
Nonfat or low-fat cottage cheese   ¼ cup
Fat-free cheese   1 oz

Other: Processed sandwich meats with 1 gram or less fat per ounce, such as deli thin, shaved meats, chipped beef♦, turkey ham   1 oz
Egg whites   2
Egg substitutes, plain   ¼ cup
Hot dogs with 1 gram or less fat per ounce♦   1 oz
Kidney (high in cholesterol)   1 oz
Sausage with 1 gram or less fat per ounce   1 oz

Count as one very lean meat and one starch exchange.

Dried beans, peas, lentils (cooked)   ½ cup

♦ = 400 mg or more sodium per exchange.

Lean Meat and Substitute List

One exchange equals 0 grams carbohydrate, 7 grams protein, 3 grams fat, and 55 calories.

One lean meat exchange is equal to any one of the following items:

Beef: USDA Select or Choice grades of lean beef trimmed of fat, such as round, sirloin and flank steak; tenderloin; roast (rib, chuck, rump); steak (T-bone, porterhouse, cubed), ground round   1 oz

Pork: Lean pork, such as fresh ham; canned, cured, or boiled ham; Canadian bacon♦; tenderloin, center loin chop   1 oz

Lamb: Roast, chop, leg   1 oz

Veal: Lean chop, roast   1 oz

Poultry: Chicken, turkey (dark meat, no skin), chicken white meat (with skin), domestic duck or goose (well-drained of fat, no skin)   1 oz

Fish:
Herring (uncreamed or smoked)   1 oz
Oysters   6 medium
Salmon (fresh or canned), catfish   1 oz
Sardines (canned)   2 medium
Tuna (canned in oil, drained)   1 oz

Game: Goose (no skin), rabbit   1 oz

Cheese:
4.5%–fat cottage cheese   ¼ cup
Grated Parmesan   2 tbsp
Cheeses with 3 grams or less fat per ounce   1 oz

Other:
Hot dogs with 3 grams or less fat per ounce♦   1½ oz
Processed sandwich meat with 3 grams or less fat per ounce, such as turkey pastrami or kielbasa   1 oz
Liver, heart (high in cholesterol)   1 oz

Medium-Fat Meat and Substitutes List

One exchange equals 0 grams carbohydrate, 7 grams of protein, 5 grams fat, and 75 calories.

One medium-fat meat exchange is equal to any one of the following items.

Beef: Most beef products fall into this category (ground beef, meatloaf, corned beef, short ribs, prime grades of meat trimmed of fat, such as prime rib)   1 oz

Pork: Top loin, chop, Boston butt, cutlet   1 oz

Lamb: Rib roast, ground   1 oz

Veal: Cutlet (ground or cubed, unbreaded)   1 oz

Poultry: Chicken dark meat (with skin), ground turkey or ground chicken, fried chicken (with skin)   1 oz

Fish: Any fried fish product   1 oz

Cheese: With 5 grams or less fat per ounce
Feta   1 oz
Mozzarella   1 oz
Ricotta   ¼ cup (2 oz)

Other:
Egg (high in cholesterol, limit to 3 per week)   1
Sausage with 5 grams or less fat per ounce   1 oz
Soy milk   1 cup
Tempeh   ¼ cup
Tofu   4 oz or ½ cup

High-Fat Meat and Substitutes List

One exchange equals 0 grams carbohydrate, 7 grams protein, 8 grams fat, and 100 calories.

Remember, these items are high in saturated fat, cholesterol, and calories, and may raise blood cholesterol levels if eaten on a regular basis. One high-fat meat exchange is equal to any one of the following items.

Pork: Spareribs, ground pork, pork sausage   1 oz

Cheese: All regular cheeses, such as American♦, cheddar, Monterey Jack, Swiss   1 oz

Other: Processed sandwich meats with 8 grams or less fat per ounce, such as bologna, pimiento loaf, salami   1 oz
Sausage, such as bratwurst, Italian, knockwurst, Polish, smoked   1 oz
Hot dog (turkey or chicken)♦   1 (10/lb)
Bacon   3 slices (20 slices/lb)

Count as one high-fat meat plus one fat exchange.

Hot dog (beef, pork, or combination)♦   1 (10/lb)
Peanut butter (contains unsaturated fat)   2 tbsp

♦ = 400 mg or more sodium per exchange.

FAT LIST

Fats are divided into three groups, based on the main type of fat they contain: monounsaturated, polyunsaturated, and saturated. Small amounts of monounsaturated and polyunsaturated fats in the foods we eat are linked with good health benefits. Saturated fats are linked with heart disease and cancer. In general, one fat exchange is:

- 1 teaspoon of regular margarine or vegetable oil
- 1 tablespoon of regular salad dressings
- 1 tablespoon of regular salad dressings

Nutrition Tips

1. All fats are high in calories. Limit serving sizes for good nutrition and health.
2. Nuts and seeds contain small amounts of fiber, protein, and magnesium.
3. If blood pressure is a concern, choose fats in the unsalted form to help lower sodium intake, such as unsalted peanuts.

Selection Tips

1. Check the Nutrition Facts on food labels for serving sizes. One fat exchange is based on a serving size containing 5 grams of fat.
2. When selecting regular margarine, choose those with liquid vegetable oil as the first ingredient. Soft margarines are not as saturated as stick margarines. Soft margarines are healthier choices. Avoid those listing hydrogenated or partially hydrogenated fat as the first ingredient.
3. When selecting low-fat margarines, look for liquid vegetable oil as the second ingredient. Water is usually the first ingredient.
4. When used in smaller amounts, bacon and peanut butter are

counted as fat choices. When used in larger amounts, they are counted as high-fat meat choices.

5. Fat-free salad dressings are on the Other Carbohydrates list and the Free Foods list.

6. See the Free Foods list for nondairy coffee creamers, whipped topping, and fat-free products,

Monounsaturated Fats List		Saturated Fats List	
One fat exchange equals 5 grams fat and 45 calories.		One fat exchange equals 5 grams of fat and 45 calories.	
Avocado, medium	⅛ (1 oz)	Bacon, cooked	1 slice (20 slices/lb)
Oill (canola, olive, peanut)	1 tsp	Bacon, grease	1 tsp
Olives: ripe (black)	8 large	Butter: stick	1 tsp
green, stuffed♦	10 large	whipped	2 tsp
Nuts		reduced-fat	1 tbsp
almonds, cashews	6 nuts	Chitterlings, boiled	2 tbsp (½ oz)
mixed (50% peanuts)	6 nuts	Coconut, sweetened, shredded	2 tbsp
peanuts	10 nuts	Cream, half and half	2 tbsp
pecans	4 halves	Cream cheese: regular	1 tbsp (½ oz)
Peanut butter, smooth or crunchy	2 tsp	reduced-fat	2 tbsp (1 oz)
Sesame seeds	1 tbsp	Fatback or salt pork†	
Tahini paste	2 tsp	Shortening or lard	1 tsp
		Sour cream: regular	2 tbsp
		reduced-fat	3 tbsp

♦ = 400 mg or more sodium per exchange.

† Use a piece 1 in x 1 in x ¼ in if you plan to eat the fatback cooked with vegetables. Use a piece 2 in x 1 in x ½ in when eating only the vegetables with the fatback removed.

Polyunsaturated Fats List
One fat exchange equals 5 grams fat and 45 calories.

Margarine: stick, tub, or squeeze	1 tsp	Salad dressing: regular♦	1 tbsp
lower-fat (30% to 50% vegetable oil)	1 tbsp	reduced-fat	2 tbsp
		Miracle Whip S Dressing*:	
Mayonnaise: regular	1 tsp	regular	2 tsp
reduced-fat	1 tbsp	reduced fat	1 tbsp
Nuts, walnuts, English	4 halves	Seeds: pumpkin, sunflower	1 tbsp
Oil (corn, safflower, soybean)	1 tsp		

♦ = 400 mg or more sodium per exchange.

* Saturated fats can raise blood cholesterol levels.

FREE FOODS LIST

A *free food* is any food or drink that contains less than 20 calories or less than 5 grams of carbohydrate per serving. Foods with a serving size listed should be limited to three servings per day. Be sure to spread them out throughout the day. If you eat all three servings at one time, it could affect your blood glucose level. Foods listed without a serving size can be eaten as often as you like.

Fat-Free or Reduced-Fat Foods

Cream cheese, fat-free	1 tbsp
Creamers, nondairy, liquid	1 tbsp
Creamers, nondairy, powdered	1 tbsp
Mayonnaise, fat-free	1 tbsp
Mayonnaise, reduced-fat	1 tsp
Margarine, fat-free	4 tbsp
Margarine, reduced fat	1 tsp
Miracle Whip®, nonfat	1 tbsp
Miracle Whip®, reduced-fat	1 tsp
Nonstick cooking spray	
Salad dressing, fat-free	1 tbsp
Salad dressing, fat-free, Italian	2 tbsp
Salsa	¼ cup
Sour cream, fat-free, reduced-fat	1 tbsp
Whipped topping, regular or light	2 tbsp

Drinks

Bouillon, broth, consommé٭
Bouillon or broth, low-sodium
Carbonated or mineral water
Cocoa powder, unsweetened   1 tbsp
Coffee
Club soda
Diet soft drinks, sugar-free
Drink mixes, sugar-free
Tea
Tonic water, sugar-free

Sugar-Free or Low-Sugar Foods

Candy, hard, sugar-free	1 candy
Gelatin dessert, sugar-free	
Gelatin, unflavored	
Gum, sugar-free	
Jam or jelly, low-sugar or light	2 tsp
Sugar substitutes*	
Syrup, sugar-free	2 tbsp

*Sugar substitutes, alternatives, or replacements that are approved by the Food and Drug Administration (FDA) are safe to use. Common brand names include: Equal® (aspartame), Sprinkle Sweet® (saccharin), Sweet One® (acesulfame K), Sweet-10® (saccharin), Sugar Twin® (saccharin), Sweet 'n Low® (saaccharin).

Seasonings

Be careful with seasonings that contain sodium or are salts, such as garlic or celery salt, and lemon pepper.

Flavoring extracts
Garlic
Herbs, fresh or dried
Pimiento
Spices
Tabasco® or hot pepper sauce
Wine, used in cooking
Worcestershire sauce

Condiments

Catsup	1 tbsp
Horseradish	
Lemon juice	
Lime juice	
Mustard	
Pickles, dill◆	1½ large
Soy sauce, regular or light◆	
Taco sauce	1 tbsp
Vinegar	

◆ = 400 mg or more of sodium per choice

COMBINATION FOODS LIST

Many of the foods we eat are mixed together in various combinations. These combination foods do not fit into any one exchange list. Often it is hard to tell what is in a casserole dish or prepared food item. This is a list of exchanges for some typical combination foods. This list will help you fit these foods into your meal plan. Ask your dietitian for information about any other combination foods you would like to eat.

Food Entrees	Serving Size	Exchanges per Serving
Tuna noodle casserole, lasagna, spaghetti with meatballs, chili with beans, macaroni and cheese◆	1 cup (8 oz)	2 carbohydrates, 2 medium-fat meats
Chow mein (without noodles or rice)	2 cups (16 oz)	1 carbohydrate, 2 lean meats
Pizza, cheese, thin crust◆	¼ of 10 in (5 oz)	2 carbohydrates, 2 medium-fat meats, 1 fat
Pizza, meat topping, thin crust◆	¼ of 10 in (5 oz)	2 carbohydrates, 2 medium-fat meats, 2 fats
Pot pie◆	1 (7 oz)	2 carbohydrates, 1 medium-fat meat, 4 fats
Frozen entrées		
Salisbury steak with gravy, mashed potato◆	1 (11 oz)	2 carbohydrates, 3 medium-fat meats, 3–4 fats
Turkey with gravy, mashed potato dressing◆	1 (11 oz)	2 carbohydrates, 2 medium-fat meats, 2 fats
Entrée with less than 300 calories◆	1 (8 oz)	2 carbohydrates, 3 lean meats

Soups

Bean◆	1 cup	1 carbohydrate, 1 very lean meat
Cream (made with water)◆	1 cup (8 oz)	1 carbohydrate, 1 fat
Split pea (made with water)◆	½ cup (4 oz)	1 carbohydrate
Tomato (made with water)◆	1 cup (8 oz)	1 carbohydrate
Vegetable beef, chicken noodle, or other broth type◆	1 cup (8 oz)	1 carbohydrate

◆ = 400 mg or more sodium per exchange.

FAST FOODS*

Food	Serving Size	Exchanges Per Serving
Burritos with beef◆	2	4 carbohydrates, 2 medium-fat meats, 2 fats
Chicken nuggets◆	6	1 carbohydrate, 2 medium-fat meats, 1 fat
Chicken breast and wing, breaded and fried◆	1 each	1 carbohydrate, 4 medium-fat meats, 2 fats
Fish sandwich/tartar sauce◆	1	3 carbohydrates, 1 medium-fat meat, 3 fats
French fries, thin	20–25	2 carbohydrates, 2 fats
Hamburger, regular	1	2 carbohydrates, 2 medium-fat meats
Hamburger, large◆	1	2 carbohydrates, 3 medium-fat meats, 1 fat
Hot dog with bun◆	1	1 carbohydrate, 1 high-fat meat, 1 fat
Individual pan pizza◆	1	5 carbohydrates, 3 medium-fat meats, 3 fats
Soft-serve cone	1 medium	2 carbohydrates, 1 fat
Submarine sandwich◆	1 sub (6 in)	3 carbohydrates, 1 vegetable, 2 medium-fat meats, 1 fat
Taco, hard shell◆	1 (6 oz)	2 carbohydrates, 2 medium-fat meats, 2 fats
Taco, soft shell◆	1 (3 oz)	1 carbohydrate, 1 medium-fat meat, 1 fat

◆ = 400 mg or more of sodium per serving.
*Ask at your fast-food restaurant for nutrition information about your favorite fast foods.

USING FOOD LABELS

Nutrition facts on food labels can help you with food choices. These labels are required by law for most foods and are based on standard serving sizes. However, these serving sizes may not always be the same as the serving sizes in this book.

- Check the serving size on the label. Is it nearly the same size as the food exchange? You may need to adjust the size of the serving to fit your meal plan.
- Look at the grams of carbohydrate in the serving size. (One starch, fruit, milk, or other carbohydrate has about 15 grams of carbohydrate.) So, if 1 cup of cereal has 30 grams of carbohydrate, it will count as 2 starch choices in your meal plan. You may need to adjust the size of the serving so it contains the number of carbohydrate choices you have for a meal or a snack.
- Look at the grams of protein in the serving size. (One meat choice has 7 grams of protein.) If the food has more than 7 grams of protein in a serving, you can figure out the number of meat choices by dividing the grams of protein by 7. Meats generally contain fat, too.
- Look at the grams of fat in the serving size. (One fat choice has 5 grams of fat.) If one waffle has 15 grams of carbohydrate and 5 grams of fat, it counts as 1 starch choice and 1 fat choice.
- Look at the number of calories in the serving size. If there are less than 20 calories per serving, it is a free food. However, if it has more than 20 calories, follow the steps listed above to count the food choices.

Exchange List

GLOSSARY

Alcohol—An ingredient in a variety of beverages, including beer, wine, liqueurs, cordials, and mixed or straight drinks. Pure alcohol itself yields about 7 calories per gram.

Calorie—A unit used to express the heat or energy value of food. Calories come from carbohydrate, protein, fat, and alcohol.

Carbohydrate—One of the three major energy sources in foods. The most common carbohydrates are sugars and starches. Carbohydrates yield about 4 calories per gram. Carbohydrates are found in foods from the Milk, Vegetable, Fruit, and Starch exchange lists.

Certified Diabetes Educators (CDE)— Health educators who specialize in diabetes and have passed the Certification Examination for Diabetes Educators are certified by the American Association of Diabetes Educators. These educators stay up-to-date on diabetes care and can help you with your diabetes management.

Cholesterol—A fatlike substance normally found in blood. A high level of cholesterol in the blood has been shown to be a major risk factor for developing heart disease. Dietary cholesterol is found in all animal products, but is especially high in egg yolks and organ meats. Eating foods high in dietary cholesteral and saturated fat tends to raise the level of blood cholesterol. Foods of plant origin such as fruits, vegetables, grains, and dried beans and peas contain no cholesterol. Cholesterol is found in foods from the Milk, Meat, and Fat exchange lists.

Dietitian—A registered dietitian (RD) is recognized by the medical profession as the primary provider of nutritional care, education, and counseling. The initials RD after a dietitian's name ensure that he or she has met the standards of The American Dietetic Association. Look for these credentials when you seek advice on nutrition.

Exchange—Foods grouped together on a list according to similarities in food values. Measured amounts of foods within the group may be exchanged or traded in planning meals. A single exchange contains approximately equal amounts of carbohydrate, protein, fat, and calories.

Fat—One of the three major energy sources in food. A concentrated source of calories—about 9 calories per gram. Fat is found in foods from the Fat and Meat lists. Some kinds of milk also have fat; some foods from the Starch list also contain fat.

*Saturated fat—Type of fat that tends to raise blood cholesterol levels. It comes primarily from animals and is usually hard at room temperature. Examples of saturated fats are butter, lard, meat fat, solid shortening, palm oil, and coconut oil.

*Polyunsaturated fat—Type of fat that is usually liquid at room temperature and is found in vegetable oils. Safflower, sunflower, corn, and soybean oils contain amounts of polyunsaturated fats. Polyunsaturated fats, such as corn oil, can help lower high blood cholesterol levels when they are part of a lower-fat diet.

*Monounsaturated fat—Type of fat that is liquid at room temperature and is found in vegetable oils, such as canola and olive. Monounsaturated fats can help lower high blood cholesterol levels when they are part of a lower-fat diet.

Fiber—An indigestible part of certain foods. Fiber is important in the diet as roughage, or bulk. Fiber is found in foods from the Starch, Vegetable, and Fruit exchange lists.

Gram—A unit of mass and weight in the metric system. An ounce is about 30 grams.

Insulin—A hormone made by the body that helps the body use food. Also, a commercially prepared injectable substance used by people who do not make enough of their own insulin.

Meal Plan—A guide showing the number of food exchanges to use in each meal and snack to control distribution of carbohydrates, proteins, fats, and calories throughout the day.

Minerals—Substances essential in small amounts to build and repair body tissue and/or control functions of the body. Calcium, iron, magnesium, phosphorus, potassium, sodium, and zinc are minerals.

Nutrients—Substances in food necessary for life. Carbohydrates, proteins, fats, minerals, vitamins, and water are nutrients.

Protein—One of the three major nutrients in food. Protein provides about 4 calories per gram. Protein is found in foods from the Milk and Meat exchange lists. Smaller amounts of protein are found in foods from the Vegetable and Starch lists.

Sodium—A mineral needed by the body to maintain life, found mainly as a component of salt. Many individuals need to cut down the amount of sodium (and salt) they eat to help control high blood pressure.

Starch—One of the two major types of carbohydrate. Foods consisting mainly of starch come from the Starch list.

Sugars—One of the two major types of carbohydrate. Foods consisting mainly of naturally present sugars are those from the Milk, Vegetable, and Fruit lists. Added sugars include common table sugar and the sugar alcohols (sorbitol, mannitol, etc.).

Triglycerides—Fats normally present in the blood that are made from food.

Gaining too much weight or consuming too much fat, alcohol, or carbohydrates may increase the blood triglycerides.

Vitamins—Substances found in food, needed in small amounts to assist in body processes and functions. These include vitamins A, D, E, the B-complex, C, and K.

To choose a maintenance calorie level, refer back to Table 11.1 in Chapter 11. Select a meal plan close to your needs, then use the exchanges to plan your own meals. For example, if you are a 40-year-old woman, who is 5 feet 6 inches tall with a mild activity level, your maintenance needs would be 1,735 calories per day. You would choose the 1,700-calorie meal plan. Practice using the exchanges until you feel comfortable picking the foods that you like to fit into your plan.

1,200-Calorie Meal Plan

(calories listed in parentheses)

EXCHANGE	EXAMPLE

Breakfast

EXCHANGE	EXAMPLE
1—fruit (60)	1 small banana
1—starch (80)	¾ cup cornflakes
1—skim milk (90)	1 cup skim milk
Free food	Coffee

Total breakfast calories = 230

Lunch

EXCHANGE	EXAMPLE
2—lean meats (110)	½ cup tuna (water-pack)
2—starches (160)	2 slices whole wheat bread
1—vegetable (25)	Lettuce with sliced tomato
1—fat (45)	1 tbsp reduced-fat mayonnaise
Free food	Iced tea

Total lunch calories = 340

Dinner

EXCHANGE	EXAMPLE
3—lean meats (165)	3 oz turkey
2—starches (160)	½ cup sweet potato, 1 plain roll
1—vegetable (25)	1 cup green beans
1—fat (45)	1 tsp margarine
Free food	Herb tea

Total dinner calories = 395

Night Snack

EXCHANGE	EXAMPLE
1—starch (80)	3 square graham crackers
1—fruit (60)	2 tbsp raisins
1—skim milk (90)	1 cup skim milk

Total night snack calories = 230

Total daily calories = 1,195, 19% fat

1,300-Calorie Meal Plan

(calories listed in parentheses)

EXCHANGE	EXAMPLE

Breakfast

1—fruit (60)	½ cup orange juice
2—starches (160)	1 English muffin
1—skim milk (90)	1 cup skim milk
Free food	Coffee, 2 tsp low-sugar jelly

Total breakfast calories = 310

Lunch

2—lean meats (110)	2 oz chicken breast
2—starches (160)	2 slices whole-wheat bread
1—vegetable (25)	Sliced carrots, cucumbers
1—fat (45)	2 tbsp reduced-fat salad dressing
Free food	Iced tea

Total lunch calories = 340

Dinner

3—lean meats (165)	3 oz salmon filet
2—starches (160)	⅔ cup brown rich
2—vegetables (50)	1 cup broccoli
1—fat (45)	1 tsp margarine
Free food	Diet lemonade

Total dinner calories = 420

Night Snack

1—starch (80)	½ bagel with 1 tbsp fat-free
1—fruit (60)	cream cheese
1—skim milk (90)	1¼ cups strawberries
	1 cup skim milk

Total night snack calories = 230

Total daily calories = 1,300, 17% fat

1,400-Calorie Meal Plan

(calories listed in parentheses)

EXCHANGE	EXAMPLE

Breakfast

EXCHANGE	EXAMPLE
1—fruit (60)	1 small banana
2—starches (160)	1 cup shredded wheat
1—skim milk (90)	1 cup skim milk
Free food	Coffee

Total breakfast calories = 310

Lunch

EXCHANGE	EXAMPLE
3—lean meats (165)	3 oz turkey
2—starches (160)	2 slices whole-wheat bread
1—vegetable (25)	Lettuce with sliced tomato
1—fat (45)	1 tsp mayonnaise
Free food	Diet soda

Total lunch calories = 395

Dinner

EXCHANGE	EXAMPLE
3—lean meats (165)	3 oz shrimp
2—starches (160)	⅔ cup brown rice
1—vegetable (25)	½ cup snow peas, mushrooms, water chestnuts
1—fat (45)	1 tsp sesame oil (to sauté shrimp)
1—fruit (60)	¾ cup blueberries
Free food	Herb tea

Total dinner calories = 455

Night Snack

EXCHANGE	EXAMPLE
1—starch (80)	3 cups popcorn (no fat added)
1—fruit (60)	1¼ cups strawberries
1—skim milk (90)	1 low-fat yogurt

Total night snack calories = 230

Total daily calories = 1,390, 18% fat

1,500-Calorie Meal Plan

(calories listed in parentheses)

EXCHANGE	EXAMPLE

Breakfast

1—fruit (60)	½ cup orange juice
2—starches (160)	1 cup sugar-frosted flakes
1—skim milk (90)	1 cup skim milk
Free food	Coffee

Total breakfast calories = 310

Lunch

3—lean meats (165)	Tuna melt (2 oz of tuna with 1 oz
2—starches (160)	Alpine lace cheese on 1 En-
1—vegetable (25)	glish muffin)
1—fat (45)	Sliced tomato
Free food	1 tsp margarine
	Iced tea

Total lunch calories = 395

Dinner

3—lean meats (165)	3 oz chicken breast
2—starches (160)	1 corn on cob, 1 roll
2—vegetables (50)	1 cup string beans
1—fat (45)	1 tsp olive oil (sauté chicken)
1—fruit (60)	⅓ cantaloupe
Free food	Diet lemonade

Total dinner calories = 480

Night Snack

2—starches (160)	2 slices raisin toast with 1 tbsp
	fat-free cream cheese
1—fruit (60)	1 peach
1—skim milk (90)	1 cup skim milk

Total night snack calories = 310

Total daily calories = 1,495, 17% fat

1,600-Calorie Meal Plan

(calories listed in parentheses)

EXCHANGE	EXAMPLE

Breakfast

EXCHANGE	EXAMPLE
1—fruit (60)	½ grapefruit
2—starches (160)	1 bagel
Free food	1 tbsp fat-free cream cheese
1—skim milk (90)	1 cup skim milk
Free food	Coffee

Total breakfast calories = 310

Lunch

EXCHANGE	EXAMPLE
3—lean meats (165)	3 oz turkey pastrami (less than 3 g fat per oz)
2—starches (160)	2 slices bread
1—vegetable (25)	Large salad
1—fat (45)	1 tbsp French dressing
1—fruit (60)	1 nectarine

Total lunch calories = 455

Dinner

EXCHANGE	EXAMPLE
3—lean meats (165)	3 oz lamb chop (remove excess fat)
2—starches (160)	1 baked potato, 1 roll
2—vegetables (50)	1 cup broccoli
2—fat (90)	2 tsp margarine
1—fruit (60)	½ cup apple cider

Total dinner calories = 525

Night Snack

EXCHANGE	EXAMPLE
2—starches (160)	30 fat free tortilla chips with salsa
1—fruit (60)	1 apple
1—skim milk (90)	1 cup skim milk

Total night snack calories = 310

Total daily calories = 1,600, 19% fat

1,700-Calorie Meal Plan

(calories listed in parentheses)

EXCHANGE	EXAMPLE

Breakfast

1—fruit (60)	½ cup orange juice
2—starches (160)	½ cup granola (low-fat)
1—skim milk (90)	1 cup skim milk
Free food	Coffee

Total breakfast calories = 310

Lunch

3—lean meats (165)	3 oz tuna fish salad
2—starches (160)	2 slices bread
1—vegetables (25)	Carrots, cucumbers
2—fat (90)	2 tsp mayonnaise
1—fruit (60)	17 grapes
Free food	Iced tea

Total lunch calories = 500

Dinner

3—lean meats (165)	3 oz roasted turkey
2—starches (160)	1 cup sweet potato
2—vegetables (50)	1 cup green beans
2—fat (90)	2 tsp margarine
2—fruits (120)	1 large pear
Free food	Diet soda

Total dinner calories = 585

Night Snack

2—starches (160)	6 graham crackers
1—fruit (60)	12 cherries
1—skim milk (90)	1 cup low-fat yogurt

Total night snack calories = 310

Total daily calories = 1,705, 20% fat

1,800-Calorie Meal Plan

(calories listed in parentheses)

EXCHANGE	EXAMPLE

Breakfast

EXCHANGE	EXAMPLE
1 —fruit (60)	½ cup grapefruit juice
2—starches (160)	1 bagel
1—fat (45)	1 tbsp cream cheese
1—skim milk (90)	1 cup skim milk
Free food	Coffee

Total breakfast calories = 355

Lunch

EXCHANGE	EXAMPLE
3—lean meats (165)	3 oz roast beef (less than 3 g fat per oz)
2—starches (160)	2 slices bread
1—vegetables (25)	1 cup tomato juice
Free food	Tossed salad
2—fat (90)	2 tbsp salad dressing
2—fruits (120)	1½ cups pineapple
Free food	Herb tea

Total lunch calories = 560

Dinner

EXCHANGE	EXAMPLE
3—lean meats (165)	3 oz Cajun catfish
2—starches (160)	⅔ cup rice
2—vegetables (50)	1 cup spinach with garlic
2—fat (90)	2 tsp olive oil (to sauté spinach and cook fish)
2—fruits (120)	1½ cup mandarin oranges
Free food	Diet soda

Total dinner calories = 585

Night Snack

EXCHANGE	EXAMPLE
2—starch (160)	1 granola bar (fat-free)
1—fruit (60)	2 tbsp raisins
1—skim milk (90)	1 cup yogurt

Total night snack calories = 310

Total Daily Calories = 1,810, 21% fat

1,900-Calorie Meal Plan

(calories listed in parentheses)

EXCHANGE	EXAMPLE

Breakfast

1—fruit (60)	1 banana
2—starches (160)	1 cup cream of wheat
1—skim milk (90)	1 cup skim milk
1—fat	1 tsp margarine
Free food	Coffee

Total breakfast calories = 355

Lunch

3—lean meats (165)	3 oz chicken salad
2—starches (160)	2 slices of bread
1—vegetables (25)	Celery, carrots, cucumber
2—fat (90)	2 tsp mayonnaise (to make
2—fruits (120)	chicken salad)
Free food	1 sliced mango
	Diet lemonade

Total lunch calories = 560

Dinner

3—lean meats (165)	3 oz meatballs (made with extra
	lean meat)
3—starches (240)	1½ cups spaghetti
2—vegetables (50)	1 cup tomato sauce
Free food	Tossed salad
2—fat (90)	2 tbsp salad dressing
2—fruits (120)	1 slice watermelon,
	½ cup fruit juice to mix with 4 oz seltzer

Total dinner calories = 665

Night Snack

2—starches (160)	4 rice cakes
1—fruit (60)	1 tbsp (100% fruit) fruit spread
1—skim milk (90)	1 cup skim milk

Total night snack calories = 310

Total daily calories = 1,890, 20% fat

2,000-Calorie Meal Plan

(calories listed in parentheses)

EXCHANGE	EXAMPLE

Breakfast

EXCHANGE	EXAMPLE
1—fruit (60)	½ cup pineapple juice
2—starches (160)	2 slices whole-wheat toast
1—skim milk (90)	1 cup skim milk
1—fat (45)	1 tsp margarine
Free food	Coffee

Total breakfast calories = 355

Lunch

EXCHANGE	EXAMPLE
3—lean meats (165)	3 oz cheese (low-fat) melted on
3—starches (240)	a bagel, 1 cup tomato soup
2—vegetables (50)	1 cup mixed vegetables
2—fat (90)	(no corn, peas)
	2 tsp margarine
2—fruits (120)	16 dried apricot halves
Free food	Diet soda

Total lunch calories = 665

Dinner

EXCHANGE	EXAMPLE
3—lean meats (165)	1 veal chop
3—starches (240)	1 cup noodles
2—vegetables (50)	1 cup sautéed mushrooms, onions,
	tomatoes, and zucchini
2—fat (90)	2 tsp olive oil to cook vegetables
2—fruits (120)	and noodles
Free food	⅔ cantaloupe
	Iced tea

Total dinner calories = 665

Night Snack

EXCHANGE	EXAMPLE
2—starches (160)	⅓ cup chocolate pudding
1—fruit (60)	1 sliced banana
1—skim milk (90)	1 cup skim milk

Total night snack calories = 310

Total daily calories = 1,995, 19% fat

2,100-Calorie Meal Plan

(calories listed in parentheses)

EXCHANGE	EXAMPLE

Breakfast

EXCHANGE	EXAMPLE
1—fruit (60)	½ cup orange juice
2—starches (160)	2 waffles (reduced-fat)
Free food	Diet syrup for waffles, coffee
1—skim milk (90)	1 cup skim milk
1—fat (45)	1 tsp margarine

Total breakfast calories = 335

Lunch

EXCHANGE	EXAMPLE
4—lean meats (220)	4 oz ground round
3—starches (240)	1 hamburger bun, 3 oz (16–25)
2—vegetables (50)	French fries
	Sliced tomato, fried onions
2—fat (90)	1 tsp oil to cook onions, 1 fat used for fries
2—fruits (120)	2 plums, 1 peach
Free food	Ketchup for fries/burger, club soda

Total lunch calories = 720

Dinner

EXCHANGE	EXAMPLE
4—lean meats (220)	4 oz baked flounder
3—starches (240)	1 cup couscous
2—vegetables (50)	½ cup roasted red peppers, ½ cup mushrooms
2—fat (90)	2 tsp olive oil to cook vegetables and flounder
2—fruits (120)	6 dates
Free food	Iced tea

Total dinner calories = 720

Night Snack

EXCHANGE	EXAMPLE
2—starches (160)	2 cups granola (low-fat)
1—fruit (60)	1½ cup strawberries
1—skim milk (90)	1 cup skim milk

Total night snack calories = 310

Total daily calories = 2,105, 21% fat

2,200-Calorie Meal Plan

(calories listed in parentheses)

EXCHANGE	EXAMPLE

Breakfast

1—fruit (60)	½ cup orange juice
2—starches (160	1 English muffin
Free food	Coffee
1—skim milk (90)	1 cup skim milk
1—fat (45)	1 tsp margarine

Total breakfast calories = 355

Lunch

4—medium-fat meats (300)	3 oz fish sticks, 2 tbsp Parmesan cheese (for macaroni)
3—starches (240)	1 cup macaroni, 1 roll
2—vegetables (50)	Salad, sliced tomato, cucumber
2—fat (90)	2 tsp margarine for macaroni, roll
2—fruits (120)	1 frozen fruit bar, ⅓ cup cranberry juice
Free food	club soda mix with cranberry juice

Total lunch calories = 800

Dinner

4—lean meats (220)	4 oz T-bone steak
3—starches (240)	3 oz boiled red potatoes
2—vegetables (50)	1 cup green beans
2—fat (90)	2 tsp margarine
2—fruits (120)	2 nectarines
Free food	Herb tea

Total dinner calories = 720

Night Snack

2—starches (160)	¹⁄₁₂ slice angel food cake
1—fruit (60)	1 cup blueberries
1—skim milk (90)	1 cup skim milk

Total night snack calories = 310

Total daily calories = 2,185, 21% fat

2,300-Calorie Meal Plan

(calories listed in parentheses)

EXCHANGE	EXAMPLE

Breakfast

EXCHANGE	EXAMPLE
2—fruits (120)	⅔ cup cranberry juice
2—starches (160)	1 bagel
1—fat (45)	1 tbsp cream cheese
1—skim milk (90)	1 cup skim milk
Free food	Coffee

Total breakfast calories = 415

Lunch

EXCHANGE	EXAMPLE
4—medium-fat meats (300)	12 chicken nuggets
3—starches (240)	Nuggets use up 2 starches, 1 cup chicken noodle soup
2—vegetables (50)	1 cup broccoli
2—fat (90)	Nuggets use up 2 fats
2—fruits (120)	1 granola bar, fat-free

Total lunch calories = 800

Dinner

EXCHANGE	EXAMPLE
4—medium-fat meats (300)	4 oz salmon baked with lemon and 2 tsp olive oil*
3—starches (240)	1 cup rice
2—vegetables (50)	Asparagus
2—fat (90)	2 tsp margarine
2—fruits (120)	1½ cups pineapple

Total dinner calories = 800   *Salmon is lean meat but adding the olive oil increases fat content to medium-fat.

Night Snack

EXCHANGE	EXAMPLE
2—starches (160)	1 cup frosted miniwheats
1—fruit (60)	1 sliced peach
1—skim milk (90)	1 cup skim milk

Total night snack calories = 310

Total daily calories = 2,325 calories, 25% fat

2,400 Calorie-Meal Plan

(calories listed in parentheses)

EXCHANGE	EXAMPLE

Breakfast

2—fruits (120)	⅔ cup grape juice
3—starches (240)	1½ cups oatmeal
1—skim milk (90)	1 cup skim milk
1—fat (45)	1 tsp margarine
Free food	Coffee

Total breakfast calories = 495

Lunch

4—medium-fat meats (300)	4 oz meatloaf
3—starches (240)	1 cup mashed potatoes, 1 roll
2—vegetables (50)	1 cup zucchini
2—fat (90)	2 tsp margarine
2—fruits (120)	2 frozen fruit bars
Frcc food	Diet soda

Total lunch calories = 800

Dinner

4—medium-fat meats (300)	4 oz monkfish with 2 tsp margarine*
3—starches (240)	1 cup corn, 1 roll
2—vegetables (50)	1 cup stewed tomatoes
2—fat (90)	2 tsp margarine
2—fruits (120)	2 slices watermelon
Free food	Iced tea

Total dinner calories = 800

*Monkfish is lean meat. Add 2 tsp margarine to make fish medium-fat.

Night Snack

3—starches (160)	6 graham crackers
1—fruits (60)	4 dried apple rings
1—skim milk (90)	1 cup skim milk

Total night snack calories = 310

Total daily calories = 2,405, 24% fat

2,500-Calorie Meal Plan

(calories listed in parentheses)

EXCHANGE	EXAMPLE

Breakfast

2—fruits (120)	1 cup grapefruit juice
3—starches (240)	3 waffles reduced-fat
Free food	Diet syrup, coffee
1—skim milk (90)	1 cup skim milk
1—fat (45)	1 tsp margarine

Total breakfast calories = 495

Lunch

4—medium-fat meats (300)	4 oz turkey burger
3—starches (240)	1 hamburger bun, ½ cup split pea soup
2—vegetables (50)	1 cup carrots
2—fat (90)	2 tsp margarine
2—fruits (120)	2 slices honeydew melon
Free food	Diet fruit punch

Total lunch calories = 800

Dinner

4—medium-fat meats (300)	4 oz prime rib
3—starches (240)	1 large baked potato, 1 roll
3—vegetables (75)	Sautéed greens
2—fat (90)	1 tsp olive oil; 1 tsp margarine
2—fruits (120)	17 grapes; ⅓ cup fruit juice
Free food	Club soda—mix with fruit juice

Total dinner calories = 825

Night Snack

3—starches (160)	1 cup fat-free frozen yogurt
2—fruits (120)	2 cups blueberries
1—skim milk (90)	1 cup skim milk

Total night snack calories = 370

Total daily calories = 2,490, 23% fat

2,600-Calorie Meal Plan

(calories listed in parentheses)

EXCHANGE	EXAMPLE

Breakfast

2—fruits (120)	1 cup orange juice
3—starches (240)	1½ cups grits
1—skim milk (90)	1 cup skim milk
1—fat (45)	1 tsp margarine
Free food	Coffee

Total breakfast calories = 495

Lunch

4—medium-fat meats (300)	Cheese omelette (2 eggs with 2 oz mozzarella cheese)
3—starches (240)	2 slices rye toast, ½ cup hash browns (uses 1 fat also)
3—vegetables (75)	Onions, mushrooms, and pepper (add to omelette)
2—fat (90)	2 tsp margarine (to sauté vegetables and cook omelette)
2—fruits (120)	1½ grapefruit sections
Free food	Herb tea

Total lunch calories = 825

Dinner

4—medium-fat meats (300)	4 oz veal cutlet
4—starches (320)	2 cups spaghetti
3—vegetables (75)	1½ cups tomato sauce
2—fat (90)	2 tsp olive oil to cook veal
2—fruits (120)	½ cup pudding (made with skim milk)
Free food	Diet soda

Total dinner calories = 905

Night Snack

3—starch (160)	¾ cup sherbet/sorbet
2—fruits (120)	2 sliced peaches
1—skim milk (90)	2 cups of decaf cappucino with steamed skim milk

Total night snack calories = 370

Total daily calories = 2,595, 23% fat

2,700 Calorie Meal Plan

(calories listed in parentheses)

EXCHANGE	EXAMPLE

Breakfast

2—fruits (120)	⅔ cup cranberry juice
3—starches (240)	2 pancakes (omit fat), 2 slices of toast
Free food	Diet syrup, coffee
1—skim milk (90)	1 cup skim milk
1—fat (45)	Fat used for 2 pancakes

Total breakfast calories = 495

Lunch

4—medium-fat meats (300)	Chicken breast and wing, breaded and fried
3—starches (240)	2 corn on cob, 1 starch used for chicken
3—vegetables (75)	1½ cups summer squash
2—fat (90)	Fats used for chicken
2—fruits (120)	½ cup fresh fruit salad topped with 1 sliced kiwi
Free food	Diet lemonade

Total lunch calories = 825

Dinner

4—medium-fat meats (300)	16 oz or 2 cups of lasagna
4—starches (320)	Lasagna uses up 4 starches
2—vegetables (50)	1 cup sautéed greens with garlic
3—fat (135)	3 tsp olive oil to cook greens
2—fruits (120)	12 oz apple cider

Total dinner calories = 925

Night Snack

3—starches (240)	½ cup sweetened Cheerios
2—fruits (120)	1 cup blueberries, 1½ cups strawberries
1—skim milk (90)	1 cup skim milk

Total night snack calories = 450

Total daily calories = 2,695, 23% fat

2,800-Calorie Meal Plan

(calories listed in parentheses)

EXCHANGE	EXAMPLE

Breakfast

2—fruits (120)	½ cup orange juice, 2 tbsp raisins
3—starches (240)	1 cup granola with ¼ cup Grape-Nuts
1—skim milk (90)	1 cup low-fat milk—take off 1 fat
1—fat (45)	Fat used for low-fat milk instead of skim milk
Free food	Coffee

Total breakfast calories = 495

Lunch

4—medium-fat meats (300)	4 oz corn beef
3—starches (240)	2 slices rye, 1 cup chicken noodle soup
2—vegetables (50)	Cabbage salad
2—fat (90)	2 tbsp thousand island dressing (on sandwich)
2—fruits (120)	1 cup applesauce
1—skim milk (90)	1 cup skim milk

Total lunch calories = 890

Dinner

4—medium-fat meats (300)	3 oz shrimp sautéed in garlic, 3 tsp olive oil, 2 tbsp Parmesan*
4—starches (320)	2 cups spaghetti
3—vegetables (75)	1½ cups escarole
3—fat (135)	3 tsp olive oil for escarole and spaghetti
2—fruits (120)	½ cup sherbet
Free food	Diet soda

Total dinner calories = 950   *Shrimp is very lean meat; added olive oil makes it mediuim-fat meat.

Night Snack

3—starches (240)	6 cookies (fat-free)
2—fruits (120)	⅔ cup cranberry juice with ½ cup club soda
1—skim milk (90)	1 cup skim milk

Total night snack calories = 450

Total daily calories = 2,785, 23% fat

2,900-Calorie Meal Plan

(calories listed in parentheses)

EXCHANGE	EXAMPLE

Breakfast

EXCHANGE	EXAMPLE
2—fruits (120)	½ cup orange juice, 2 tbsp raisins
3—starches (240)	½ cup bran cereal, 2 slices whole wheat toast
1—skim milk (90)	1 cup skim milk
2—fat (90)	2 tsp margarine
Free food	Coffee

Total breakfast calories = 540

Lunch

EXCHANGE	EXAMPLE
4—medium-fat meats (300)	Tuna salad (4 oz tuna* with 2 tsp mayonnaise)
3—starches (240)	1 cup tomato soup, 2 slices bread
3—vegetables (75)	Salad, carrots, and celery
3—fat (135)	3 tbsp French dressing
2—fruits (120)	1 cup fresh fruit salad
1—skim milk (90)	1 cup skim milk

Total lunch calories = 960

*Tuna is a lean meat—mayonnaise can be added to make it medium fat meat.

Dinner

EXCHANGE	EXAMPLE
4—medium-fat meats (300)	3 oz veal cutlet with 1 oz mozzarella cheese
4—starches (320)	1 cup linguine, 2 slices Italian bread
3—vegetables (75)	1½ cups snap peas
3—fat (135)	3 tsp margarine
2—fruits (120)	24 cherries

Total dinner calories = 950

Night Snack

EXCHANGE	EXAMPLE
3—starch (240)	9 graham crackers
2—fruits (120)	1 small banana, 1 cup blueberries
1—skim milk (90)	8 oz low-fat yogurt

Total night snack calories = 450

Total daily calories = 2,900, 24% fat

3,000-Calorie Meal Plan

(calories listed in parentheses)

EXCHANGE	EXAMPLE

Breakfast

EXCHANGE	EXAMPLE
2—fruits (120)	⅔ cup cran-raspberry juice
3—starches (240)	3 fat-free waffles
Free food	Diet syrup, coffee
1—milk (90)	1 cup skim milk
2—fat (90)	2 tsp margarine

Total breakfast calories = 540

Lunch

EXCHANGE	EXAMPLE
4—medium-fat meats (300)	Chicken salad (4 oz chicken* with 2 tsp mayonnaise)
3—starches (240)	2 slices bread, 1 cup chicken noodle soup
3—vegetables (75)	Lettuce, tomato, cucumbers
3—fat (135)	3 tbsp French dressing
3—fruits (180)	¾ cup pudding
1—skim milk (90)	1 cup skim milk

Total lunch calories = 1,020

*Chicken without skin is lean meat—mayo can be added to make it medium-fat.

Dinner

EXCHANGE	EXAMPLE
4—medium-fat meats (300)	2 cups macaroni and cheese
4—starches (320)	4 starches used in macaroni and cheese
3 vegetables (75)	1 cup stewed tomatoes, ½ cup zucchini, salad
3—fat (135)	2 tsp margarine, 1 tbsp French dressing
3—fruits (180)	1½ cups frozen yogurt

Total dinner calories = 1,010

Night Snack

EXCHANGE	EXAMPLE
3—starches (240)	6 cookies (fat-free)
2—fruits (120)	½ cup pudding
1—skim milk (90)	1 cup skim milk

Total night snack calories = 450

Total daily calories = 3,020, 25% fat

APPENDIX III

Nutrient Values of Common Foods

The tables are based on software programs provided by Nutritionist IV Diet Analysis™ from First DataBank, San Bruno, CA.

This information is collected and developed from sources believed to be reliable and correct. However, the knowledge base is under ongoing development and should not be considered complete. The authors of this software have undertaken no independent examination, investigation, or verification of information provided by original sources. Therefore, First DataBank assumes no liability and denies any responsibility for incorrect information resulting from the use of their database or their software.

Nutrient Values of Common Foods

Food	Portion/Weight		Calories	Fat	Protein	Carbo-hydrate
		(g)		(g)	(g)	(g)
Beverages						
Apple Cider	1 cup	248	124	0.3	0.3	34.2
Beer—Light	1 fl ounce	30	8	0.0	0.1	0.4
Beer—Regular	1 fl ounce	30	12	0.0	0.1	1.1
Cocktail—Bloody Mary	1 fl ounce	30	23	0.0	0.2	1.0
Cocktail—Daiquiri	1 fl ounce	30	56	0.0	0.0	2.1
Cocktail—Gin and Tonic	1 fl ounce	30	22	0.0	0.0	2.1
Cocktail—Wine Coolers	1 cup	238	117	1.4	0.7	15.2
Cocoa From Mix—						
Aspartame Sweetened	1 cup	255	63	0.5	5.1	11.2
Coffee—Brewed	1 fl ounce	30	0	0.0	0.0	0.1
Cordials/Liqueur—54 Proof	1 fl ounce	34	97	0.0	0.0	11.5
Fruit Punch Drink—Canned	1 fl ounce	31	14	0.0	0.0	3.7
Gatorade—Thirst Quenching						
Drink	1 fl ounce	30	7	0.0	0.0	1.9
Hot Cocoa Mix—Rich Chocolate—						
Carnation	1 serving	28	110	1.0	1.0	24.0
Juice Apple—Canned or Bottled	1 cup	248	117	0.3	0.2	29.0
Juice—Cranberry—Bottled	1 cup	253	144	0.3	0.0	36.4
Juice—Grape—Frozen—						
Concentrate—Diluted	1 cup	245	125	0.2	0.5	31.3
Juice—Grapefruit—Frozen—						
Diluted	1 cup	247	101	0.3	1.4	24.0
Juice—Orange—Frozen—						
Concentrate—Diluted	1 cup	242	109	0.2	1.7	26.1
Juice—Pineapple—Canned	1 cup	250	140	0.2	0.8	34.5
Lemonade—Frozen Concentrate—						
Diluted	1 cup	248	99	0.0	0.3	26.0
Soda—Club—Carbonated	1 fl ounce	30	0	0.0	0.0	0.0
Soda—Cola Type—Carbonated	1 fl ounce	31	12	0.0	0.0	3.2
Soda—Ginger Ale—Carbonated	1 fl ounce	31	10	0.0	0.0	2.7
Soda—Lemon Lime/7Up—						
Carbonated	1 fl ounce	31	12	0.0	0.0	3.2
Soda—Tonic Water/Quinine—						
Carbonated	1 fl ounce	31	10	0.0	0.0	2.7
Tea—Brewed	1 fl ounce	30	0	0.0	0.0	0.1
Tea—Lemon—Snapple	1 cup	237	110	0.0	0.0	27.0
Tomato Juice—Canned	1 cup	237	40	0.1	1.8	10.0

Nutrient Values of Common Foods (cont.)

Food	Portion/Weight	Calories	Fat	Protein	Carbo-hydrate
	(g)		(g)	(g)	
Vegetable Juice—V8—Regular	1 cup	242	48	0.0	0.0	9.7
Whiskey/Gin/Rum/Vodka—						
80 proof	1 fl ounce	28	64	0.0	0.0	0.0
Wine—Table—All Varieties	1 fl ounce	30	20	0.0	0.1	0.4
Breads						
Bagel—Cinnamon/Raisin—3.5"	1 item	71	195	1.2	7.0	39.2
Bagel—Plain—3.5"	1 item	71	195	1.1	7.5	37.9
Biscuit—Buttermilk	1 Item	35	127	5.8	2.2	17.0
Bread—Crisp—Whole Grain—Wasa	1 slice	6	21	0.0	0.5	4.5
Bread—French	1 slice	25	68	0.8	2.2	13.0
Bread—Italian	1 slice	30	81	1.1	2.6	15.0
Bread—Melba Toast—Wheat	1 slice	5	16	0.0	1.0	3.0
Bread—Mixed Grain	1 slice	26	65	1.0	2.6	12.1
Bread—Pita—White	1 item	60	165	0.7	5.5	33.4
Bread—Pita—Whole Wheat	1 item	64	170	1.7	6.3	35.2
Bread—Pumpernickel	1 slice	32	80	1.0	2.8	15.2
Bread—Raisin	1 slice	26	71	1.1	2.1	13.6
Bread—Rye	1 slice	32	82	1.1	2.7	15.5
Bread—Sourdough	1 slice	25	68	0.8	2.2	13.0
Bread—Stick—Plain—Keebler	1 item	3	15	0.0	0.5	3.0
Bread—Wheat—Low Cal	1 slice	23	45	0.5	2.1	10.0
Bread—White—Commercial Preparation	1 slice	25	66	0.9	2.1	12.4
Bread—Whole Wheat—Soft—Enriched	1 slice	28	68	1.2	2.7	12.7
Cornbread	1 piece	51	127	3.6	3.1	20.2
Cracker—Animal—Ralston	1 item	2	8	0.2	0.1	1.5
Cracker—Cheese/Peanut Butter Sandwich	1 item	7	31	1.7	0.7	4.0
Cracker—Graham—Honey	1 item	7	29	0.7	0.5	5.4
Cracker—Hi Ho—Reduced-Fat—Sunshine	1 item	3	14	0.5	0.2	2.1
Cracker—Hi Ho—Whole Wheat—Sunshine	1 item	3	16	0.9	0.3	2.0
Cracker—Matzo—Plain	1 item	28	112	0.4	2.8	23.7
Cracker—Pretzel Chip—Original—Mr. Phipps	1 item	2	7	0.2	0.1	1.3
Cracker—Ritz	1 item	3	18	1.0	0.2	2.1

Food	Portion/Weight	Calories	Fat	Protein	Carbo-hydrate
	(g)	(g)	(g)	(g)	
Cracker—Saltines	1 item	3	13	0.4	0.3	2.2
Cracker—Snack Mix—Cheese—Ritz	1 ounce	28	130	6.0	2.0	18.0
Cracker—Tater Crisp—Original—Mr. Phipps	1 item	1	5	0.2	0.1	0.9
Cracker—Wheat Thins—Original Nabisco	1 item	2	8	0.4	0.1	1.2
Cracker—Wheat Thins—Reduced Fat—Nabisco	1 item	2	6	0.2	0.1	1.2
Cracker—Wheat—Wheatsworth—Nabisco	1 item	3	16	0.7	0.4	2.0
Croissant—Apple/Butter	1 item	57	145	5.0	4.2	21.1
Croissant—Butter	1 item	57	231	12.0	4.7	26.1
Croutons	1 cup	30	122	2.0	3.6	22.1
French Toast—Frozen	1 piece	59	126	3.6	4.4	18.9
Muffin—Blueberry—Fat-Free—Entenmann's	1 item	57	120	0.0	2.0	26.0
Muffin—Blueberry—From Mix	1 item	50	150	4.4	2.6	24.4
Muffin—Corn—Commercial Preparation	1 item	57	174	4.8	3.4	29.0
Muffin—English—Plain	1 item	57	134	1.0	4.4	26.2
Pancakes—Low-Fat—Frozen—Aunt Jemima	1 piece	33	43	0.5	1.3	11.0
Pancakes—Original—Frozen—Aunt Jemima	1 piece	33	66	1.0	2.0	13.3
Pancakes—Plain—From Mix	1 item	38	83	2.9	3.0	11.0
Pancakes—Whole Wheat—From Mix	1 item	44	91	2.9	3.7	12.9
Pizza Crust—Fresh—Contadina	1 serving	59	170	2.5	5.0	31.0
Pretzel—Dutch—Mister Salty—Nabisco	1 item	16	60	0.5	1.5	12.5
Roll—Crescents—Pillsbury	1 item	29	100	5.5	2.0	11.0
Roll—Dinner—Whole Wheat	1 item	28	75	1.3	2.5	14.5
Roll—Hamburger—Low-Calorie	1 item	43	84	0.9	3.6	18.1
Roll—Hamburger—Mixed-Grain	1 item	43	113	2.6	4.1	19.2
Roll—Hot Dog—Low-Calorie	1 item	43	84	0.9	3.6	18.1
Roll—Hot Dog—Plain	1 item	43	123	2.2	3.7	21.6
Roll—Kaiser	1 item	57	167	2.5	5.6	30.0

Nutrient Values of Common Foods (cont.)

Food	Portion/Weight	Calories	Fat	Protein	Carbo-hydrate
	(g)	(g)	(g)	(g)	
Roll—Submarine/Hoagie—					
Enriched	1 item 135	400	8.0	11.0	72.0
Stuffing—Bread—Home Recipe	1 cup 232	390	16.7	8.8	51.5
Waffle—Nutri-Grain—Multi-Bran—					
Kellogg	1 item 39	90	3.0	2.5	16.0
Waffle—Special K—Eggo—					
Kellogg	1 item 29	70	0.0	3.0	14.5
Waffles—Enriched—From Mix—					
Egg and Milk	1 item 75	205	8.0	7.0	27.0
Waffles—Plain—Frozen	1 item 35	87	2.7	2.1	13.5
Breakfast Cereal					
All Bran—Kellogg	1 cup 60	160	2.0	8.0	44.0
Cap'N Crunch—Crunchberries—					
Quaker	1 cup 35	133	2.0	1.3	29.3
Cap'N Crunch—Peanut Butter—					
Quaker	1 cup 36	147	3.3	2.7	28.0
Cheerios—General Mills	1 cup 30	110	2.0	3.0	23.0
Corn Flakes—Ralston	1 cup 25	97	0.1	2.0	21.6
Cream of Wheat/Iron—Quick-					
Cooked	1 cup 240	133	0.4	3.8	27.3
Crispix	1 cup 32	120	0.1	2.3	27.9
Froot Loops	1 cup 28	111	0.5	1.6	25.0
Frosted Flakes	1 cup 35	133	0.1	1.6	31.6
Fruitful Bran	1 cup 42	139	0.7	3.2	33.5
Granola—Nature Valley	1 cup 113	503	19.6	11.5	75.5
Honey Nut Cheerios	1 cup 28	104	0.7	3.1	22.4
Instant Oats—Cinnamon					
Graham—Quaker	1 item 40	150	2.5	4.0	30.0
Life	1 cup 44	172	2.5	8.0	29.6
Low Fat Granola—Kellogg	1 cup 110	420	6.0	10.0	86.0
Mini Wheats—Frosted	1 cup 47	161	0.5	3.9	38.6
Muslix—Crunchy Golden	1 cup 64	259	5.3	6.1	48.0
Nutri Grain—Golden Wheat—					
Kellogg	1 cup 40	133	0.7	4.0	32.0
Oats—Rolled—Regular—Quick-					
Cooked	1 cup 234	145	2.3	6.1	25.3
Puffed Rice	1 cup 14	54	0.1	0.9	12.6
Puffed Wheat	1 cup 12	46	0.2	1.8	9.4

Nutrient Values of Common Foods (cont.)

Food	Portion/Weight		Calories	Fat	Protein	Carbo-hydrate
		(g)	(g)	(g)	(g)	
Raisin Bran	1 cup	50	157	0.6	3.5	39.0
Raisin Squares—Kellogg	1 cup	73	240	1.3	5.3	58.7
Rice Krispies	1 cup	28	105	0.1	2.1	24.1
Shredded Wheat'N Bran— Spoon Size	1 cup	55	194	0.6	7.0	43.4
Shredded Wheat—Spoon Size	1 cup	47	170	0.6	4.8	39.3
Special K	1 cup	21	79	0.1	3.6	16.0
Wheat Germ—Toasted	1 cup	113	432	12.1	32.9	56.0
Wheaties—General Mills	1 cup	30	110	1.0	3.0	24.0
Combination Food						
Beef Pot pie	1 slice	210	500	31.9	16.4	36.5
Burrito—Bean and Cheese	1 item	93	189	5.9	7.5	27.5
Cheese Soufflé	1 cup	95	205	15.9	9.6	5.8
Cheeseburger—Bacon/ Condiments	1 item	195	608	36.8	32.0	37.1
Cheeseburger—Plain	1 item	102	319	15.1	14.8	31.8
Chili Con Carne With Beans— Canned	1 cup	255	322	14.2	22.5	27.2
Corn Dog—Plain	1 item	175	460	18.9	16.8	55.8
Corned Beef Hash—Canned	1 cup	220	398	24.9	19.4	23.5
Enchilada—Cheese	1 item	163	319	18.8	9.6	28.5
Fajita—Beef	1 serving	158	290	12.4	11.9	32.6
Fajita—Chicken	1 serving	158	287	9.3	15.3	35.7
Falafil—Prepared—Fantastic Foods	1 cup	106	250	4.0	15.0	42.0
Hamburger—Single Meat— Plain—Large	1 item	137	425	22.9	22.6	31.7
Hot Dog—Plain With Bun— Generic	1 item	98	242	14.5	10.4	18.0
Macaroni and Cheese—Baked— Home Recipe	1 cup	200	430	22.2	16.8	40.2
Meatloaf—Beef/Pork—With Celery and Onion	1 serving	100	197	11.0	17.0	6.1
Nachos—With Cheese	1 serving	113	346	18.9	9.1	36.3
Pizza—Cheese—Baked	1 slice	63	140	3.2	7.7	20.5
Pizza—Cheese/Meat/Vegetable	1 slice	79	184	5.4	13.0	21.3
Pizza—Pepperoni—Baked	1 slice	71	181	7.0	10.1	19.9
Pork/Beans With Frankfurters— Canned	1 cup	257	365	16.9	17.3	39.6

Nutrient Values of Common Foods (cont.)

Food	Portion/Weight	Calories	Fat	Protein	Carbo-hydrate
	(g)	(g)	(g)	(g)	
Pork/Beans—Canned—Baked	1 cup	253	268	3.9	13.1	50.5
Ravioli—Cheese—Fresh—						
Contadina	1 cup	87	280	12.0	13.0	31.0
Ravioli—Light—Cheese—						
Fresh—Contadina	1 cup	88	240	5.0	13.0	35.0
Salad—Chicken	1 cup	205	502	36.2	26.0	17.4
Salad—Coleslaw	1 cup	120	82	3.1	1.6	14.9
Salad—Pasta—Homestyle—Kraft	1 cup	188	480	32.0	8.0	82.0
Salad—Potato	1 cup	250	358	20.5	6.7	27.9
Salad—Taco	1 serving	198	279	14.8	13.2	23.6
Sandwich—BLT—With Mayon-						
naise	1 item	148	282	15.6	6.8	28.8
Sandwich—Club	1 item	315	590	20.8	35.6	41.7
Sandwich—Steak	1 item	204	459	14.1	30.3	52.0
Sandwich—Submarine—	1 item	216	410	13.0	28.6	44.3
Roast Beef						
Sandwich—Submarine—With						
cold cuts	1 item	228	456	18.6	21.8	51.0
Spaghetti/Tomato/Meatballs—						
Home Recipe	1 cup	248	330	122.0	19.0	39.0
Taco	1 item	171	369	20.6	20.7	26.7
Dairy Products						
Cheese Spread—American—						
Processed	1 ounce	28	82	6.0	4.7	2.5
Cheese—Amer—White—						
Singles—Healthy Choice	1 slice	21	30	0.0	5.0	2.0
Cheese—American—Light—Kraft	1 ounce	28	70	4.0	6.0	2.0
Cheese—American—Processed—						
Slice—Kraft	1 ounce	28	110	9.0	5.0	0.5
Cheese—Blue	1 ounce	28	98	8.1	6.0	0.7
Cheese—Brie	1 ounce	28	93	7.8	5.8	0.1
Cheese—Cheddar—Inch Cubes	1 item	17	60	5.7	4.3	0.2
Cheese—Cheddar—Light &						
Lively—Kraft	1 ounce	28	70	4.0	6.0	2.0
Cheese—Cheddar/Wine—						
Cracker Barrel	1 ounce	28	100	7.0	4.0	3.0
Cheese—Colby	1 ounce	28	110	9.0	6.7	0.7

Nutrient Values of Common Foods (cont.)

Food	Portion/Weight	Calories	Fat	Protein	Carbo-hydrate
	(g)		(g)	(g)	(g)
Cheese—Colby—Reduced-Fat—Kraft	1 ounce	28	80	5.0	9.0	0.0
Cheese—Cottage–1% Low-Fat	1 cup	226	164	2.3	28.0	6.2
Cheese—Cottage–4% Fat—Small Curd	1 cup	210	217	9.5	26.2	5.6
Cheese—Cottage—Fat-Free	1 cup	226	140	0.0	26.0	8.0
Cheese—Cream	1 ounce	28	97	9.8	2.1	0.8
Cheese—Cream—Soft—Philadelphia Light	1 tbsp	16	35	2.5	1.5	1.0
Cheese—Cream—Whipped—Philadelphia	1 tbsp	10	36	3.7	0.7	0.3
Cheese—Cream/Strawberries—Philadelphia	1 tbsp	16	50	4.5	0.5	2.5
Cheese—Feta—Ounce	1 ounce	28	73	6.0	4.0	1.2
Cheese—Goat—Hard	1 ounce	28	128	10.1	8.7	0.6
Cheese—Goat—Soft	1 ounce	28	76	6.0	5.3	0.3
Cheese—Gruyère	1 ounce	28	116	9.1	8.4	0.1
Cheese—Monterey Jack	1 ounce	28	105	8.5	6.9	0.2
Cheese—Mozzarella—Made From Skim Milk	1 ounce	28	71	4.5	6.8	0.8
Cheese—Mozzarella—Made From Whole Milk	1 ounce	28	79	6.1	5.5	0.6
Cheese—Muenster	1 ounce	28	103	8.4	6.6	0.3
Cheese—Neufchatel—Philadelphia	1 ounce	28	70	6.0	3.0	0.5
Cheese—Parmesan—Grated	1 tbsp	5	22	1.5	2.1	0.2
Cheese—Provolone	1 ounce	28	98	7.5	7.2	0.6
Cheese—Ricotta—Fat-Free	1 cup	248	190	1.6	33.9	9.9
Cheese—Ricotta—Low-Fat	1 cup	248	257	7.4	36.8	10.8
Cheese—Ricotta—Made With Part Skim Milk	1 cup	246	85	19.5	28.0	12.6
Cheese—Ricotta—Made With Whole Milk	1 cup	246	428	31.9	27.7	7.5
Cheese—String—Moo Town Snack—Sargento	1 piece	24	70	5.0	7.8	0.5
Cheese—String—Moo Town—Light—Sargento	1 piece	24	60	3.0	7.0	0.5
Cheese—Swiss	1 ounce	28	105	7.7	8.0	1.0

Nutrient Values of Common Foods (cont.)

Food	Portion/Weight	Calories	Fat	Protein	Carbo-hydrate
	(g)	(g)	(g)	(g)	(g)
Cheese—Swiss—Light & Lively—Kraft	1 ounce	28	70	3.0	6.0	2.0
Cream—Coffee—Table—Light—Fluid	1 cup	240	469	46.3	6.5	8.8
Cream—Half & Half—Milk and Cream—Fluid	1 cup	242	315	27.8	7.2	10.4
Cream—Sour—Cultured	1 cup	230	493	48.2	7.3	9.8
Cream—Whipped—Imitation—Pressurized	1 cup	70	184	15.6	0.7	11.2
Cream—Whipping—Heavy—Unwhipped—Fluid	1 cup	238	821	88.1	4.9	6.6
Creamer—Nondairy—Powder—Coffeemate	1 tsp	2	10	0.5	0.0	1.0
Creamer—No-Fat—Irish/French Vanilla—Coffeemate	1 tbsp	15	25	0.0	0.0	6.0
Creamer—No-Fat—Nondairy—Liquid—Coffeemate	1 tbsp	15	10	0.0	0.0	2.0
Creamer—Nondairy—Coffeemate—Liquid	1 tbsp	15	16	1.0	0.0	2.0
Milk—Buttermilk—Cultured	1 cup	245	99	2.2	8.1	11.7
Milk—Chocolate—1% Fat	1 cup	250	158	2.5	8.1	26.1
Milk—Chocolate—2% Fat	1 cup	250	179	5.0	8.0	26.0
Milk—Chocolate—Whole—Vitamin D	1 cup	250	208	8.5	7.9	25.9
Milk—Condensed—Sweetened—Canned	1 cup	306	982	26.6	24.2	166.0
Milk—Eggnog—Commercial	1 cup	254	342	19.0	9.7	34.4
Milk—Low-Fat 1%	1 cup	244	102	2.6	8.0	11.7
Milk—Low-Fat 2%	1 cup	244	121	4.7	8.1	11.7
Milk—Skim	1 cup	245	85	0.4	8.4	11.9
Milk—Whole—Regular—(3.3% Fat)	1 cup	244	150	8.2	0.0	11.4
Milkshake—Chocolate—Thick	1 item	300	356	8.1	9.2	63.5
Milkshake—Vanilla—Thick	1 item	313	350	9.5	12.1	55.6
Sour Cream—Fat-Free—Knudsen	1 tbsp	16	17	0.0	1.0	3.0
Sour Cream—Light—Knudsen	1 tbsp	16	20	1.3	1.0	1.0
Yogurt—Fruit Flavors—Fat-Free—Yoplait	1 cup	227	214	0.0	7.0	21.4

Nutrient Values of Common Foods (cont.)

Food	Portion/Weight	Calories	Fat	Protein	Carbo-hydrate
		(g)	(g)	(g)	(g)
Yogurt—Fruit Flavors—Light— Yoplait	1 cup	227	120	0.0	7.0	21.4
Yogurt—Fruit Flavors—Low-Fat— Milk Solids Added	1 cup	227	239	3.2	11.0	42.2
Yogurt—Plain—Nonfat— Milk Solids Added	1 cup	227	127	0.4	13.0	17.4
Yogurt—Plain—Whole Milk— No Solids	1 cup	227	139	7.4	7.9	10.6
Yogurt—Vanilla—Low-Fat— Dannon	1 cup	227	210	3.0	1.0	36.0
Yogurt—Vanilla—Weight Watchers	1 cup	227	90	0.0	8.0	14.0
Desserts					
Brownie—Dark Chocolate Fudge—Prepared From Mix	1 item	42	190	8.0	2.0	27.0
Brownie—With Frosting/Nuts— Large	1 item	56	227	9.1	2.7	35.8
Cake—Angel Food—Prepared	1 slice	28	73	0.2	1.7	16.4
Cake—Carrot/Icing—Home Recipe	1 slice	111	484	29.3	5.1	52.4
Cake—Chocolate—With Chocolate Frosting	1 slice	64	235	10.5	2.6	34.9
Cake—Gingerbread—Prepared From Mix	1 slice	67	207	6.8	2.7	34.0
Cake—Pound—Free & Light— Sara Lee	1 slice	28	70	0.0	1.0	17.0
Cake—Strawberry Shortcake	1 serving	175	344	8.9	4.8	61.2
Cake—Yellow—From Mix	1 slice	63	202	5.9	3.0	34.3
Cheesecake—Commercial Preparation	1 slice	80	257	18.0	4.4	20.4
Cheesecake—No-Bake-Type— From Mix	1 slice	99	271	12.6	5.5	35.1
Cookie—Animal Cracker	1 item	3	11	0.4	0.2	1.9
Cookie—Chocolate Chip— From Mix	1 item	16	79	4.1	0.9	10.3
Cookie—Chocolate Chip— Home Recipe	1 item	16	78	4.5	0.9	9.3
Cookie—Fig Bar	1 item	16	55	1.2	0.6	11.3

Nutrient Values of Common Foods (cont.)

Food	Portion/Weight	Calories	Fat	Protein	Carbo-hydrate
	(g)	(g)	(g)	(g)	
Cookie—Fortune	1 item	8	30	0.2	0.3	6.7
Cookie—Gingersnap	1 item	7	29	0.7	0.4	5.4
Cookie—Macaroon	1 item	24	97	3.1	0.9	17.3
Cookie—Peanut Butter—From Mix	1 item	10	50	2.6	0.8	5.9
Cookie—Peanut Butter—Keebler	1 item	17	80	4.0	1.0	10.0
Cookie—Reduced-Fat—Chips Ahoy—Nabisco	1 item	11	50	2.0	0.7	7.7
Cookie—Reduced-Fat—Oreo—Nabsico	1 item	11	46	1.7	0.7	8.0
Cookie—Sandwich—Chocolate Cream Filling	1 item	10	47	2.1	0.5	7.0
Cookie—Sandwich—Chocolate/Vanilla	1 item	10	50	2.3	0.5	7.0
Cookie—Shortbread	1 item	7	35	1.8	0.5	4.8
Cookie—Sugar Wafer Vanilla—Sunshine	1 item	9	43	2.0	0.3	6.0
Cookie—Sugar—From Mix	1 item	20	98	4.8	0.9	13.1
Cookie—Tea Biscuit	1 item	3	11	0.4	0.2	1.9
Cookie—Vanilla Wafer	1 item	4	18	0.6	0.2	3.0
Danish Pastry—Lemon	1 item	71	263	13.1	3.8	33.9
Danish Pastry—Nut	1 item	65	280	16.4	4.6	29.7
Danish Pastry—Plain	1 item	57	250	13.6	4.1	29.1
Doughnut—Cake	1 item	45	198	10.8	2.3	23.4
Doughnut—Cake—Chocolate Icing	1 item	43	204	13.3	2.2	20.6
Doughnut—Cake—Glazed	1 item	45	192	10.3	2.3	22.9
Doughnut—French Cruller—Glazed	1 item	41	169	7.5	1.3	24.4
Doughnut—Old-Fashioned	1 item	47	108	10.8	2.4	23.4
Doughnut—Yeast—Jelly Filling	1 item	85	280	15.9	5.0	33.1
Eclair—Custard With Chocolate Icing	1 item	100	262	15.7	6.4	24.2
Frozen Yogurt—Chocolate—Soft Serve	1 cup	144	230	8.6	5.8	35.9
Frozen Yogurt—Fruit Varieties	1 cup	226	216	2.0	7.0	41.8

Food	Portion/Weight	Calories	Fat	Protein	Carbo-hydrate
Nutrient Values of Common Foods (cont.)					
	(g)		(g)	(g)	(g)
Frozen Yogurt—Vanilla—					
Soft Serve	1 cup	144	229	8.1	5.8	34.8
Fruit Pie—Fried	1 item	85	266	14.4	2.4	33.0
Gelatin Dessert—Prepared	1 cup	270	159	0.0	3.2	37.8
Gelatin—Jello—Sugar-Free—					
Prepared	1 cup	240	16	0.0	2.0	0.0
Granola Bar	1 item	25	109	4.2	2.4	16.0
Ice Cream Cone—Sugar	1 item	10	40	0.4	0.8	8.4
Ice Cream Cone—Wafer	1 item	4	16	0.3	0.3	3.2
Ice Cream Sundae—Caramel	1 item	155	304	9.3	7.3	49.3
Ice Cream Sundae—Hot Fudge	1 item	158	284	8.6	5.6	47.7
Ice Cream Sundae—Strawberry	1 item	153	268	7.9	6.3	44.6
Ice Cream—Chocolate	1 cup	132	285	14.5	5.0	37.2
Ice Cream—French Vanilla	1 cup	86	185	11.2	3.5	19.1
Ice Cream—Strawberry	1 cup	132	253	11.1	4.2	36.4
Ice Cream—Truly Free—					
Chocolate—Baskin-Robbins	1 cup	236	160	0.0	10.0	30.0
Ice Cream—Truly Free—					
Vanilla—Baskin-Robbins	1 cup	236	160	0.0	8.0	30.0
Ice Cream—Vanilla—					
Haagen-Dazs	1 cup	212	540	36.0	10.0	42.0
Ice Milk—Vanilla—Hardened	1 cup	132	184	5.6	5.0	30.0
Ice Milk—Vanilla—Soft Serve	1 cup	176	222	4.6	8.6	38.4
Pie—Apple—2 Crusts—Baked	1 cup	192	492	21.3	4.2	73.2
Pie—Boston Cream—					
Commercial Preparation	1 slice	92	232	7.8	2.2	39.5
Pie—Coconut Custard—1					
Crust—Baked	1 cup	179	421	22.4	10.7	44.6
Pie—Lemon Meringue—1					
Crust—Baked	1 cup	188	479	19.2	7.0	70.9
Pie—Pecan—1 Crust—Baked	1 cup	179	748	41.0	9.1	91.8
Pie—Pumpkin—1 Crust—Baked	1 cup	179	378	20.0	7.2	43.9
Popsicle	1 item	95	70	0.0	0.0	18.0
Pudding Pops—Chocolate—					
Frozen	1 item	47	71	2.2	1.9	11.9
Pudding Pops—Vanilla—Frozen	1 item	47	74	2.1	1.9	12.6
Pudding—Rice—With Raisins	1 cup	265	440	14.8	13.7	65.6

Nutrient Values of Common Foods (cont.)

Food	Portion/Weight	Calories	Fat	Protein	Carbo-hydrate
	(g)		(g)	(g)	(g)
Pudding—Vanilla—Fat-Free— Sugar-Free—Jell-O	1 cup	16	50	0.0	0.0	12.0
Pudding—Vanilla—Ready to Eat	1 cup	226	294	8.1	5.2	49.5
Sherbet—Orange	1 cup	193	270	3.8	2.2	58.7
Toaster Pastries/Pop Tarts	1 item	52	196	5.8	1.9	35.2
Twinkie—Hostess	1 item	43	143	4.2	1.3	25.6
Twinkie—Lite—Hostess	1 item	43	110	2.0	2.0	21.0
Eggs						
Egg—Fried in Butter—Whole— Large	1 item	46	91	6.9	6.2	0.6
Egg—Hard-Cooked—No Shell— Large	1 item	50	77	5.3	6.3	0.6
Egg—Raw—White—Large	1 item	33	16	0.0	3.5	0.3
Egg—Raw—Yolk—Large	1 item	17	59	5.1	2.8	0.3
Egg—Scrambled/Milk/Butter	1 item	60	99	7.3	6.7	1.3
Egg Substitute—Liquid	1 cup	251	211	8.3	30.1	1.6
Fast Foods						
Baked Potato—Plain—Wendy's	1 serving	284	310	0.0	7.0	71.0
Banana Split—Dairy Queen	1 item	369	510	11.0	9.0	93.0
Bean Burrito—Taco Bell	1 item	198	390	12.0	13.0	58.0
Beef Burrito—Taco Bell	1 item	206	432	19.0	22.0	48.0
Big Beef Burrito Supreme— Taco Bell	1 item	255	525	25.0	25.0	41.7
Burrito Supreme—Taco Bell	1 item	248	440	19.0	18.0	50.0
Burrito—Light Bean—Taco Bell	1 item	198	330	6.0	14.0	55.0
Burrito—Light Chicken Supreme— Taco Bell	1 item	248	410	10.0	18.0	62.0
Burrito—Light Chicken— Taco Bell	1 item	170	290	6.0	12.0	45.0
Burrito—Light Supreme— Taco Bell	1 item	248	350	8.0	20.0	50.0
Cheeseburger—Bacon Double— Burger King	1 item	221	640	39.0	44.0	29.0
Cheeseburger—Bacon Jr— Wendy's	1 serving	170	440	25.0	22.0	33.0
Cheeseburger—Double— Burger King	1 item	213	600	36.0	41.0	29.0

Nutrient Values of Common Foods (cont.)

Food	Portion/Weight	Calories	Fat	Protein	Carbo-hydrate
		(g)	(g)	(g)	(g)
Cheeseburger—Jr Deluxe—Wendy's	1 serving	390	20.0	18.0	36.0
		179			
Cheeseburger—Jr—Wendy's	1 serving	320	13.0	18.0	34.0
		129			
Cheeseburger—Single—Everything—Wendy's	1 serving	510	29.0	30.0	36.0
		237			
Cheeseburger—Whopper Jr—Burger King	1 item	460	28.0	23.0	29.0
		180			
Cheeseburger—Whopper—Burger King	1 item	730	46.0	27.0	45.0
		294			
Chicken Nuggets—6 Piece—Wendy's	1 serving	280	20.0	14.0	12.0
		94			
Chicken Sandwich Breaded—Wendy's	1 serving	450	20.0	26.0	43.0
		208			
Chicken Sandwich Grilled—Wendy's	1 serving	290	7.0	24.0	35.0
		177			
Chicken Tenders—Burger King	1 item	41	2.0	2.7	2.3
		15			
Chili—Small—Wendy's	1 serving	190	6.0	19.0	20.0
		227			
Chili—Large—Wendy's	1 serving	290	9.0	28.0	31.0
		340			
Cinnamon Twist—Taco Bell	1 serving	139	6.0	1.0	19.5
		35			
Cookie—Chocolate Chip—Wendy's	1 item	270	11.0	4.0	38.0
		57			
Croissant—Egg and Cheese—Burger King	1 item	369	24.7	12.8	24.3
		127			
Croissant—Sausage—Egg—Cheese—Burger King	1 item	530	41.0	20.0	21.0
		159			
French Fries Biggie—Wendy's	1 serving	420	20.0	6.0	58.0
		159			
French Fries—Medium—Wendy's	1 serving	340	17.0	5.0	48.0
		130			
French Fries—Small—Wendy's	1 serving	240	12.0	3.0	33.0
		91			
French Toast Sticks—Burger King	1 serving	500	27.0	4.0	60.0
		141			
Frosty Dairy Dessert—Large—Wendy's	1 serving	570	17.0	15.0	95.0
		405			
Frosty Dairy Dessert—Medium—Wendy's	1 serving	460	13.0	12.0	76.0
		324			
Frosty Dairy Dessert—Small—Wendy's	1 serving	340	10.0	9.0	57.0
		243			
Hamburger Single/Everything—Wendy's	1 serving	440	23.0	26.0	36.0
		219			

Nutrient Values of Common Foods (cont.)

Food	Portion/Weight	Calories	Fat	Protein	Carbo-hydrate
		(g)	(g)	(g)	(g)
Hamburger—Burger King	1 item	129	330	15.0	20.0	28.0
Hamburger—Double Whopper—Burger King	1 item	351	870	56.0	46.0	45.0
Hamburger—Jr—Wendy's	1 serving	117	270	9.0	15.0	34.0
Hamburger—Plain Single—Wendy's	1 item	133	350	15.0	24.0	31.0
Hamburger—Whopper Jr—Burger King	1 item	168	420	24.0	21.0	29.0
Hamburger—Whopper—Burger King	1 item	270	640	39.0	27.0	45.0
Ice Cream Cone—Chocolate Dip—Dairy Queen	1 item	156	330	16.0	6.0	40.0
Ice Cream Cone—Vanilla—Regular—Dairy Queen	1 item	213	340	10.0	9.0	53.0
Ice Cream Sundae—Chocolate—Dairy Queen	1 item	177	300	7.0	6.0	54.0
KFC—Chicken—Breast—Original Recipe	1 serving	137	360	20.0	33.0	12.0
KFC—Chicken—Breast/Wing—Skin—Rotisserie	1 item	176	335	18.7	40.0	1.0
KFC—Chicken—Thigh—Original Recipe	1 serving	92	260	17.0	19.0	9.0
KFC—Chicken—Thigh/Leg—Without Skin—Rotisserie	1 item	117	217	12.2	27.0	0.0
KFC—Chicken—Thigh/Leg—With Skin—Rotisserie	1 item	146	333	23.7	3.0	1.0
KFC—Chicken—Breast—Without Wing Skin—Rotisserie	1 item	117	199	5.9	37.0	0.0
KFC—Extra Tasty Crispy Chicken—Breast	1 piece	168	470	28.0	31.0	25.0
KFC—Extra Tasty Crispy Chicken—Thigh	1 piece	118	370	25.0	19.0	18.0
KFC—Extra Tasty Crispy Chicken—Wing	1 piece	55	200	13.0	10.0	10.0
KFC—Kentucky Nuggets	1 piece	16	47	3.0	2.7	2.5
McDonald's—Apple Bran Muffin	1 item	75	180	0.5	4.0	40.0
McDonald's—Bacon Egg & Cheese Biscuit	1 serving	152	450	27.0	17.0	33.0

Nutrient Values of Common Foods (cont.)

Food	Portion/Weight	Calories	Fat	Protein	Carbo-hydrate
	(g)	(g)	(g)	(g)	
McDonald's—Big Mac Hamburger	1 item	215	510	26.0	25.0	42.0
McDonald's—Biscuit	1 serving	76	260	13.0	4.0	32.0
McDonald's—Cheese Danish	1 item	105	410	22.0	7.0	47.0
McDonald's—Cheeseburger	1 item	122	320	13.0	15.0	36.0
McDonald's—Chicken Fajita	1 item	82	190	8.0	11.0	20.0
McDonald's—Chicken McNuggets— 9 Piece	1 serving	165	450	27.0	28.0	24.0
McDonald's—Cinnamon and Raisin Danish	1 item	105	430	22.0	5.0	56.0
McDonald's—Cookie— McDonaldland	1 package	56	260	9.0	4.0	41.0
McDonald's—Egg McMuffin	1 item	137	290	13.0	17.0	27.0
McDonald's—Filet O Fish	1 item	145	360	16.0	14.0	41.0
McDonald's—French Fries— Large	1 serving	147	450	22.0	6.0	57.0
McDonald's—French Fries— Medium	1 serving	97	320	17.0	4.0	36.0
McDonald's—French Fries— Small	1 serving	68	210	10.0	3.0	26.0
McDonald's—French Fries— Super Size	1 serving	176	540	26.0	8.0	68.0
McDonald's—Hamburger	1 item	108	270	9.0	12.0	35.0
McDonald's—Hash Browns	1 serving	53	130	8.0	1.0	14.0
McDonald's—Hot Cakes—Plain	1 serving	150	280	4.0	8.0	54.0
McDonald's—Hot Cakes With Syrup and Margarine (2)	1 serving	222	560	14.0	8.0	100.0
McDonald's—Hot Fudge Frozen Yogurt Sundae	1 serving	179	290	5.0	8.0	54.0
McDonald's—McGrilled Chix Classic (Plain)	1 item	188	250	3.0	24.0	33.0
McDonald's—Quarter Pounder Cheeseburger	1 item	199	520	29.0	28.0	37.0
McDonald's—Quarter Pounder Hamburger	1 item	171	420	20.0	23.0	36.0
McDonald's—Sausage and Egg Biscuit	1 item	170	520	35.0	16.0	33.0
McDonald's—Sausage McMuffin With Egg	1 item	163	440	29.0	19.0	27.0

Nutrient Values of Common Foods (cont.)

Food	Portion/Weight	Calories	Fat	Protein	Carbo-hydrate
		(g)	(g)	(g)	(g)
McDonald's—Scrambled Eggs (2)	1 serving 102	170	12.0	13.0	1.0
McDonald's—Shake—Chocolate—Small	1 serving 293	350	6.0	13.0	62.0
McDonald's—Shake—Strawberry—Small	1 serving 293	340	5.0	12.0	63.0
McDonald's—Shake—Vanilla—Small	1 serving 293	310	5.0	12.0	54.4
McDonald's—Vanilla Low-Fat Frozen Yogurt Cone	1 item 90	120	0.5	4.0	24.0
Mexican Pizza—Taco Bell	1 serving 223	574	38.0	19.0	39.7
Nacho Cheese Sauce—Taco Bell	1 serving 28	51	4.0	2.0	2.5
Nachos Bellgrande—Taco Bell	1 serving 287	633	34.0	22.0	60.6
Nachos Supreme—Taco Bell	1 item 145	364	18.0	12.0	41.0
Nachos—Taco Bell	1 serving 106	345	18.0	7.0	37.5
Onion Rings	1 item 10	34	1.9	0.5	3.9
Pie—Dutch Apple—Burger King	1 slice 113	310	15.0	3.0	39.0
Pintos and Cheese—Taco Bell	1 serving 128	190	9.0	9.0	19.0
Pizza—Cheese—Hand-Tosssed—Pizza Hut	1 slice 108	235	7.0	13.0	29.0
Pizza—Cheese—Pan—Pizza Hut	1 slice 108	261	11.0	12.0	28.0
Pizza—Cheese—Thin Crust—Pizza Hut	1 slice 87	205	8.0	11.0	21.0
Pizza—Italian Sausage—Pan—Pizza Hut	1 slice 116	293	15.0	12.0	27.0
Pizza—Meat Lovers—Hand-Tossed—Pizza Hut	1 slice 130	314	11.0	17.0	29.0
Pizza—Meat Lovers—Pan—Pizza Hut	1 slice 130	340	18.0	16.0	28.0
Pizza—Pepperoni Lovers—Pan—Pizza Hut	1 slice 123	332	17.0	15.0	28.0
Pizza—Pepperoni—Pan—Pizza Hut	1 slice 104	265	12.0	11.0	28.0
Pizza—Pepperoni—Personal Pan—Pizza Hut	1 item 255	637	28.0	27.0	69.0
Pizza—Super Supreme—Pan—Pizza Hut	1 slice 143	323	17.0	15.0	28.0
Pizza—Super—Hand-Tossed—	1 slice 143	296	13.0	16.0	30.0

Pizza Hut

Nutrient Values of Common Foods (cont.)

Food	Portion/Weight	Calories	Fat	Protein	Carbo-hydrate
	(g)	(g)	(g)	(g)	
Pizza—Supreme—Personal Pan—Pizza Hut	1 item	317	722	34.0	33.0	70.0
Pizza—Veggie Lovers—Hand-Tossed—Pizza Hut	1 slice	133	216	6.0	11.0	30.0
Pizza—Veggie Lovers—Pan—Pizza Hut	1 slice	133	243	10.0	10.0	29.0
Potato Baked—Bacon and Cheese—Wendy's	1 serving	380	530	18.0	17.0	77.0
Potato Baked—Broccoli and Cheese—Wendy's	1 serving	411	460	14.0	9.0	79.0
Potato Baked—Chili and Cheese—Wendy's	1 serving	439	610	24.0	21.0	82.0
Refried Beans—Wendy's	1 serving	54	80	3.0	4.0	14.0
Salad—Light Taco With Chips—Taco Bell	1 item	535	680	25.0	35.0	81.0
Salad—Light Taco Without Chips—Taco Bell	1 item	464	330	9.0	30.0	35.0
Soft Taco—Taco Bell	1 item	99	220	11.0	12.0	19.0
Subway—Club Sandwich—On Italian Roll	1 item	227	693	22.0	46.0	83.0
Subway—Cold Cut Combo SW—On Wheat	1 item	233	883	41.0	48.0	88.0
Subway—Ham and Cheese SW—On Italian Roll	1 item	213	643	18.0	38.0	81.0
Subway—Meatball SW—On Italian Roll	1 item	241	918	44.0	42.0	96.0
Subway—Roast Beef SW—On Italian Roll	1 item	213	689	23.0	42.0	84.0
Subway—Turkey Breast SW—Wheat Roll	1 item	219	674	20.0	42.0	88.0
Taco Bell—Combination Burrito	1 item	198	407	16.0	18.0	46.0
Taco Bellgrande—Taco Bell	1 item	163	355	23.1	18.3	17.7
Taco Salad With Salsa/No Shell—Taco Bell	1 serving	530	520	31.4	30.6	30.0
Taco Salad With Salsa/Shell—Taco Bell	1 serving	535	860	55.0	32.0	64.0
Taco—Light Chicken Soft—Taco Bell	1 item	120	180	5.0	9.0	26.0

Nutrient Values of Common Foods (cont.)

Food	Portion/Weight		Calories	Fat	Protein	Carbo-hydrate
		(g)	(g)	(g)	(g)	
Taco—Light Soft Supreme—Taco Bell	1 item	128	200	5.0	14.0	23.0
Taco—Light Soft—Taco Bell	1 item	99	180	5.0	13.0	19.0
Taco—Light Supreme—Taco Bell	1 item	106	160	5.0	13.0	14.0
Taco—Taco Bell	1 item	78	180	11.0	10.0	11.0
Fats and Oils						
Butter—Regular	1 tsp	5	35	4.1	0.0	0.0
Butter—Whipped	1 tsp	4	27	3.1	0.0	0.0
Cooking Spray—Unflavored—Pam	1 serving	0	0	0.0	0.0	0.0
Margarine—Extra Light—Promise	1 tbsp	14	50	6.0	0.0	0.0
Margarine—Regular—Unspecified Oils	1 tsp	5	33	3.8	0.0	0.0
Margarine—Whipped	1 tbsp	9	64	7.3	0.1	0.1
Mayonnaise—Fat-Free—Kraft	1 tbsp	16	10	0.0	0.0	2.0
Mayonnaise—Low-Calorie/Diet	1 tbsp	16	37	3.1	0.1	2.6
Molly McButter	1 serving	1	8	0.0	0.0	2.0
Oil—Vegetable—Canola—Heart Beat—Nucoa	1 tbsp	14	120	14.0	0.0	0.0
Oil—Vegetable—Olive	1 tbsp	14	119	13.5	0.0	0.0
Oil—Vegetable—Sesame	1 tbsp	14	120	13.6	0.0	0.0
Salad Dressing—Blue Cheese	1 tbsp	15	77	8.0	0.7	1.1
Salad Dressing—Blue Cheese—Low-Calorie	1 tbsp	16	15	1.2	0.8	0.4
Salad Dressing—Caesar	1 tbsp	15	70	7.0	0.0	1.0
Salad Dressing—Fat-Free—Catalina—Kraft	1 tbsp	18	22	0.0	0.0	5.5
Salad Dressing—French	1 tbsp	16	67	6.4	0.1	2.7
Salad Dressing—French—Low-Calorie—USDA	1 tbsp	16	21	1.0	0.0	3.5
Salad Dressing—Italian	1 tbsp	15	68	7.1	0.1	1.5
Salad Dressing—Italian—Low-Calorie—USDA	1 tbsp	15	15	1.5	0.0	0.7
Salad Dressing—Miracle Whip—Free—Kraft	1 tbsp	16	20	0.0	0.0	5.0
Salad Dressing—Miracle Whip—Kraft	1 tbsp	14	70	7.0	0.0	2.0

Nutrient Values of Common Foods (cont.)

Food	Portion/Weight		Calories	Fat	Protein	Carbo-hydrate
		(g)		(g)	(g)	(g)
Salad Dressing—Ranch Style	1 tbsp	15	54	5.7	0.4	0.6
Salad Dressing—Russian	1 tbsp	15	75	7.8	0.3	1.6
Salad Dressing—Russian—Low Calorie	1 tbsp	16	23	0.7	0.1	4.5
Salad Dressing—Thousand Island	1 tbsp	16	58	5.6	0.1	2.4
Salad Dressing—Thousand—Low Calorie	1 tbsp	15	24	1.6	0.1	2.5
Shortening—Baking—Soy/Palm/Cottonseed	1 tbsp	13	113	12.8	0.0	0.0
Fish						
Bluefish—Broiled	1 serving	117	186	6.4	30.1	0.0
Clams—Breaded—Fried	1 serving	85	172	9.5	12.1	8.8
Cod—Atlantic—Cooked—Dry Heat	1 serving	85	89	0.7	19.4	0.0
Crab—Steamed—Pieces	1 cup	155	150	2.4	30.0	0.0
Crab Cake	1 item	60	93	4.5	12.1	0.3
Fish Sticks—Breaded—Frozen—Cooked	1 item	28	76	3.4	4.4	6.7
Haddock—Breaded—Fried	1 serving	85	199	9.7	16.5	10.6
Haddock—Broiled	1 serving	85	95	0.8	20.6	0.0
Lobster—Boiled or Steamed	1 ounce	28	27	0.2	5.8	0.4
Lobster Newburg	1 cup	250	485	26.5	46.3	12.8
Monkfish—Broiled	1 ounce	28	27	0.6	5.3	0.0
Mussels—Atlantic/Pacific—Meat Only	1 ounce	28	27	0.6	4.1	0.9
Oysters—Breaded—Fried	1 item	15	28	1.8	1.3	1.7
Roughy—Orange—Broiled	1 ounce	28	25	0.3	5.4	0.0
Salmon—Cooked—Moist Heat	1 serving	85	156	6.5	23.3	0.0
Salmon—Pink—Canned—Solids and Liquids	1 serving	85	118	5.1	16.8	0.0
Salmon—Smoked	1 serving	85	99	3.7	15.5	0.0
Shrimp—Cooked—Moist Heat	1 serving	85	84	0.9	17.8	0.0
Shrimp—French Fried	1 serving	85	206	10.4	18.2	9.8
Sole/Flounder—Cooked—Dry Heat	1 serving	85	99	1.3	20.5	0.0
Squid—Cooked—Fried	1 serving	85	149	6.4	15.2	6.6
Surimi	1 serving	85	84	0.8	12.9	5.8
Swordfish—Cooked—Dry Heat	1 serving	85	132	4.4	21.6	0.0
Trout—Broiled	1 serving	85	162	7.2	22.6	0.0

Nutrient Values of Common Foods (cont.)

Food	Portion/Weight	Calories	Fat	Protein	Carbo-hydrate
	(g)	(g)	(g)	(g)	
Tuna—Light—Canned in Oil—Drained	1 ounce	28	56	2.3	8.3	0.0
Tuna—White—Canned in Water	1 serving	85	116	2.1	22.7	0.0
Tuna—Yellow—Broiled	1 ounce	28	39	0.4	8.5	0.0
Fruits						
Apples—Raw—With Skin—2 3/4" Diameter	1 item	138	81	0.5	0.3	21.0
Applesauce—Canned—Sweetened—USDA	1 cup	255	194	0.5	0.5	50.8
Applesauce—Canned—Unsweetened—USDA	1 cup	244	105	0.1	0.4	27.5
Apricots—Dried—Sulfured—Uncooked	1 cup	130	309	0.6	4.8	80.3
Avocado—Raw—California	1 item	173	306	30.0	3.7	12.0
Banana—Raw—Peeled	1 item	114	105	0.6	1.2	26.7
Blackberries—Raw	1 cup	144	74	0.6	1.0	18.4
Blueberries—Raw	1 cup	145	81	0.6	1.0	20.5
Cherries—Sweet—Raw	1 item	7	4	0.1	0.1	1.1
Dates—Domestic—Natural and Dry—Whole	1 item	8	22	0.0	0.2	6.1
Fruit Cocktail—Canned in Heavy Syrup	1 cup	255	186	0.2	1.0	48.2
Fruit Cocktail—Canned—Light Syrup Pack	1 cup	252	144	0.2	1.0	37.6
Grapefruit—Pink and Red—Raw	1 item	246	73	0.3	1.4	18.4
Grapes—Raw—Slip Skin (American)Type	1 cup	92	58	0.3	0.6	15.8
Mango—Raw	1 item	207	135	0.6	1.1	35.2
Melons—Cantaloupe—Raw—Cubed Pieces	1 cup	160	56	0.5	1.4	13.4
Melons—Honeydew—Raw—Cubed Pieces	1 cup	170	59	0.2	0.8	15.6
Orange—Raw—All Common Varieties—Whole	1 item	131	61	0.2	1.2	15.4
Peaches—Canned—Heavy Syrup Pack	1 cup	256	189	0.3	1.2	51.0
Peaches—Canned—Juice Pack	1 cup	248	109	0.1	1.6	28.7

Nutrient Values of Common Foods (cont.)

Food	Portion/Weight	Calories	Fat	Protein	Carbo-hydrate
	(g)	(g)	(g)	(g)	
Peaches—Canned—Light Syrup	1 cup	251	136	0.1	1.1	36.5
Peaches—Raw—Whole	1 item	87	37	0.1	0.6	9.7
Pears—Canned—Heavy Syrup Pack	1 cup	255	189	0.3	0.5	48.9
Pears—Canned—Light Syrup Pack	1 cup	251	143	0.1	0.5	38.1
Pears—Raw—Bartlett—With Skin	1 item	166	97	0.7	0.7	25.1
Pineapple—Canned—Heavy Syrup Pack	1 cup	255	199	0.3	0.9	51.5
Pineapple—Canned—Light Syrup Pack	1 cup	252	131	0.3	0.9	33.9
Pineapple—Raw—Diced	1 cup	155	76	0.7	0.6	19.2
Plums—Raw	1 cup	292	160	1.8	2.3	38.0
Prunes—Dried—Uncooked—USDA	1 cup	161	385	0.8	4.2	101.0
Raisins—Seedless	1 cup	145	435	0.7	4.7	115.0
Raspberries—Raw	1 cup	123	60	0.7	1.1	14.2
Strawberries—Frozen—Sweetened—Whole	1 cup	255	199	0.4	1.3	53.5
Strawberries—Raw	1 cup	149	44	0.6	0.9	10.5
Tangerines—Raw—Peeled	1 item	84	37	0.2	0.5	9.4
Watermelon—Raw	1 cup	160	51	0.7	1.0	11.5
Grains and Snacks						
Couscous—Cooked	1 cup	179	200	0.3	6.8	41.6
Noodles—Chow Mein—Chinese	1 cup	45	237	13.8	3.8	25.9
Noodles—Egg—Enriched—Cooked	1 cup	160	213	2.4	7.6	39.7
Noodles—Egg—Spinach—Enriched—Cooked	1 cup	160	211	2.5	8.1	38.8
Pasta—Macaroni—Cooked—Firm Stage—Hot	1 cup	130	190	1.0	7.0	39.0
Pasta—Noodles—Ramen—Oriental	1 cup	227	207	8.6	5.9	30.7
Pasta—Spaghetti—Cooked—Al Dente	1 cup	130	190	1.0	7.0	39.0
Pasta—Vegetable Spirals—Cooked	1 cup	134	172	0.2	6.1	35.7

Nutrient Values of Common Foods (cont.)

Food	Portion/Weight	Calories	Fat	Protein	Carbo-hydrate
	(g)	(g)	(g)	(g)	
Popcorn—Butter Flavor—Pop Secret	1 cup	8	37	2.5	0.8	4.0
Popcorn—Butter Flavor—Pop Secret Light	1 cup	5	21	0.8	0.5	3.3
Popcorn—Carmen Coated	1 cup	35	152	4.5	1.3	27.8
Popcorn—Cheese Flavor	1 cup	11	57	3.7	1.0	5.7
Popcorn—Plain—Popped	1 cup	10	40	0.5	1.3	8.0
Popcorn—Popped—Oil and Salt	1 cup	11	55	3.1	1.0	6.3
Pretzel—Dutch—Twisted	1 item	17	65	1.0	2.0	13.0
Pretzel—Thin—Twisted	1 item	6	24	0.2	0.6	4.8
Rice Cakes—Regular	1 item	9	35	0.3	0.7	7.6
Rice—Brown—Medium Grain—Cooked	1 cup	195	218	1.6	4.5	45.8
Rice—Fried	1 cup	177	204	1.1	4.3	43.7
Rice—White—Medium Grain—Enriched—Cooked	1 cup	186	242	0.4	4.4	53.2
Taco Shell—Baked	1 item	13	60	2.9	0.9	8.1
Tortilla Chips—Nacho Cheese Flavor	1 ounce	28	141	7.3	2.2	17.7
Tortilla Chips—White—Guiltless Gourmet	1 ounce	28	110	1.0	3.0	22.0
Tortilla—Corn	1 item	25	55	0.6	1.4	11.7
Tortilla—Flour	1 item	35	114	2.5	3.0	19.5
Meats					
Bacon Bits	1 tbsp	6	26	1.6	1.9	1.7
Bacon—Pork—Broiled/Pan-Fried/Roasted	1 slice	6	36	3.1	1.9	0.0
Beef—Bottom Round Roast—Cooked—Lean	1 serving	85	161	6.3	24.5	0.0
Beef—Bottom Round Roast—Lean and Fat	1 serving	85	211	12.7	22.6	0.0
Beef—Corned—Canned	1 serving	85	212	12.7	23.0	0.0
Beef—Ground—Patty—Broiled—Extra Lean	1 item	85	218	13.9	21.6	0.0
Beef—Ground—Patty—Broiled—Medium Lean	1 item	85	231	15.7	21.0	0.0

Nutrient Values of Common Foods (cont.)

Food	Portion/Weight	Calories	Fat	Protein	Carbo-hydrate
		(g)	(g)	(g)	(g)
Beef—Ground—Patty—Broiled— Regular	1 item	85	246	17.6	20.5	0.0
Beef—Pot Roast—Chuck—Blade Cut—Cooked	1 serving	85	213	11.1	26.4	0.0
Beef—Rib Roast—Broiled—Lean and Fat	1 serving	85	291	23.3	18.9	0.0
Beef—Rib Roast—Broiled— Lean Only	1 serving	85	195	10.6	23.2	0.0
Beef—Steak—Sirloin—Broiled— Lean and Fat	1 serving	85	219	13.1	23.6	0.0
Beef—Steak—Sirloin—Broiled— Lean Only	1 serving	85	166	6.1	25.8	0.0
Beef—Steak—Top Round— Broiled—Lean Only	1 serving	85	153	4.2	26.9	0.0
Beef—Steak—Top Round— Broiled—Lean/Fat	1 serving	85	184	8.2	25.6	0.0
Beef—Tenderloin Steak—Broiled	1 serving	85	179	8.5	24.0	0.0
Bologna—Beef—Light— Oscar Meyer	1 slice	28	60	4.0	3.0	2.0
Bologna—Cured Pork—4" by ⅛" Slice	1 slice	23	56	4.6	3.5	0.2
Bratwurst—Pork—Cooked— Link	1 item	85	256	22.0	12.0	1.8
Frankfurter—No Bun—Beef and Pork	1 item	57	182	16.6	6.4	1.5
Frankfurter—Light—Low-Fat— Ball Park	1 item	57	140	12.0	7.0	1.0
Ham—Boiled—Regular— Luncheon Meat	1 slice	28	51	3.0	5.0	0.9
Italian Sausage—Pork—Link	1 item	67	216	17.2	13.4	1.0
Kielbasa—Pork and Beef	1 slice	26	80	7.1	3.5	0.6
Knockwurst—Pork and Beef— Link	1 item	68	209	18.9	8.1	1.2
Lamb Chop—Rib—Broiled— Lean and Fat	1 serving	85	307	25.2	18.8	0.0
Lamb Chop—Rib— Broiled—Lean Only	1 serving	85	200	11.0	23.6	0.0
Lamb—Ground—Broiled	1 serving	85	241	16.7	21.0	0.0

Nutrient Values of Common Foods (cont.)

Food	Portion/Weight	Calories	Fat	Protein	Carbo-hydrate
	(g)	(g)	(g)	(g)	
Lamb—Leg—Roasted—Lean and Fat	1 serving	85	219	14.0	21.7	0.0
Lamb—Leg—Roasted—Lean Only	1 serving	85	162	6.6	24.1	0.0
Pepperoni—Pork/Beef ⅛" Slice	1 slice	6	27	2.4	1.2	0.2
Pork Chop—Loin—Broiled—Lean and Fat	1 item	82	197	10.7	23.5	0.0
Pork Chop— Loin—Broiled—Lean Only	1 item	74	149	6.0	22.3	0.0
Pork—Canadian Bacon—Grilled	1 slice	23	43	2.0	5.6	0.3
Pork—Center Loin—Roasted—Lean and Fat	1 item	84	197	11.3	22.1	0.0
Pork—Center Loin—Roasted—Lean Only	1 slice	72	173	9.4	20.5	0.0
Pork—Tenderloin—Roasted—Lean Only	1 ounce	28	46	1.4	8.0	0.0
Salami—Cooked—Beef—4" by ⅛" Slice	1 slice	23	60	4.8	3.5	0.7
Sausage—Pork—Link—Cooked	1 item	13	48	4.1	2.6	0.1
Sausage—Pork—Patty—Cooked	1 item	27	99	8.4	5.3	0.3
Veal—All Cuts—Lean and Fat—Cooked	1 serving	85	196	9.7	25.6	0.0
Veal—All Cuts—Lean Only—Cooked	1 serving	85	167	5.6	27.1	0.0
Veal—Ground—Broiled	1 serving	85	146	6.4	20.7	0.0
Veal—Leg—Lean and Fat—Breaded—Fried	1 serving	85	194	7.8	23.2	8.4
Nuts and Seeds					
Nut—Almonds—Shelled—Chopped	1 cup	130	766	67.9	26.0	26.5
Nut—Cashew Oil Roasted	1 cup	130	749	62.7	21.0	37.1
Nut—Coconut Shredded—Premium Baker's	1 tbsp	8	30	2.0	0.0	3.0
Nut—Filbert/Hazel—Dried—Chopped	1 cup	115	727	72.0	15.0	17.6
Nut—Macadamia—Oil Roasted	1 cup	134	962	103.0	9.7	17.3
Nut—Mixed—Oil Roasted	1 cup	142	876	80.0	23.8	30.4

Nutrient Values of Common Foods (cont.)

Food	Portion/Weight	Calories	Fat	Protein	Carbo-hydrate
	(g)	(g)	(g)	(g)	
Nut—Peanuts—All Types—					
Oil Roasted	1 cup	144	837	71.0	37.9	27.3
Nut—Pistachio—Dry Roasted	1 cup	128	776	67.6	19.1	35.2
Peanut Butter—Chunk Style	1 tbsp	16	94	8.0	3.9	3.5
Peanut Butter—Old-Fashioned	1 tbsp	16	95	8.1	4.2	2.7
Peanut Butter—Smooth Type	1 tbsp	16	94	8.0	3.9	3.3
Seed—Sunflower—Dried	1 cup	144	821	71.4	32.8	27.0
Trail Mix—Regular	1 cup	150	693	44.1	20.7	67.3
Poultry					
Chicken Frankfurter	1 item	45	116	8.8	5.8	3.1
Chicken—Breast—No Skin—Fried	1 item	172	322	8.1	57.5	0.9
Chicken—Breast—No Skin—Roast/Broil	1 item	174	284	6.1	53.4	0.0
Chicken—Breast—Roast—Deli—Healthy Choice	1 slice	9	8	0.0	1.7	0.3
Chicken—Breast—With Skin—Fried in Batter	1 item	280	728	37.0	69.6	25.2
Chicken—Breast—With Skin—Fried in Flour	1 item	196	435	17.4	62.4	3.2
Chicken—Leg—No Skin—Roast/Broil	1 item	96	181	8.0	25.7	0.0
Chicken—Leg—Roast/Broil	1 item	115	264	15.3	29.6	0.0
Chicken—Thigh—Fried—Flour Coated	1 item	62	162	9.3	16.6	2.0
Chicken—Thigh—Meat/Skin—Batter Fried	1 item	86	238	14.2	18.6	7.8
Chicken—Thigh—Meat/Skin—Roast/Broil	1 item	62	153	9.6	15.5	0.0
Chicken—Thigh—No Skin—Roast/Broil	1 item	52	109	5.7	13.5	0.0
Chicken—Wing—Fried—Flour Coated	1 item	32	103	7.1	8.4	0.8
Chicken—Wing—Meat/Skin—Batter Fried	1 item	49	159	10.7	9.7	5.4
Turkey Bologna	1 slice	28	56	4.3	3.9	0.3

Nutrient Values of Common Foods (cont.)

Food	Portion/Weight	Calories	Fat	Protein	Carbo-hydrate
	(g)	(g)	(g)	(g)	
Turkey Salami	1 slice	28	55	3.9	4.7	0.2
Turkey—Breast—Roasted—Deli—Healthy Choice	1 slice	9	10	0.3	1.7	0.3
Turkey—Dark Meat—No Skin—Roasted	1 cup	140	262	10.1	40.0	0.0
Turkey—Ground—Cooked	1 ounce	28	66	3.7	7.8	0.0
Turkey—Ham—Honey Cured—Louis Rich	1 slice	28	23	0.7	3.7	0.7
Turkey—Light Meat—No Skin—Roasted	1 cup	140	220	4.5	41.9	0.0
Turkey—Sausage—Links—Louis Rich	1 item	29	45	3.0	5.5	0.0
Soups					
Black Bean—Canned—Prepared—Water	1 cup	247	116	1.5	5.6	19.8
Cheese—Canned—Condensed—Prepared	1 cup	247	156	10.5	5.4	10.5
Chicken Noodle—Canned—With Water	1 cup	241	74	2.5	4.1	9.4
Clam Chowder—Manhattan Style—Water	1 cup	244	78	2.2	2.2	12.2
Clam Chowder—New England—With Milk	1 cup	248	164	6.6	9.5	16.6
Cream of Mushroom—Canned—With Water	1 cup	244	129	9.0	2.3	9.3
Lentil With Ham—Canned—Ready to Eat	1 cup	248	139	2.8	9.3	20.2
Minestrone—Canned—Prepared—Water	1 cup	241	81	2.5	4.3	11.2
Tomato—Canned—Prepared With Milk	1 cup	248	161	6.0	6.1	22.3
Tomato—Canned—Prepared With Water	1 cup	244	85	1.9	2.1	16.6
Vegetable With Beef—Canned	1 cup	251	158	3.8	11.2	20.4
Vegetarian—Canned—Prepared—Water	1 cup	241	72	1.9	2.1	12.0

Nutrient Values of Common Foods (cont.)

Food	Portion/Weight	Calories	Fat	Protein	Carbo-hydrate
		(g)	(g)	(g)	(g)
Sugars and Sweets					
Apple Butter	1 tbsp	20	37	0.2	0.1	9.1
Candy—After Eight Mints—Fondant	1 item	20	37	0.2	0.1	9.1
Candy—Caramels—Plain/Chocolate	1 piece	6	21	0.2	0.1	5.2
Candy—Chocolate—Semisweet	1 cup	170	811	50.5	7.1	108.0
Candy—Crunch—Fun Size—Nestlé	1 item	11	50	2.5	0.5	6.3
Candy—Gum Drops	1 item	4	13	0.0	0.0	3.5
Candy—Hard	1 item	6	22	0.0	0.0	5.9
Candy—Jelly Beans	1 item	3	6	0.0	0.0	2.6
Candy—Kisses With Almonds—Hershey's	1 piece	5	26	1.7	0.5	2.4
Candy—Kisses—Chocolate—Hershey's	1 piece	5	26	1.5	0.4	2.8
Candy—Licorice	1 cup	220	807	1.1	0.0	205.0
Candy—Life Savers	1 item	2	7	0.0	0.0	1.9
Candy—M&M—Peanut	1 piece	49	9	0.5	0.2	1.2
Candy—Milk Chocolate With Almonds	1 item	44	231	15.1	4.0	23.4
Candy—Milk Chocolate Plain	1 item	44	226	13.5	3.0	26.1
Candy—Peanut Butter Cup	1 piece	17	92	5.4	2.2	8.7
Candy—Reese's Pieces	1 piece	1	3	0.2	0.1	0.5
Candy—Skittles	1 piece	62	4	0.0	0.0	1.1
Candy—York Peppermint Patty	1 item	43	149	3.9	1.3	33.6
Chocolate Chips—Real—Semi-sweet—Baker's	1 item	1	2	0.1	0.0	0.3
Fudge—Chocolate Marshmallow/Nuts	1 piece	22	96	4.3	0.7	15.1
Honey—Strained/Extracted	1 tbsp	21	63	0.0	0.1	17.3
Jam/Preserves—Regular	1 tbsp	20	48	0.0	0.1	12.9
Jam/Preserves—Strawberry—Low-Calorie	1 tsp	6	8	0.0	0.0	2.0
Marshmallows	1 item	7	22	0.0	0.1	5.9
Sugar—Brown—Packed	1 cup	220	827	0.0	0.0	214.0
Sugar—White—Granulated	1 cup	200	774	0.0	0.0	200.0

Nutrient Values of Common Foods (cont.)

Food	Portion/Weight	Calories	Fat	Protein	Carbo-hydrate
	(g)	(g)	(g)	(g)	
Syrup—Chocolate Fudge—Thick	1 tbsp	21	72	2.8	0.9	12.4
Syrup—Chocolate—Quik—Nestlé	1 tbsp	19	55	0.3	0.0	12.5
Syrup—Pancake—Low-Calorie	1 tbsp	20	32	0.0	0.0	8.7
Syrup—Pancake—Regular	1 tbsp	20	56	0.0	0.0	14.9
Syrup—Strawberry—Quik—Nestlé	1 tbsp	13	36	0.0	0.0	9.0
Topping—Butterscotch	1 tbsp	21	51	0.0	0.3	13.5
Topping—Nuts in Syrup	1 tbsp	21	83	4.5	0.9	10.9
Vegetables					
Artichoke Hearts—Marinated—Quarters	1 item	14	10	1.0	0.0	1.0
Asparagus—Cooked—Drained—Cuts/Tips	1 cup	180	45	1.0	5.0	8.0
Beans—Baked Beans—Canned	1 cup	254	236	1.1	12.2	52.1
Beans—Green—Cut—Frozen—Green Giant	1 cup	124	37	0.0	0.8	7.5
Beans—Kidney—All Types—Canned	1 cup	256	207	0.8	13.3	38.1
Beans—Lima—Frozen—Boiled—Drained	1 cup	170	170	0.6	10.3	32.0
Beans—Navy—Canned	1 cup	262	296	1.1	19.7	53.6
Beans—Refried	1 cup	253	271	2.7	15.8	46.8
Beans—Snap—Green—Raw—Boiled	1 cup	125	43	0.4	2.4	9.9
Beets—Sliced—Canned—Drained	1 cup	170	52	0.2	1.6	12.2
Broccoli—Raw—Boiled—Drained—Chopped	1 cup	156	43	0.6	4.7	7.9
Broccoli—Raw—Chopped	1 cup	88	24	0.3	2.6	4.6
Broccoli—with Cheese Sauce—Green Giant	1 cup	168	105	3.8	4.5	13.5
Brussels Sprouts—Frozen—Boiled	1 cup	155	65	0.6	5.6	12.9
Cabbage—Common—Raw—Shredded	1 cup	70	17	0.2	1.0	3.8
Cabbage—Domestic—Boiled—Drained	1 cup	150	33	0.7	1.5	6.7
Carrot—Baby—Raw—2 ¾"	1 item	10	3	0.1	0.1	0.8
Carrot—Raw—Scraped—Shredded	1 cup	110	47	0.2	1.1	11.2

Nutrient Values of Common Foods (cont.)

Food	Portion/Weight	Calories	Fat	Protein	Carbo-hydrate
	(g)	(g)	(g)	(g)	
Carrot—Raw—Scraped—Whole	1 item	72	31	0.1	0.7	7.3
Carrots—Boiled—Drained—Sliced	1 cup	156	70	0.3	1.7	16.3
Cauliflower—Raw—Boiled—Drained	1 cup	124	28	0.6	2.3	5.1
Celery—Pascal—Raw—Stalk	1 item	40	6	0.1	0.3	1.5
Chestnuts—Water—Canned—La Choy	1 cup	11	75	0.2	1.4	18.6
Corn—Sweet—Canned—Cream Style	1 cup	256	184	1.1	4.5	46.4
Corn—Sweet—Canned—Drained	1 cup	164	133	1.6	4.3	30.5
Corn—Sweet—Frozen Kernels—Boiled	1 cup	164	133	0.1	5.0	33.7
Cucumber—Raw	1 cup	225	29	0.3	1.2	6.6
Eggplant—Raw	1 cup	82	21	0.2	0.8	5.0
Lentils—Whole—Cooked	1 cup	198	230	0.8	17.9	39.9
Lettuce—Iceberg—Raw—Chopped	1 cup	55	7	0.1	0.6	1.2
Lettuce—Romaine—Raw—Shredded	1 cup	56	8	0.1	0.9	1.3
Mixed Vegetables—Frozen—Boiled	1 cup	182	107	0.3	5.2	23.8
Mushrooms—Raw—Chopped	1 cup	70	17	0.3	1.5	3.3
Olives—Green—Pickled—Canned—Medium	1 cup	3	3	0.5	0.0	0.0
Onions—Mature—Raw—Chopped	1 cup	160	60	0.3	1.9	13.8
Onions—Young Green—Top and Bulb	1 item	6	0.1	0.0	0.1	0.4
Peas—Green—Frozen—Boiled	1 cup	160	125	0.4	8.2	22.8
Peas—Sugar Snap—Frozen—Green Giant	1 cup	136	75	0.0	4.5	15.0
Peppers—Sweet—Raw	1 item	74	20	0.1	0.7	4.8
Pickle—Dill—Cucumber—Medium Sized	1 item	65	5	0.0	0.0	1.0
Pickle—Sweet/Gherkin—Small—Whole	1 item	15	20	0.0	0.0	5.0
Potato—Baked—Flesh and Skin	1 cup	235	257	0.2	5.4	59.4

Nutrient Values of Common Foods (cont.)

Food	Portion/Weight	Calories	Fat	Protein	Carbo-hydrate
		(g)	(g)	(g)	(g)
Potato—Baked—Flesh and Skin Whole	1 item	202	220	0.2	4.7	51.0
Potato—Baked—Flesh Only	1 cup	255	237	0.3	5.0	54.9
Potato—French Fried—Heated in Oven	1 cup	57	186	10.7	2.0	21.5
Potato—Mashed—From Dry—With Milk	1 cup	210	166	4.6	4.2	27.5
Potato—Mashed—From Raw—With Milk	1 cup	210	162	1.2	4.1	36.9
Potato—Mashed—Home Recipe—Milk/Butter	1 cup	211	223	8.9	4.0	35.1
Rutabagas—Boiled—Drained—Mashed	1 cup	240	93	0.5	3.1	21.0
Sauerkraut—Canned	1 cup	236	44	0.3	2.2	10.1
Soybeans—Boiled	1 cup	172	298	15.4	28.6	17.1
Spinach—Creamed—Frozen—Green Giant	1 cup	218	160	6.0	8.0	20.0
Spinach—Raw—Boiled—Drained	1 cup	180	41	0.5	5.4	6.8
Spinach—Raw—Chopped	1 cup	56	12	0.2	1.6	2.0
Squash—Winter—Baked—Mashed	1 cup	205	80	1.3	1.8	17.9
Squash—Zucchini—Raw—Boiled	1 cup	180	28	0.1	1.2	7.1
Sweet Potato—Baked—Peeled	1 item	114	117	0.1	2.0	27.7
Sweet Potato—Candied	1 piece	105	144	3.4	0.9	29.3
Tomato Paste—Canned	1 cup	262	220	2.3	9.9	49.3
Tomato Puree—Canned	1 cup	250	102	0.3	4.2	25.1
Tomato—Diced	1 cup	180	37	0.6	1.5	8.4
Tomato—Red—Canned—Stewed	1 cup	255	66	0.4	2.4	10.5
Tomato—Red—Ripe—Raw	1 cup	221	46	0.7	1.9	10.2
Tomato—Sun-Dried	1 cup	54	139	1.6	7.6	30.1

Metric Conversion Charts

Temperature Conversion

Formulas for conversion

Fahrenheit to Celsius: subtract 32, multiply by 5, then divide by 9; for example:

$$212°F - 32 = 180$$
$$180 \times 5 = 900$$
$$900 \div 9 = 100°C$$

Celsius to Fahrenheit: multiply by 9, the divide by 5, then add 32; for example:

$$100°C \times 9 = 900$$
$$900 \div 5 = 180$$
$$180 + 32 = 212°F$$

Temperatures (Fahrenheit to Celsius)

-10°F = -23°C	coldest part of freezer
0°F = -17°C	freezer
32°F = 0°C	water freezes
68°F = 20°C	room temperature
85°F = 29°C	
100°F = 38°C	

115°F = 46°C	water simmers
135°F = 57°C	water scalds
140°F = 60°C	
150°F = 66°C	
160°F = 71°C	
170°F = 77°C	
180°F = 82°C	water simmers
190°F = 88°C	
200°F = 95°C	
205°F = 96°C	water simmers
212°F = 100°C	water boils, at sea level
225°F = 110°C	
250°F = 120°C	very low (or slow) oven
275°F = 135°C	very low (or slow) oven
300°F = 150°C	low (or slow) oven
325°F = 165°C	low (or moderately slow) oven
350°F = 180°C	moderate oven
375°F = 190°C	moderate (or moderately hot) oven
400°F = 205°C	hot oven
425°F = 220°C	hot oven
450°F = 230°C	very hot oven
475°F = 245°C	very hot oven
500°F = 260°C	extremely hot oven/broiling
525°F = 275°C	extremely hot oven/broiling

Liquid Measures Conversion

For foods such as yogurt, applesauce, or cottage cheese that are not quite liquid, but not quite solid, use fluid measures for conversion.

Both systems, the U.S. standard and metric, use spoon measures. The sizes are slightly different, but the difference is not significant in general cooking. (It may, however, be significant in baking.)

Tbs = tablespoon   tsp = teaspoon

Spoons, cups pints, quarts	Fluid oz	Milliliters (ml), deciliters (dl) and liters (l); rounded off
1 teaspoon (tsp)	⅙ oz	5 ml
3 tsp (1 Tbs)	½ oz	15 ml
1 Tbs	1 oz	¼ dl (or 1 Tbs)
4 Tbs (¼ c)	2 oz	½ dl (or 4 Tbs)
⅓ c	2⅔ oz	¾ dl
½ c	4 oz	1 dl
¾ c	6 oz	1¾ dl
1 c	8 oz	250 ml (or ¼ L)
2 c (1 pint)	16 oz	500 ml (or ½ L)
4 c (1 quart)	32 oz	1 L
4 qt (1 gallon)	128 oz	3¾ L

Solid Measure Conversion

Converting solid measures between U.S. standard and metric systems is not as straightforward as it might seem. The density of the substance being measured makes a big difference in the volume to weight conversion. For example, 1 tablespoon of flour is ¼ ounce and 8.75 grams whereas 1 tablespoon of butter or shortening is ½ ounce and 15 grams. The following chart is intended as a guide only; some experimentation may be necessary to achieve success.

Formulas for conversion

ounces to grams: multiply ounces by 28.35

grams to ounces: multiply grams figure by .035

ounces	pounds	grams	kilograms
1		30	
4	¼	115	
8	½	225	
9		250	¼
12	¾	430	
16	1	450	
18		500	½
	2¼	1000	1
	5		2¼
	10		4½

Linear Measures Conversion

Pan sizes are very different in countries that use metrics versus the U.S. standard. This is more significant in baking than in general cooking.

Formulas for conversion

inches to centimeters: multiply the inch by 2.54

centimeters to inches: multiple the centimeter by 0.39

inches	cm	inches	cm
½	1½	9	23
1	2½	10	25
2	5	12 (1 ft.)	30
3	8	14	35
4	10	15	38½
5	13	16	40
6	15	18	45
7	18	20	50
8	20	24 (2 ft.)	60

Index

ABOUT THE AUTHORS

Steven R. Peikin was born in Philadelphia, where he attended Temple University and Jefferson Medical College of Thomas Jefferson University. After medical school he trained at the University of California, San Francisco, the National Institutes of Health, and Massachusetts General Hospital, and he became board certified in internal medicine and gastroenterology. Dr. Peikin was an honorary fellow at the University of Liverpool, United Kingdom. He is presently Professor of Medicine and Head of Gastroenterology at the Robert Wood Johnson Medical School at Camden, New Jersey, and Cooper Hospital/University Medical Center. He is internationally known for his research on gastrointestinal hormones and the control of food intake.

Liz Zorzanello Emery received her B.S. in Foods and Nutrition from Drexel University in Philadelphia and her M.S. in Health Education from St. Joseph's University in Philadelphia. She has been Instructor of Nutrition at Drexel University and Philadelphia Community College. She is currently employed as a Registered Dietitian with Novartis Nutrition.